# Keep Your Brain Young

## A Health & Diet Program for Your Brain, Including 150 Recipes

**Dr. Fraser Smith,** BA, ND
**with Dr. Ellie Aghdassi,** PhD, RD

Robert
ROSE

*For complete cataloguing information, see page 369.*

**Disclaimer**
This book is a general guide only and should never be a substitute for the skill, knowledge, and
experience of a qualified medical professional dealing with the facts, circumstances, and symptoms of
a particular case.

The nutritional, medical, and health information presented in this book is based on the research,
training, and professional experience of the authors, and is true and complete to the best of their
knowledge. However, this book is intended only as an informative guide for those wishing to know more
about health, nutrition, and medicine; it is not intended to replace or countermand the advice given
by the reader's personal physician. Because each person and situation is unique, the author and the
publisher urge the reader to check with a qualified health-care professional before using any procedure
where there is a question as to its appropriateness. A physician should be consulted before beginning
any exercise program. The author and the publisher are not responsible for any adverse effects or
consequences resulting from the use of the information in this book. It is the responsibility of the reader
to consult a physician or other qualified health-care professional regarding his or her personal care.

The recipes in this book have been carefully tested by our kitchen and our tasters. To the best of our
knowledge, they are safe and nutritious for ordinary use and users. For those people with food or other
allergies, or who have special food requirements or health issues, please read the suggested contents of
each recipe carefully and determine whether or not they may create a problem for you. All recipes are
used at the risk of the consumer.

We cannot be responsible for any hazards, loss or damage that may occur as a result of any recipe use.

For those with special needs, allergies, requirements or health problems, in the event of any doubt,
please contact your medical adviser prior to the use of any recipe.

Design and production: Kevin Cockburn/PageWave Graphics Inc.
Editors: Bob Hilderley, Senior Editor, Health; and Sue Sumeraj, Recipes
Copy editor: Kelly Jones
Proofreader: Sheila Wawanash
Indexer: Gillian Watts
Illustrations: Kveta/Three in a Box

Cover and chapter opener image: © iStockphoto.com/tombaky

The publisher gratefully acknowledges the financial support of our publishing program by the
Government of Canada through the Canada Book Fund.

Published by Robert Rose Inc.
120 Eglinton Avenue East, Suite 800, Toronto, Ontario, Canada M4P 1E2
Tel: (416) 322-6552 Fax: (416) 322-6936
www.robertrose.ca

Printed and bound in Canada

1  2  3  4  5  6  7  8  9  MI  22  21  20  19  18  17  16  15  14

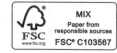

# CONTENTS

*continued on next page*

## Part 5: Menu Plans and Recipes for a Healthy Brain

# Feeding the Brain

**This book is a how-to guide for individuals who want to prevent aging-related diseases.**

It is a fact of life: we are all going to age. And some of us are going to experience aging-related diseases, such as Alzheimer's or Parkinson's disease, that affect our thinking, motion, and mood. We can readily find information on how to keep our heart healthy and our joints pain free. We can even find ways to rejuvenate our skin. But most everyone agrees that none of these things matter much if our mind begins to fail, our memories get lost, and our ability to solve even simple problems begins to deteriorate. Wouldn't we all jump at the chance to protect ourselves from the mental symptoms caused by neurological diseases, to repair any existing damage, and to enhance our quality of life as we age?

Thanks to the efforts of medical research scientists and clinicians, North Americans are living longer than ever before. Forty million Americans and five million Canadians are now over the age of 65. One in 10 of the people in this demographic has Alzheimer's. That's almost five million people. By 2050, epidemiologists predict that 16 million North Americans will have Alzheimer's. Add vascular dementia and Parkinson's disease to these numbers and you see that aging-related diseases are becoming epidemic.

Even as we find ways to maintain our bodies well into our 80s or even 90s, we are still stricken with many kinds of aging diseases related to the central nervous system. Some conditions are more frequent now than they were a generation ago, perhaps because of environmental factors, but also possibly because doctors are able to diagnose diseases more effectively. Still, only half of all cases of Alzheimer's have been reported.

In their most stark presentations, aging processes of the brain can rob people of their ability to take care of themselves or even recognize loved ones. Very commonly, these diseases can severely limit human performance and, to some extent, the ability to continue to be contributing and useful members of society (which the elderly most certainly can be and should be). Many of the people who are entering their senior years now are questioning the conventional wisdom that to age means to accept diminishing mental capacity. Although older generations may not have the learning ease of small children, they are looking for the key to maintaining their intellect and their ability to solve problems at home and at work. Yes, more people are working for more years. Retirement has become less desirable. These people have science on their side — in the sense that new discoveries in neuroplasticity (the way that the brain can remodel itself to adapt to aging, injury, and everyday demands) and nutritional sciences suggest that there are numerous ways to stay young mentally. This book is a how-to guide for individuals who want to prevent aging-related diseases.

It is also a guide for individuals with progressive neurodegenerative conditions and their caregivers in improving quality of life. Although many aging-related diseases are genetically predetermined to some degree, or are often well established before they are detected, the rational approach is to do everything possible to achieve optimal functioning of our brain, and to remove all negative disturbances to our health. The brain has regenerative capabilities, but these alone cannot reverse illness. The right thing to do is to prevent damage.

And that is the spirit in which this book is written — that it is preferable to use the best information we have now to take a proactive approach, instead of waiting passively for the perfect cure to come along. In many cases, there is no time to wait, but in all cases, it is always a wise decision to take actions that improve our well-being. The results of doing so can be useful, and sometimes remarkable.

This book offers the promise of protecting, repairing, and enhancing your mental health while coincidentally improving your general physical well-being. This is not a promise to reverse aging or cure aging-related diseases, but it is an insurance policy on improved health, mental and physical. Wouldn't we all have much to gain by taking out an insurance policy on the fitness of our mind?

The good news is that we can protect our brain from the forces of aging by eating foods that create a nutritional shield against disease. By following a simple step-by-step dietary program, one enhanced with nutritional supplements and regular exercise, both physical and mental, we can extend the term of our life insurance policy. This program is relatively simple, but it is well supported by evidence-based scientific research and clinical practice. Besides, the recipes in this diet program are easy to prepare and the meals taste great. Following this program empowers us all to grow older more gracefully … and more slowly.

**Dr. Fraser Smith, BA, ND**
Assistant Dean for Naturopathic Medicine, Associate Professor, College of Professional Studies, National University of Health Sciences, Lombard, Illinois

**Dr. Ellie Aghdassi, PhD, RD**
Program Manager, Toronto Dementia Research Alliance, Assistant Professor, Dalla Lana School of Public Health, University of Toronto, Toronto, Ontario

# Quick Guide to the Healthy Brain Diet Program

The Healthy Brain Diet Program presented in this book has 12 steps that are complementary and accumulative. It is best to start by laying a nutritional foundation and move toward the menu plan and recipes. Let's preview the 12 steps before exploring them in greater depth. There is nothing too difficult to understand here. All you need, in Dr. Linus Pauling's words, is a willingness to "live longer and feel better."

**1** **Lay a good nutritional foundation:** One sure way to keep dementia at bay is to cultivate general good health, eating the right foods in the right amounts. Follow the guidelines for general good health established by the U.S. Department of Agriculture (USDA) and Health Canada.

**2** **Restore the determinants of good health:** Sleep well, drink adequate amounts of water, expose yourself to sunlight, exercise regularly, lower stress, and maintain social interactions — these are the determinants of good health that apply to dementia. Addressing these factors will help prevent the onset of brain disease and help improve the quality of life in full-blown cases of dementia.

**3** **Energize the brain:** The brain is the hungriest kind of tissue in the body. Eat an energy-rich, low-glycemic-index diet that fuels the brain steadily without spikes in blood sugar levels. Spiking blood sugar damages neurons moment by moment.

**4** **Prevent plaques:** Eat heart-healthy foods to keep the arteries, capillaries, and blood supply to the brain free of plaques formed by deposits of damaged LDH ("bad") cholesterol particles. Plaques can reduce oxygen supply to the brain and eventually cause ischemia and stroke.

**5** **Reduce inflammation:** Limit pro-inflammatory foods in your diet and substitute anti-inflammatory foods. The risk of atherosclerosis and brain damage can be reduced because plaque is less likely to form or rupture.

**6** **Protect your brain against free radicals:** Damage to the brain tissues and cells by oxidative stress and free radicals can be mitigated through a diet rich in antioxidant foods, chiefly plant foods known as phytonutrients.

**(7) Detoxify your body:** Support the body's detoxification mechanisms by eating foods that lower the toxic load throughout the body. When detoxification is weak, harmful compounds accumulate in the body — compounds that can sometimes damage the nervous system. When the body's detoxification system is working properly, we have more protection from disease processes that lead to neurologic aging.

**(8) Eat more omega-3 essential fatty acids:** Surround the brain with essential fatty acids (EFAs) by consuming more fish oil and flaxseed oil. Omega-3 fatty acids protect the meninges surrounding the brain from damage and modulate inflammation in the nervous system.

**(9) Enhance brain function with special nutrients:** Several foods and supplements can be considered brain tonics that support circulation in the brain and protect against the aging effects of oxidation.

**(10) Regenerate the brain:** A healthy part of the brain will sometimes take over functions once held by damaged areas. This regenerative function is known as neuroplasticity. Tap into the regenerative potential of the brain.

**(11) Create a care team:** Invite medical professionals, family members, and friends to help you maintain a high quality of life. People with dementia and their caregivers experience a mixture of emotions — from confusion, frustration, anger, and fear to uncertainty, depression, and grief — which tend to progress with the disease. Help is needed at every step.

**(12) Prepare to make changes:** Change can be managed, even if it is not easy. We often react to life events when new circumstances or distressing problems are thrust upon us. But many (not all) neurological degenerative conditions can be steady, slow, and cumulative — which may provide an opportunity to come to terms with many changes along the way.

## PART 1

# Understanding Brain Diseases

# How Does the Brain Work?

## Alzheimer's Disease

Elizabeth was 79 when she began to show signs of memory loss and difficulty learning new things; for example, remembering directions to a restaurant she had never visited before. Her husband, Ben, found that her mood had become unpredictable. She could swing from being giddy to feeling low-spirited, cross, and mean in the course of a day. They were both very concerned about this. They talked to their family doctor about the problem and, based on this information, and his own concerns about possible dementia, their doctor referred Elizabeth to a neurologist.

The neurologist, Dr. Alouise, did a thorough intake and had an assistant perform a number of evaluations on Elizabeth. Some of these seemed to be like children's guessing games to her, but to her surprise she sometimes had difficulty conjuring up the name of things that she knew. For instance, when shown the picture of a whisk, she could only describe it as "that thing you use to mix up an omelet" and only a few minutes later did the proper name occur to her. This seemed to happen for many objects. Other questions were asked. Dr. Alouise arranged for a brain scan and ordered some blood tests… (continued on page 22)

## Brain Basics

The brain is an extremely complex structure made of tissue and nerves that control everything we do, from voluntary actions (such as walking) to involuntary actions (such as breathing). The brain is responsible for communicating moment by moment with all other parts of the body through the central nervous system (CNS) and the peripheral nervous system (PNS). The brain is also responsible for managing our emotions and thoughts, and for nurturing our short-term and long-term memory.

Scientists are slowly discovering its secrets, but in many ways, the brain is still a new frontier, and aging-related diseases continue to challenge neurologists to fully understand them.

However, there is no need to take a course in neuroanatomy to grasp the structures and functions of the brain that relate to aging-related diseases. It is intriguing to know how our brains function normally so we can see how they sometimes do not function so well as we age.

## Neuron Function

The adult brain contains between 80 and 100 billion cells. Each cell has about 100 thousand connections to other cells. Known also as neurons, these cells fire electrochemical signals (a small electrical current) along their lining, or membrane, until this signal reaches the tip of one of the branches of another cell. There it causes the release of a chemical compound that attaches to the next neuron in the chain, leading to a new signal. These chemicals are called neurotransmitters.

## Neuron Function

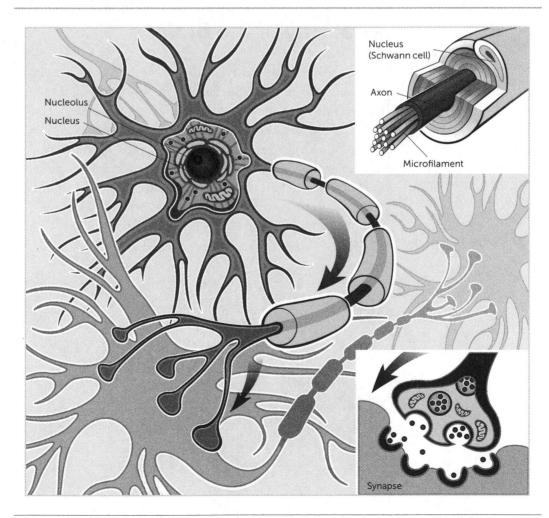

Nucleus (Schwann cell)

Axon

Microfilament

Nucleolus

Nucleus

Synapse

### Kinds of Neurotransmitters

Neurotransmitters can be excitatory (prompting a neuron to fire) or inhibitory (impeding a neuron from firing). Some of the major excitatory neurotransmitters are the chemical monoamines, including epinephrine, norepinephrine, histamine, serotonin, and dopamine. The disruption of dopamine production in the brain is a causal factor in Parkinson's disease. Some of the major inhibitory neurotransmitters are serotonin and gamma-aminobutyric acid (GABA). Other neurotransmitters include acetylcholines and amino acids.

- *Acetylcholines*
- *Amino acids:* Gamma-aminobutyric acid and glycine glutamate aspartate
- *Neuropeptides:* Oxytocin, endorphins, vasopressin
- *Monoamines:* Epinephrine, norepinephrine, histamine, serotonin, and dopamine

## Anatomy of the Brain

The parts of the brain are typically grouped by location into the forebrain, midbrain, and hindbrain. The forebrain includes the cerebrum, thalamus, and hypothalamus (part of the limbic system). The midbrain consists of the tectum and tegmentum. The hindbrain is made of the cerebellum, pons, and medulla. Often the midbrain, pons, and medulla are referred to together as the brain stem. These parts of the brain are not discrete; rather, they interact through a series of networks and feedback loops.

## Parts of the Brain

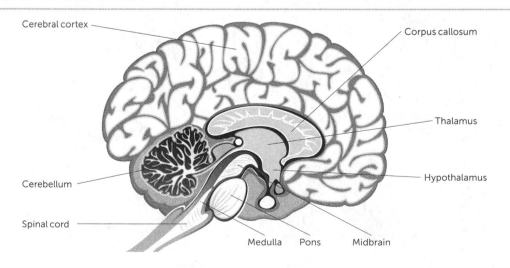

Cerebral cortex

Corpus callosum

Thalamus

Hypothalamus

Cerebellum

Spinal cord

Medulla     Pons     Midbrain

## Cerebral Lobes

The cerebral cortex is further divided into four lobes:

- *Frontal lobe:* responsible for reasoning, planning, speech, movement, emotions, and problem solving
- *Parietal lobe:* responsible for movement, orientation, recognition, and perception of stimuli
- *Occipital lobe:* responsible for visual processing
- *Temporal lobe:* responsible for perception and recognition, hearing, memory, and speech

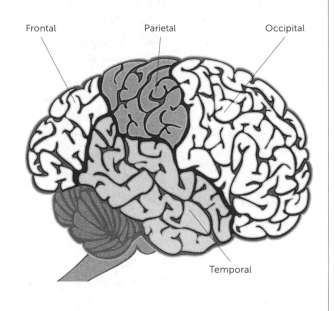

Frontal    Parietal    Occipital

Temporal

## Forebrain

The cerebrum, thalamus, and hypothalamus make up the forebrain. The pituitary gland is connected to the hypothalamus and secretes hormones that regulate homeostasis, or equilibrium, among the various body systems and the brain.

## Cerebrum

Also known as the cerebral cortex, the cerebrum is the largest part of the human brain, associated with higher brain function, such as thought and action. The cerebral cortex is composed of two hemispheres, right and left, that are connected by the corpus callosum. The right hemisphere is typically associated with creativity, holism, and pattern recognition, and the left hemisphere is associated with logic and reasoning. The cerebral cortex also has nerve cells that control muscle movement. Many of our impulses to move originate there. We also use much of this part of the brain for memory function. How we store memories is still unknown. In some neurological diseases, such as Alzheimer's disease, these functions of the cerebrum are disturbed.

**DID YOU KNOW?**

### Executive Function

The prefrontal cortex is the executive of the brain, responsible for planning, judging, decision making, and assigning tasks. The prefrontal cortex enables you to complete actions sequentially. You cannot execute all tasks at one time. In some neurological diseases, the prefrontal cortex loses this executive ability and thinking becomes confused.

## Thalamus

The thalamus acts as a processing center for the sensory information coming into the brain. All of the information gathered by our senses, which give us knowledge of our world, travels along this pathway. Our spinal cord carries signals and actual neurons (some of which are 3 feet/90 cm long) that transmit information from the brain down to and from the senses up to our central nervous system. In some neurological diseases, such as stroke (depending on where blood supply to the brain was interrupted), the thalamus is damaged and our senses become confused.

## Brain-Body Feedback Loop

The three main communication systems in the body — cardiovascular, immune, and endocrine — are governed by the brain, which instigates the circulation of hormones that feed back signals to the brain in a loop. How does this work? Using the thyroid system as an example, the hypothalamus sends thyrotropin-releasing hormone (TRH) to the pituitary gland to create more thyroid-stimulating hormone (TSH). When the thyroid successfully makes more thyroid hormone and blood levels of the hormone rise, both the pituitary and the hypothalamus are inhibited — and, for a time, less thyroid hormone is produced.

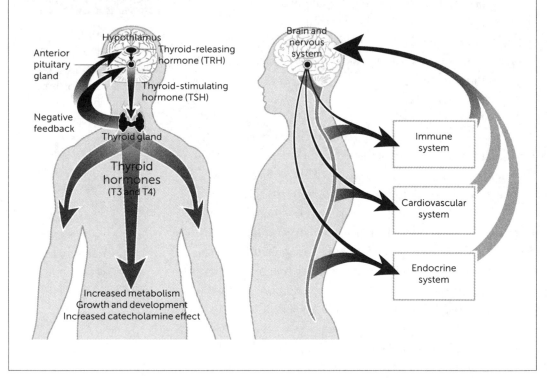

## Hypothalamus

The hypothalamus is responsible for hormone production. These hormones govern body temperature, thirst, hunger, sleep, moods, sex drive, and the release of other hormones. The hypothalamus is one of several glands, including the pituitary gland, that interact within the endocrine system. This interaction is extensive. For example, the secretion of the thyroid gland hormone is triggered by thyroid-stimulating hormone (TSH), which comes from the pituitary gland, which is under the control of the hypothalamus. In some neurological diseases, such as tumors that destroy portions of the hypothalamus or pituitary gland, endocrine function can be lost, or increase and become unbalanced.

## Limbic System

The limbic system, often referred to as the emotional brain, is found within the cerebrum. This system contains the thalamus, hypothalamus, amygdala, and hippocampus. The amygdala responds to threats by generating feelings of anxiety and emotional energy, the fight-or-flight response. The hippocampus is absolutely critical to learning and helps to "write" memories into our brain. The hippocampus actually sprouts new neurons, and the faster we learn, the more it can regenerate.

## Midbrain

The midbrain is a relay center for vision and hearing information. The midbrain includes the tectum and tegmentum, which, in turn, include the substantia nigra. The neurotransmitter dopamine is generated in the substantia nigra. This neurotransmitter is used in the regulation of movement, as in the case of Parkinson's disease. Dopamine is also involved in motivation, pleasure, desire, and reward systems in the brain.

## Hindbrain

The hindbrain, or brain stem, is responsible for basic vital life functions, such as breathing, heartbeat, and blood pressure. The brain stem is made up of the midbrain, pons, and medulla. The pons is a bridge that connects the medulla to the spinal cord and governs the autonomic system, including digestion, body temperature, and heart rate. This part of the brain is common to many other living organisms, including all animals. The brain stem is involved in cardiovascular-system control, respiratory-system control, pain-sensitivity control, alertness, awareness, and consciousness. In some neurological diseases, such as traumatic head injury, damage to the brain stem can be life threatening.

### Cerebellum

The cerebellum is similar to the cerebrum, with two hemispheres and a cortex. The cerebellum is involved with the regulation and coordination of movement, posture, and balance. The cerebellum also acts as a source of learning, memory, and control for coordinated movements. When a dancer learns a complex dance routine, the cerebellum is involved. The cerebellum not only ensures the smooth operation of the motor system, but it is also involved in the overall thought-processing system of the brain. In some neurological diseases, such as Wernicke-Korsakoff syndrome (brought on by excessive long-term alcohol consumption and deficiency of vitamin $B_1$), the cerebellum loses control of motor functions.

# Peripheral Nervous System

The peripheral nervous system (PNS) consists of the nerves and ganglia outside of the brain and spinal cord. The main function of the PNS is to connect the central nervous system (CNS) to the limbs and organs, essentially serving as a communication relay going back and forth between the brain and the extremities. Unlike the CNS, the PNS is not protected by the bone of spine and skull, or by the blood-brain barrier, leaving it exposed to toxins and mechanical injuries.

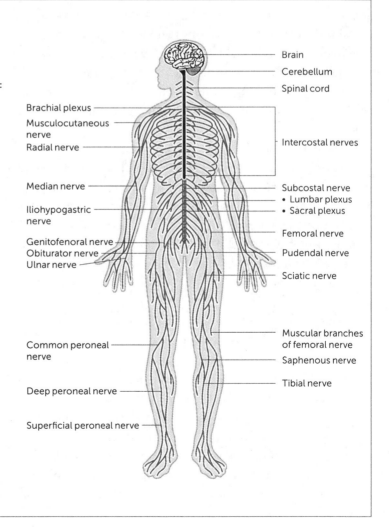

Brachial plexus
Musculocutaneous nerve
Radial nerve
Median nerve
Iliohypogastric nerve
Genitofenoral nerve
Obiturator nerve
Ulnar nerve
Common peroneal nerve
Deep peroneal nerve
Superficial peroneal nerve

Brain
Cerebellum
Spinal cord
Intercostal nerves
Subcostal nerve
• Lumbar plexus
• Sacral plexus
Femoral nerve
Pudendal nerve
Sciatic nerve
Muscular branches of femoral nerve
Saphenous nerve
Tibial nerve

# Key Neurologic Terms

*Atherosclerosis:* a condition characterized by medium-sized arteries that have developed a layer of plaque that can obstruct the vessel or lead to a blood clot.

*Atherosclerotic plaque:* an outgrowth in the inner lining of the blood vessel that is composed of cholesterol, dead white blood cells, proteins, and eventually calcium. Plaques can block arteries and stiffen the walls of arteries.

*Central nervous system:* a system composed of the brain and spinal cord, where information from the senses is transmitted to the brain, thinking and learning occurs, and control signals of muscles originates.

*Chronic:* a condition that spans a length of time. The exact criteria depend on the condition; but by definition months or years (or decades).

*Cognition:* a term referring to the mental processes involved in gaining knowledge and comprehension. These processes include thinking, knowing, remembering, judging, and problem solving.

*Dementia:* the process where thinking, memory, and the control of behavior erodes into what is usually a permanent state of disability. Dementia has various degrees of severity. The disease is progressive, but can develop slowly. This is not to be confused with delirium, which is a temporary loss of orientation to place and people, and can result in uncontrolled or even violent behavior.

*Ischemia:* this term refers to the phenomenon where the blood supply and therefore the oxygen supply to a tissue is interrupted. Ischemic events that last more than a few minutes typically lead to cell death. Ischemic events in the heart are often termed a myocardial infarction, and in the brain, a stroke (although there are several variants).

*Neurology:* the diagnosis and treatment of diseases of the nervous system.

*Neuroplasticity:* the phenomenon whereby the brain can relearn certain skills and remap, or rewrite, information and memories to new areas of the brain. This is related to the ability of the brain to spawn new cells or remodel existing connections — often in the hippocampus, a brain region critical to learning and memory that can actively grow even later in life.

*Pathology:* the study of the causes, processes, and outcomes of disease. Pathology can be directed at the study of cells, the components of cells (such as the nucleus and DNA, or deoxyribonucleic acid), tissues, and organs, as well as the effects of disease on overall functions in the body.

*Traumatic brain injury:* damage to the brain from a physical force, which can lead to loss or lowered consciousness and long-term changes in personality, mood and cognitive function. It is not a degenerative change in the sense that Alzheimer's disease is, but chronic, progressive issues in thinking and mood can occur that will intensify if not treated.

# Kinds of Neurological Diseases and Disorders

There are many different kinds of neurological diseases. The Merck manual lists more than 50 kinds, and the National Institute of Neurological Disorder and Stroke lists more than 300 associated conditions. Related conditions are typically grouped by symptoms or function, such as dementia, motor control, and seizure conditions. Some conditions, such as Parkinson's disease, overlap the categories of dementia and motor-control conditions. Progressive degenerative aging-related neurological diseases are the focus of this book.

## Dementia (Aging-Related)

- Alzheimer's disease
- Amyotrophic lateral sclerosis (ALS), also called Lou Gehrig's disease
- Cerebrovascular (vascular) dementia
- Drug-induced neurological degeneration
- Lewy body dementia
- Motor neuron disease
- Parkinson's disease
- Peripheral neuropathy

## Movement Disorders

- Dystonia
- Huntington's disease
- Parkinson's disease
- Progressive supranuclear palsy
- Multiple system atrophy (MSA)
- Tourette's syndrome
- Tremor

## Seizure Disorders

- Epilepsy
- Febrile seizures
- Temporal lobe seizures

## Traumatic Brain Injury

- Penetrating injury
- Closed head injury
- Post-concussion syndrome

## Communications (Language) Disorders

- Aphasia
- Dyslexia
- Apraxia
- Agraphia

## Demyelinating Disorders

- Multiple sclerosis
- Neuropathies
- Guillain-Barré disease

## Sleep Disorders

- Sleep apnea
- Narcolepsy

## Headache Disorders

- Migraine headaches
- Cluster headaches
- Tension headaches

## Infections

- Meningitis
- Encephalitis

**Q** **What are aging-related brain diseases?**

**A** There are many kinds of neurological diseases, from acoustic neuroma to Zellweger syndrome, but only a few that are aging-related. Aging-related diseases are characterized by the degeneration of brain cells and the progressive loss of common motor skills, thoughts, and memories.
These progressive aging-related neurological diseases are collectively known as dementia, or senility, in some sources. They are found primarily in the CNS and secondarily in the PNS.

# Do I Have Dementia?

## CASE STUDY

### Alzheimer's Disease (continued from page 12)

Elizabeth struggled through a series of tests — physical examinations, MRI scans, and cognitive questionnaires. When she returned to Dr. Alouise's office a week later, he did not have good news. Elizabeth was in the early stages of what was in all likelihood Alzheimer's disease. This was a shock for Elizabeth and her family. It sent her and her husband into a tailspin of sorts.

Dr. Alouise connected with local resources, including a chapter of an organization that supports Alzheimer's patients and their families… (continued on page 37).

## DID YOU KNOW?

**High Target**

Neurological aging diseases often target the higher centers of the brain. Alzheimer's disease robs people of their cognitive ability — and that precious storehouse of treasures, their memory.

Dementia and senility are the collective terms given to aging-related diseases caused by the gradual death of brain cells. These diseases are degenerative and share many symptoms, chiefly impairment in thought, memory, mood, and motion. Although most people with dementia are elderly, dementia is not an inevitable part of aging; instead, dementia is caused by specific brain diseases. Alzheimer's disease is the most common kind of dementia, followed by vascular dementia.

As neurologists have learned more about the way the brain functions, they have also discovered more defining symptoms of aging-related diseases. Tests have been developed to improve the diagnosis of these diseases. In many cases, early and accurate diagnosis can help protect, repair, and enhance your mental health.

# Location of Aging-Related Diseases

| Aging-Related Disease | Brain Location | Neurological Symptoms |
|---|---|---|
| Alzheimer's disease | • Forebrain: cerebrum<br>• Blood vessels: walls of the meningeal and cerebral blood vessels<br>• Thalamus | • Loss of short-term memory<br>• Declining ability to learn<br>• Social life lost<br>• Loss of self-care abilities |
| Amyotrophic lateral sclerosis | • Cerebral cortex and spinal cord | • Similar to motor neuron diseases<br>• Loss of speech, eye movement |
| Cerebrovascular dementia | • Cerebral cortex | • Similar to Alzheimer's<br>• May progress rapidly due to undetected blood vessel occlusion (ministroke) and then remain at same level of severity for some time |
| Diabetes | • Beta cells of pancreas<br>• Insulin receptors on muscle cells | • Elevated blood sugar<br>• Damage to body proteins<br>• Later-stage damage to nervous system due to chemical alteration of proteins in the entire nervous system and destruction of Schwann cells (peripheral nervous system)<br>• Multiple hormonal effects |
| Drug-induced neurological degeneration | • Any brain center<br>• Substantia nigra<br>• Cerebral cortex | • Depends on location, but may include changes in thinking, expression, or movement |
| Lewy body dementia | • Cerebral cortex<br>• Substantia nigra | • Same as Alzheimer's<br>• Movement disorders similar to Parkinson's<br>• Frightening nightmares (early)<br>• Hallucinations (later in disease) |
| Motor neuron disease | • Motor neurons of the cerebral cortex<br>• Anterior horn cells (motor cells) of the spinal cord | • Loss of muscle strength<br>• Loss of coordination<br>• Muscle spasm<br>• Muscle atrophy |

| Aging-Related Disease | Brain Location | Neurological Symptoms |
| --- | --- | --- |
| Parkinson's disease | • Midbrain: substantia nigra<br>• Endocrine system: dopamine pathways | • Exhaustion of dopamine<br>• Loss of motor functions<br>• Dementia |
| Peripheral neuropathy | • Nerve cells and their branches originating from the spinal cord | • Loss of sensation<br>• Pain<br>• Muscle atrophy |
| Sleep disorders | • Hypothalamus<br>• Limbic system<br>• Pineal gland | • Difficult falling asleep or staying asleep<br>• Lack of refreshing rapid eye movement (REM) or deeper-level 3 or 4 sleep |

# Alzheimer's Disease

Named for German physician Alois Alzheimer and also called senile dementia, Alzheimer's disease is the most common kind of dementia. An early diagnosis is important for the control of symptoms that eventually erase many memories and impede an ability to handle daily functions.

## Symptoms of Alzheimer's Disease

- Short-term memory fails
- Learning skills decline
- The naming of objects, making simple calculations, reasoning, and figuring out directions become difficult
- Social skills are lost
- Long-term memory, even of the names of family members, weakens, although moments of clarity do occur

## Amyloid Plaques

When pathologists look at the brain of a victim of Alzheimer's disease, they see amyloid plaques, a clear sign of damage. These plaques are seen primarily in the blood vessels of the cerebral cortex (the part of the brain that controls thinking and the initiation of movement) and on the walls of the meninx, the covering that surrounds the brain. Plaques slowly but surely destroy memory, thinking, and basic life skills, eventually leading to heart attack or stroke.

## Alzheimer's Progression

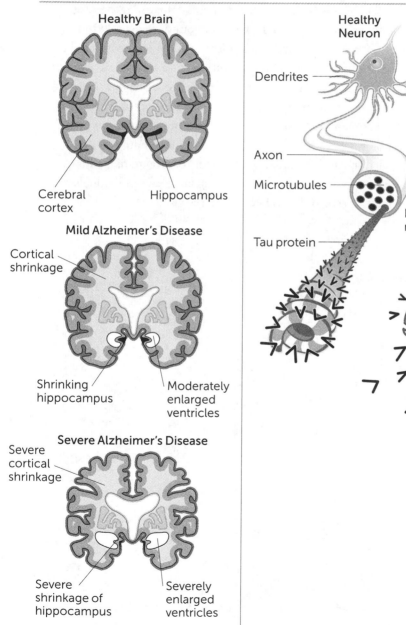

**Healthy Brain**

Cerebral cortex

Hippocampus

**Mild Alzheimer's Disease**

Cortical shrinkage

Shrinking hippocampus

Moderately enlarged ventricles

**Severe Alzheimer's Disease**

Severe cortical shrinkage

Severe shrinkage of hippocampus

Severely enlarged ventricles

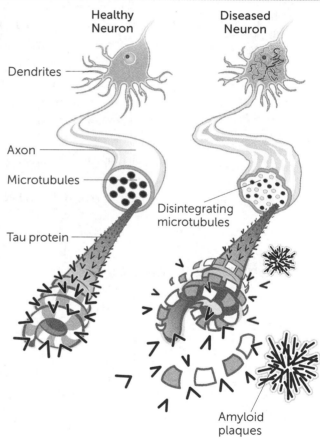

**Healthy Neuron**

**Diseased Neuron**

Dendrites

Axon

Microtubules

Tau protein

Disintegrating microtubules

Amyloid plaques

## Astrocytes

Astrocytes are the most common neuron in the brain. They form the blood-brain barrier and so control what can and cannot enter the brain from the blood supply. In Alzheimer's disease, astrocytes can develop scar tissue, from brain injury or trauma, that can reduce brain function.

## Neurofibrillary Tangles

Neurofibrillary tangles, formerly called microtubules, are stringy lesions located between neurons. They are part of the architectural skeleton of cells, including brain cells. But these "crossbeams" or "studs" of the brain are damaged by deposits of a protein called tau. Tau deposits are found in several kinds of brain disease, including Alzheimer's. It has been postulated that the neurofibrillary tangles may initially be a reaction to oxidative stress. They show up later in Alzheimer's and do not account for most of the neuron loss themselves, but their presence shows progression of the disease. The result is neuronal and synaptic loss. The areas most affected are the hippocampus (central to learning) and the associative cortex (central to reasoning). Genetic factors are also involved, causing some individuals to be more at risk for tau-related brain disease.

## Neurofibrillary Tangles

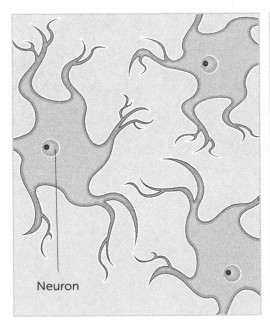

Neuron

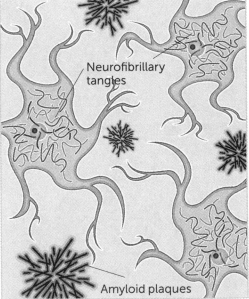

Neurofibrillary tangles

Amyloid plaques

## Aluminum Toxicity

Aluminum has been found in the lesions of Alzheimer's disease. This potentially toxic metal is found in antacids, drinking water (especially softened water), baking powder, processed foods, beer, underarm deodorant, and cookware.

## Alzheimer's Diagnosis

A diagnosis of Alzheimer's disease typically involves a physical examination and a differential diagnosis of symptoms, as well as various cognitive, functional, and global assessments. There are many other clinical tools to help diagnose Alzheimer's disease and other dementias, as recommended by the American Academy of Neurology, the American Alzheimer's Association, and the Alzheimer Society of Canada.

**DID YOU KNOW?**

**Sniff Test**
The loss of smell is a well-known early sign of dementia. Amyloid plaques accumulate in the part of the brain involved in perceiving odors, which can be a precursor to Alzheimer's disease.

## The American Academy of Neurology Recommended Tests for Dementia

- Complete blood cell count
- Electrolyte levels in the blood (potassium, sodium, chloride)
- Blood levels of glucose, nitrogen, creatinine
- Blood levels of vitamin $B_{12}$
- Liver function
- Thyroid function
- Depression screening

## Cognitive, Functional, and Global Assessments

According to the American Alzheimer's Association, the assessments marked with an asterisk are most often found in clinical settings.

**Cognitive assessments (testing thinking ability)**
- Alzheimer's Disease Assessment Scale, cognitive subsection (ADAS-cog)
- Blessed Information-Memory-Concentration Test (BIMC)
- Clinical Dementia Rating (CDR) Scale
- Mini-Mental State Examination (MMSE)*

**Functional assessments (seeing how well the person carries out skills of daily life)**
- Functional Assessment Questionnaire (FAQ)*
- Instrumental Activities of Daily Living (IADL)

- Physical Self-Maintenance Scale (PSMS)*
- Progressive Deterioration Scale (PDS)

**Global assessments (overall life and cognitive assessment)**
- Clinical Global Impression of Change (CGIC)
- Clinical Interview-Based Impression (CIBI)
- Global Deterioration Scale (GDS)

**Caregiver-based assessments**
- Behavioral Pathology in Alzheimer's Disease Rating Scale (BEHAVE-AD)
- Neuropsychiatric Inventory (NPI)*

Adapted from the American Alzheimer's Association

# Warning Signs

The Alzheimer's Association has identified 10 behavioral changes that indicate possible onset of Alzheimer's:
1. Memory loss that disrupts daily life
2. Challenges in planning or solving problems
3. Difficulty completing familiar tasks at home, at work, or at leisure
4. Confusion with time and place
5. Trouble understanding visual images and spatial relationships
6. New problems with words in speaking or writing
7. Misplacing things and losing the ability to retrace steps
8. Decreased or poor judgment
9. Withdrawal from work or social activities
10. Changes in mood and personality

### Alzheimer's Disease Assessment Scale

Here is an example of how suspected or confirmed Alzheimer's disease might be evaluated. No one tool is completely diagnostic and a clinical history and often some kind of brain imaging is part of the diagnostic workup.

The instrument covers a number of key areas such as behavior, mood, and dementia symptoms, such as delusions (faulty beliefs) or hallucinations (faulty sensory information, such as seeing things or hearing things that are not there). Each of these items is rated for how severe it is and how much it distresses the patient. A professional trained in the use of this scale creates a report after scoring it.

# Caregiver Memory Questionnaire

Name of patient: _____ Date _____

Informant: Spouse: _____ Child: _____ Other: _____

Please answer the following questions based on changes that have occurred since the patient first began to experience memory problems.

Circle "yes" only if the symptom has been present the past month. Otherwise, circle "no".

Rate the severity of the symptom (how it affects the patient)
1= Mild (noticeable, but not significant)
2= Moderate (significant, but not dramatic)
3= Severe (very marked, prominent, dramatic)

Rate the distress you experience because of that symptom
0= Not distressing
1= Minimal (slightly distressing, not a problem to cope with)
2= Mild (not very distressing, generally easy to cope with)
3= Moderate (fairly distressing, not always easy to cope with)
4= Severe (very distressing, difficult to cope with)
5= Extreme or very extreme (extremely distressing, unable to cope with

*Please answer each question honestly and carefully. Ask for assistance if you are not sure how to answer the question.*

**Delusions**
Yes   No

Does she believe that others are stealing from her or planning to harm her?
Severity:  1   2   3   Distress:  0   1   2   3   4   5

**Hallucinations**
Yes   No

Does he act as if he hears voices? Does he talk to people who are not there?
Severity:  1   2   3   Distress:  0   1   2   3   4   5

**Agitation or aggression**
Yes   No

Is she stubborn or resistive to help from others?
Severity:  1   2   3   Distress:  0   1   2   3   4   5

**Depression or dysphoria**
Yes   No

Is he sad or in low spirits. Does he cry?
Severity:  1   2   3   Distress:  0   1   2   3   4   5

**Anxiety**
Yes   No

Does she become upset when separated from you? Does she have other signs of nervousness, such as shortness of breath, sighing, unable to relax, feeling extensively tense?
Severity:  1   2   3   Distress:  0   1   2   3   4   5

**Elation or euphoria**
Yes   No

Does he appear to be *too* good or act excessively happy?
Severity:  1   2   3   Distress:  0   1   2   3   4   5

**Apathy or indifference**
Yes   No

Does she appear to be less interested in her usual activities and plans of others?
Severity:  1   2   3   Distress:  0   1   2   3   4   5

**Disinhibition**
Yes   No

Does he seem to act impulsively? Talk to strangers as if he knows them? Say things that may hurt people's feelings?
Severity:  1   2   3   Distress:  0   1   2   3   4   5

**Irritability or lability**
Yes   No

Is she impatient and cranky? Does she have trouble coping with delays or waiting for planned activities?
Severity:  1   2   3   Distress:  0   1   2   3   4   5

**Motor disturbance**
Yes   No

Does he engage in repetitive activities, such as pacing around the house, handling buttons, wrapping string, or doing other things repetitively?
Severity:  1   2   3   Distress:  0   1   2   3   4   5

**Nightime behaviors**
Yes   No

Does she awaken you during the night, rise too early in the morning, or take excessive naps during the day?
Severity:  1   2   3   Distress:  0   1   2   3   4   5

**Appetite and eating**
Yes   No

Has he lost or gained weight or had a change in the food he likes?
Severity:  1   2   3   Distress:  0   1   2   3   4   5

**Q** How does dementia progress?

**A** Alzheimer's progresses slowly through three stages, as itemized in the 2012 Johns Hopkins White Paper, *Memory: Your Personal Guide to Alzheimer's Disease and Dementia*:

*Stage 1 Symptoms*
- Forgetfulness
- Faulty judgment
- Poor insight
- Misplaced possessions

*Stage 2 Symptoms*
- Memory deteriorates
- Basic self-care skills decline
- Trouble expressing themselves
- Unable to dress, bath, cook
- Occasional delusions and hallucinations

*Stage 3 Symptoms*
- Reasoning capacity is lost
- Cannot walk
- Require full-time home or institutional care
- Susceptible to lung and urinary tract infections
- Pneumonia (most common cause of death)
- Death

# Vascular Dementia

Vascular dementia is the second-most common form of dementia. Most dementia associated with cerebrovascular changes is caused by atherosclerosis, which may in time lead to small blood clots or infarcts, hemorrhage, or transient ischemic attacks (TIAs). Atherosclerosis predisposes a person to stroke.

Atherosclerosis is characterized by a progressive narrowing of the inside of the artery, due to a buildup of plaques, leading to a lack of healthy blood flow to any downstream tissues. Emboli from the heart or lungs can travel to the brain and lodge there. Local clotting events can occlude large or small vessels. Vascular inflammation due to infection or to the use of drugs that raise blood pressure and tighten up blood vessels (such as amphetamines) can cause ischemia. These all can lead to cerebrovascular attack (CVA), or stroke, and cognitive decline.

## Symptoms of Vascular Dementia

**Ischemia:** Carotid artery stenosis or vertebral artery stenosis are conditions that involve the narrowing of the inner surface of the arteries in the neck and spine (which give the brain its blood supply). This can lead to ischemia. Intracranial vessels can also

be affected. Transient ischemic attacks are a reversible closing of the artery, and people who experience them usually show other symptoms related to a change in the brain (such as confusion, numbness of some body part, unsteadiness). They are most likely caused by a reversible clot. However, they can progress to stroke, and are a serious warning that the person is at risk of stroke.
**Stroke:** Stroke is due to a neurological deficit caused by decreased cerebral circulation.

# Parkinson's Disease

Parkinson's disease is caused by the decline of a specific type of brain cell that manufactures the neurotransmitter dopamine. Dopamine influences the function of motor neurons that control movement. A physical examination can reveal the characteristic symptoms of Parkinson's disease.

## Symptoms of Parkinson's Disease

- Rigid muscles, sometimes with a tremor that can progress to affect the face and voice
- Walking and gait can be affected
- Certain tasks that have long been done well, such as doing up buttons, become very difficult
- At an advanced stage, Parkinson's disease may result in changes to thought patterns and even a kind of dementia

## Dopamine-Containing Cells

Our brain cells are designed to move our muscles in concert. One of the key pathways for this is the corticospinal tract; the nerves in this pathway originate in the higher centers of the brain and send their axons (the extension of the nerve cell) all the way down the spinal cord. The firing of these nerves is modified by the action of other cells in the brain, including an area called the substantia nigra. This keeps the muscle contractions from being stiff, exaggerated, or jerky. In Parkinson's disease, the dopamine-containing cells that impact movement begin to die off, and as the disease progresses, the symptoms become more prominent. Dopamine-replacement medications and anti-tremor drugs can improve quality of life. Deep-brain surgery and stem cell implants have proven to prolong life.

## Parkinson's Disease

Ron was 55 years old when he first visited our clinic on referral from his family doctor. He did double duty as a professor of engineering communications at the local university and a senior editor for a mid-sized publishing company. For a few months now, Ron had been having trouble projecting his voice in the lecture hall. After one class, two students approached him hesitantly and asked if he could start using a microphone. In 20 years of teaching he had never had this complaint, but he sucked up his pride and got the AV technicians to wire him up for the next class.

During the same few months, Ron noticed that his left foot was slapping down as he walked through the halls, loud enough to make him feel self-conscious about walking. Things started to get even more strange when a business colleague he had not seen for almost a year asked him to hurry up while they were walking to a meeting. "Hurry up or we'll be late for our meeting." That same day another friend he was visiting asked if he was having back problems because he was showing such difficulty tying up his shoes.

That summer at a family picnic Ron lacked eye-hand coordination while playing badminton, and a month later, when oldtimers hockey began, he "froze" on the ice — a teammate passed the puck, but when Ron went to shoot, nothing happened. He stood there dumbfounded while his teammates asked if he was okay. Later, a teammate who had witnessed this event worried that Ron must have had a small stroke, what he called a TIA. Things were getting serious now… (continued on page 46).

# Motor Neuron Disease

Motor neuron disease refers to pathology affecting the nerves that control muscles: either those in the spinal cord or the muscles higher up in the cerebral cortex of the brain. The result is muscle wasting, which involves weakness and a loss of control of those muscles. Nerve cells have a nourishing effect on muscle fibers, and when nerves are damaged, muscles will waste away due to the lack of these chemical messengers.

## Symptoms of Motor Neuron Disease

- Fine twitches at first, which indicate spontaneous contractions of degenerating nerve fibers

- Electromyography (a measurement of electrical activity in muscles) shows evidence of a loss of nerve control of the muscle and a decrease in the number of motor units (clusters of muscle cells that work together) active during contractions
- Eventually, weak muscles that are noticeably different than still, healthy muscles become the cardinal sign

# Amyotrophic Lateral Sclerosis

Amyotrophic lateral sclerosis (ALS), also known as Lou Gehrig's disease, is one of the most common diseases of the nerves that control muscles or motor neurons. This disease affects both upper (brain) and lower (spinal cord) motor neurons — and therefore involves a degeneration of motor neurons in both areas. There is very little inflammation, and abnormalities in the neurofilaments (part of the "skeleton" of the cell) are seen in the neuron cell body.

## Symptoms of Amyotrophic Lateral Sclerosis

- ALS starts with weakness and cramps; it may begin in the hands, and is usually asymmetrical
- Mouth and throat muscles that control swallowing and speech, enervated by cranial nerves, are often affected, leading to dysarthria (difficulty speaking) and dysphagia (difficulty with swallowing)
- Muscle groups throughout the body become affected, leading eventually to almost total paralysis
- Death occurs from respiratory failure

## SOD Mutation

The body has proteins called enzymes that carry out special functions that help break down free-radical-producing compounds. One important enzyme in the cell that helps to protect the cell structures is called superoxide dismutase (SOD). SOD catalyzes the reactions of a toxic byproduct of oxygen in the body that can then be broken down to water. The altered specificity of SOD in ALS patients may lead to a reverse reaction whereby more free radicals are formed, leading to neural damage. The very enzyme (SOD) that is meant to serve as a shield to protect the nerve cell against free radicals actually leads to more free radical damage to the cell!

**Q** **I've heard that monosodium glutamate can compound the effects of ALS. How does that work?**

**A** Patients with a family history of amyotrophic lateral sclerosis should avoid monosodium glutamate (MSG). This flavoring agent can cause transient elevations in glutamate levels, which may exacerbate ALS. On the cellular level in ALS, scientists have found that glutamate transport is abnormal. Glutamate is a neurotransmitter that leads to the increased activation of nerve cells. It causes the opening of communication channels, and when sodium and calcium rush into the brain or nerve cell, there is also a release of calcium already stored in the cell. Under normal circumstances, this leads to a small electrical signal going along the nerve — a good thing. Calcium, having served its purpose, is supposed to be quickly removed from the synapse (the space in between nerve cells where neurons are only chemically, not physically, connected) by special helper cells, called astrocytes. (Sustained elevations in intracellular calcium would lead to cell death.) Astrocytes remove glutamate and convert it to glutamine. In ALS, there is a decrease in glutamate transport activity in the motor cortex and spinal cord, and perhaps also upticks in calcium inside cells.

# Neuropathies

Neuropathies present with sensory loss, muscle weakness, and atrophy, with decreased deep-tendon reflexes. Neuropathy can take on several forms within the peripheral nervous system.

- *Chemical-induced diabetes mellitus:* Neuropathy can result from the destruction of Schwann cells, which are support cells for peripheral nerves, in diabetes mellitus. High levels of sugar in the blood eventually kill these nerves.
- *Entrapment:* Neuropathy can result from pressure on a nerve, as in the case of carpal tunnel syndrome, where the median nerve is compressed.
- *Neurological degeneration:* Neuropathy can result from toxic agents, such as lead, chemotherapeutic agents, and some pharmaceuticals.
- *Nutritional deficiency:* Neuropathy can result from vitamin deficiency. For example, a loss of sensation in the hands and feet can occur in vitamin $B_{12}$ deficiency.
- *Trauma:* Neuropathy can result from trauma, where there is a direct injury to a nerve. For example, calcium deposits in the openings for nerves along the spine (these little openings are called foramina) can start to actually impinge on the nerve roots that exit the spine, and eventually lead to pain, weakness, strange sensations, or even death of the nerve.

# Sleep Disorders

Many people today do not get enough sleep. Although 8 hours is the recommended amount for many, the average is less than 7. Lack of sleep has been associated with the development of anxiety disorders. A sleep deficiency may be one of the greatest disturbances to brain health today.

Difficulty sleeping can occur at different points for various reasons. Some people find it hard to fall asleep (initial insomnia) because of anxiety or depression. Sleep patterns can be disturbed by shift work and traveling across time zones.

> **Q** A single cup of coffee keeps me awake if I have it after 5 p.m., but my spouse is able to have 3 mugs of coffee if we go out for dinner and then sleeps just fine. Why am I so sensitive?
>
> **A** People metabolize caffeine differently. Some people are slow caffeine metabolizers and others are rapid metabolizers. Part of this is due to differences in the type of enzyme that breaks down caffeine in the liver. It is called the cytochrome P450 enzyme, and different people have slightly different types.

**DID YOU KNOW?**

**Sleep Apnea**
This is a more serious cause of poor sleep quality and requires assessment by a sleep specialist. Sleep apnea occurs when respiration has ceased for 10 seconds or more, with a decrease in oxygen partial pressure (PO2). Obstructions (obesity or pharyngeal/laryngeal defects) or erratic control from the brain (central apnea) can be the cause.

# Diabetes Mellitus

In diabetes mellitus, the insulin-secreting cells of the pancreas, the beta cells, are destroyed by the body's own immune system. When these cells run out, or there are too few of them still functioning, the symptoms of the disease appear (frequent urination, thirst, hunger, and weight loss). Diabetes leads to high levels of sugar in the bloodstream. This, in turn, causes glucose to attach itself to body proteins that can alter their function.

## Effect on the Brain

In the brain, this can lead to the buildup of advanced glycation end products (AGEs), which damage neurons. High glucose levels and AGEs can increase oxidative stress and free radical products. Blood vessel integrity can decrease and atherosclerosis is accelerated. The support cells of the nerves, the Schwann cells, are also damaged by high glucose levels, which cause a sugar called sorbitol to form in the cell. Sorbitol crystalizes and leads to Schwann cell death.

## Traumatic Brain Injury

One complex and very serious type of dysfunction of the brain is that related to traumatic brain injury (TBI). There are many causes of TBI, including motor vehicle accidents, concussions in contact sports, and exposure of military personnel to blasts, such as those from improvised explosive devices. TBI can be due to a penetrating injury to the head (such as a gunshot wound) or a closed injury (blast or blunt trauma that does not break the skull open).

### Prolonged and Insidious Aftereffects

The immediate aftereffects of TBI can in themselves lead to damage to the brain and loss of function. For example, a large blood clot or a large amount of bleeding in the brain can cause pressure to rise (inside the closed compartment of the skull) and lead to brain damage or death. Another classic example is when a child is hit on the head with a baseball and becomes lethargic later on that day. Insidiously, blood is pooling on top of or just inside the brain, and the pressure increase is eventually lethal unless treated promptly at an emergency room.

Concussions received in sports are increasingly recognized as a cause of declining cognition, and even dementia symptoms decades later. Due to the large numbers of veterans who have received TBI in Afghanistan and Iraq (and while this certainly happened in previous conflicts, the large number of landmines and other ordinance directed at these military personnel has resulted in many brain injuries, amputations, etc.), scientists and clinicians are paying closer attention to the diagnosis and management of the aftereffects of TBI.

While many facets of the management and treatment of TBI are beyond this book, we wish to draw attention to the fact that the chronic (across decades sometimes, but often weeks or months) nature of TBI shares features with brain degenerative conditions. We hope that the general health measures in this book, combined with the best that medicine — both conventional and complementary — have to offer, will bring relief to many of these TBI sufferers.

# What Causes Dementia?

## CASE STUDY

### Alzheimer's Disease (continued from page 22)

During the next 2 years following her diagnosis, Elizabeth's symptoms began to progress. She stopped driving the car after becoming disoriented and lost in a local street in her subdivision. She took to writing very specific notes about people and phone calls to make on the calendar on the kitchen wall. But this was not enough and her neurologist prescribed Aricept to boost her cognitive function.

At that time, Elizabeth also began to consult with a naturopathic doctor, Dr. Besson, who carefully took a history of her symptoms and treatments she received from other practitioners. He was careful to avoid any naturopathic treatments that would interfere with medical treatments. Elizabeth started on a regimen of high-quality fish oils, ginkgo biloba extract, something called phosphatidylserine, and vitamin E. She also began to do tai chi, and to change her diet to include far more vegetables and fruits and less canned food. She found that between the medical and naturopathic treatments, she had regained some clarity. During this period of her life, she was aware of the encroaching dementia, but she was enjoying a good quality of life. Although she did not resume driving, she did become more active again in her life. She got involved in some of the groups at her church, and kept social dates with her friends… (continued on page 64)

## Atherosclerosis

There is no single cause for dementia or for any of the common aging-related diseases, although sometimes the symptoms are caused by an inherited factor or a physical trauma. For the most part, these conditions involve an interplay of genetics, environment, and lifestyle. They also tend to be systemic, focused primarily on the vascular system, with atherosclerosis and inflammation the chief factors in aging-related diseases. Unfortunately, our society consumes a diet that promotes atherosclerosis and inflammation in many people; fortunately, specific foods can help you avoid these related conditions.

# Causes of Dementia

Research has been focused on these possible causes of aging-related brain diseases. No single cause has been found, although some causes contribute more to the onset and course of the disease than others and some causes are linked or associated.

- Atherosclerosis
- Inflammation
- Oxygen depravation
- Oxidative stress
- Neurotoxins

- Glucose damage
- Protein deposition
- Physiological stress
- Poor sleep hygiene
- Nutrient deficiencies

Atherosclerosis remains the chief factor in developing Alzheimer's disease, which, in turn, is the most common cause of dementia. The primary cause of aging of the vascular system is not age itself, but a process of slowly accumulating damage. This damage process is called atherosclerosis. Damage to the vascular system of the brain can degrade performance. As this blood vessel disease progresses, cognitive performance declines. Death from myocardial infarction or stroke is possible if vascular problems are not treated as an emergency in the short term, and if lifestyle is not changed in the long term.

## Silent Aging

Some people age more quickly in appearance than others but show no signs of aging-related disease, while others appear healthy even as their memory, their cognitive ability, and their enjoyment of life decline faster than normal. There are several reasons for this "silent aging." One is that our skin, hair, and general energy level can remain youthful even while our vascular system begins to undergo degenerative changes. The delicate tissues that make up the brain, heart, kidney, and other organs can accrue damage slowly over time. While not dramatic, these small amounts of damage can have a cumulative effect.

## Plaque Formation

In atherosclerosis, a slowly growing plaque attaches to the inside lining of the arteries. The plaque itself is composed of cholesterol, rancid fats, and dead white blood cells. This is usually capped off with a substance called fibrin, which is a bit like scar tissue or repair tissue. Most people are familiar with the concept that coronary arteries may become partially blocked — or sometimes completely blocked — as they grow older. This blockage can cause a heart attack or stroke. Although atherosclerosis can be delayed or prevented, heart attacks and strokes are common occurrences.

**Q A**   **What is the blood-brain barrier?**

The system of blood circulation to the brain starts with some fairly large and flexible arteries that go through the neck and spine and connect to the base of the brain. From there, these become major cerebral arteries. Much like a tree, these arteries branch off, many times over, and eventually become a huge collection of small blood vessels, called capillaries, which is where much of the oxygen transfer happens. These capillaries are tightly sealed up in certain regions, and they resist entry of some molecules from the bloodstream into the brain, forming the so-called blood-brain barrier.

**DID YOU KNOW?**

**Metabolic Activity**

An adult's brain is composed of approximately 80 to 100 billion neurons. This involves a massive amount of metabolic activity and energy expenditure. The brain is dependent on a vast network of blood vessels to keep it functioning without overheating. This vast circulatory system not only supplies oxygen to the brain and respiratory system, but also glucose and other nutrients to the gut.

# Inflammation

Pain, heat, redness, and swelling are the hallmarks of inflammation, and any injury, ranging from a bee sting to a brain trauma, can become inflamed. Inflammation is triggered by the immune system: pro-inflammatory hormones direct white blood cells to eliminate infection and damaged tissue. These agents are matched by anti-inflammatory compounds that remove the threat and start the healing process.

## Acute Inflammation

Acute inflammation that rises and recedes indicates a balanced immune system, but inflammation that does not recede is problematic. The immune system gets stuck on "high alert" even when there is no immediate danger. The inflammation cascade of pain, heat, redness, and swelling becomes chronic and the body loses its equilibrium, or homeostasis.

# Arterial Plaque Development and Rupture

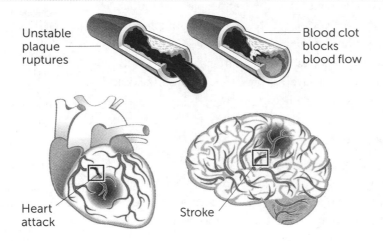

Unstable plaque ruptures

Blood clot blocks blood flow

Heart attack

Stroke

**Q**
**A**

**How is cardiovascular inflammation diagnosed?**

Currently, there are numerous ways to gain insight into inflammation in the body. General measures include an observation of symptoms and a measurement of blood levels of C-reactive protein (a pro-inflammatory marker). There are also other markers, such as lipoprotein-associated phospholipase A2 (Lp-PLA2), which tells us something about how aggressive low-density lipoprotein (LDL, or "bad") molecules might be in driving the inflammatory process.

## Chronic Inflammation

Chronic inflammation has been attributed to diet and stress. For most people, the modern high-carbohydrate diet causes some level of inflammation, especially so when compounded by food allergies and toxins. As we get older, foods that never bothered us before, like dairy and wheat products, may trigger chronic low-grade indigestion or other seemingly minor symptoms that put our immune system on guard. Constant exposure to noxious chemicals and airborne irritants can also disturb the immune system.

## Role of Inflammation in Atherosclerosis

In atherosclerosis, chronic inflammation causes plaques to become unstable, flaky, and easy to break open (because the hard cap of scar tissue peels off). Inflammation can activate a blood clot when the plaque ruptures. In turn, this blood clot will block the flow of blood to whatever tissue that artery was supposed to feed. If it is in the heart, doctors call this a myocardial infarction or a heart attack. If it is in the brain, it is called an ischemic attack or a stroke.

## Plaque Physiology

*Cholesterol deposition in the blood*
*(cholesterol, rancid fats, dead white blood cells,*
*and fibrin in the blood)*

## Inflammation

*(accelerates growth of plaque from blood vessel*
*and eventually leads to instability)*

*Plaque rupture and blood clot forms*

*Myocardial infarction (heart attack) or ischemia (stroke)*

## Cholesterol Control

There is a correlation between a high cholesterol level and atherosclerosis. For many years, a primary aim of medical strategies to both treat and prevent heart disease (and atherosclerosis in general) has been to reduce the cholesterol that circulated as a part of the particles called low-density lipoproteins (LDL), known as "bad" cholesterol, and to increase high-density lipoproteins (HDL), known as "good" cholesterol, to prevent plaque buildup. High levels of LDL particles can lead to more vascular aging because of the damage they cause. High levels of HDL tend to be protective. However, high inflammation can disable the protective elements in HDL, rendering it as potentially dangerous as LDL.

As oxidation of LDL increases, so too does the danger to the artery. Smaller LDL particles that are present in higher numbers create more chances for collisions with the inside lining of the artery. Some forms of LDL are more atherogenic than others. Cholesterol is a needed component of brain cells and muscles; scarce cholesterol levels can lead to ill health.

## Cholesterol Checkup

As long as your cholesterol levels are normal, you need only check them every few years. If you have abnormal cholesterol levels, your doctor will want to check them more frequently. In the United States and a few other countries, cholesterol is measured in milligrams per deciliter of blood, abbreviated as mg/dL. In Canada and most European countries, it's measured in millimoles per liter of blood, abbreviated as mmol/L. Aim for the cholesterol numbers on page 42.

Aim for the cholesterol numbers on page 42.

## DID YOU KNOW?

### New Guidelines

Recently, in the United States, guidelines for the treatment of high LDL cholesterol readings have begun to shift. The most current recommendations from the American College of Cardiology (ACC) and American Heart Association (AHA), developed in conjunction with the National Heart, Lung, and Blood Institute (NHLBI), downplay LDL as a stand-alone indicator for treatment. The new guidelines incorporate other risk factors. Factors such as diabetes and family history of heart disease are more strongly considered. Critics say that this simply doubles the market for patients who will be put on statin drugs. Advocates applaud it as a more nuanced approach that individualizes treatment. Canada has not adopted these guidelines, but the topic in general has become an area of intense focus in the medical literature.

# Total Cholesterol

| Total cholesterol (U.S. and some other countries) | Total cholesterol* (Canada and most of Europe) | |
|---|---|---|
| Below 200 mg/dL | Below 5.2 mmol/L | Desirable |
| 200–239 mg/dL | 5.2–6.2 mmol/L | Borderline high |
| 240 mg/dL and above | Above 6.2 mmol/L | High |

# LDL Cholesterol

| LDL cholesterol (U.S. and some other countries) | LDL cholesterol* (Canada and most of Europe) | |
|---|---|---|
| Below 70 mg/dL | Below 1.8 mmol/L | Ideal for people at very high risk of heart disease |
| Below 100 mg/dL | Below 2.6 mmol/L | Ideal for people at risk of heart disease |
| 100–129 mg/dL | 2.6–3.3 mmol/L | Near ideal |
| 130–159 mg/dL | 3.4–4.1 mmol/L | Borderline high |
| 160–189 mg/dL | 4.1–4.9 mmol/L | High |
| 190 mg/dL and above | Above 4.9 mmol/L | Very high |

# High Cholesterol

| HDL cholesterol (U.S. and some other countries) | HDL cholesterol* (Canada and most of Europe) | |
|---|---|---|
| Below 40 mg/dL (men) Below 50 mg/dL (women) | Below 1 mmol/L (men) Below 1.3 mmol/L (women) | Poor |
| 40–49 mg/dL (men) 50–59 mg/dL (women) | 1–1.3 mmol/L (men) 1.3–1.5 mmol/L (women) | Better |
| 60 mg/dL and above | 1.6 mmol/L and above | Best |

*Canadian and European guidelines differ slightly from American guidelines. These conversions are based on American guidelines.

Adapted from http://www.mayoclinic.com/health/cholesterol-levels/CL00001

### Full Lipid Profile

Knowing these figures is a good start — but it is important to know that some types of LDL are far more aggressive, or atherogenic, than others. Their size, number, and components can make them more dangerous to the blood vessel. Many cardiologists now order advanced lipid testing to gain insight into these important details. Measuring and then improving the lipid profile may help to delay the onset of Alzheimer's and other forms of dementia.

## Oxygen Deprivation

When there is impaired circulation to the brain, the neurons suffer. Brief episodes of oxygen deprivation, or hypoxia, can stun and even kill brain cells. If the blood supply is interrupted for too long, more than a few minutes, brain cells will start to die.

Some people with advanced atherosclerosis accumulate small infarcts. These are little blockages of small blood vessels in the brain. Unfortunately, no big catastrophe occurs to signal that part of the brain function has been lost. It does not present like a stroke, yet slowly but surely, this process takes its toll over time. Memory, thinking, and reaction times gradually diminish. If severe enough, multi-infarct dementia will develop.

Interestingly, mild hypoxia can prepare the brain to survive more drastic episodes, but on balance, there is nothing to be gained by the loss of blood flow to the brain, and oxygen deprivation will, in time, undermine its function.

## Oxidative Stress and Free Radicals

Oxidative stress plays a role in the development of neurodegenerative diseases, including ALS, Parkinson's disease, and Alzheimer's disease. Oxidation involves removing electrons from an atom or molecule, a change that can be destructive. We need oxygen to live, but high concentrations of it are toxic.

Our body converts food into energy by breaking the carbon-to-carbon bonds in food molecules and using oxygen as a necessary element in extracting the potential energy contained in these carbon bonds. This metabolic process, although absolutely necessary for the maintenance of our cells, also generates dangerous byproducts, notably free radicals. Free radicals are unstable atoms or molecules that seek to achieve stability by

**DID YOU KNOW?**

**Mixed Dementia**

A number of Alzheimer's disease patients also have vascular disease of the brain, which is referred to as mixed dementia. And although there are specific structural and biochemical aspects of Alzheimer's disease that make it distinct, at the end of the day, degenerative brain diseases begin to share common features. The deterioration of cerebral blood vessels is another symptom that can be a causal factor.

stripping electrons from other molecules. In their wake, they create more unstable molecules that then attack their neighbors in domino-like chain reactions. By the time a free radical chain fizzles out, it may have ripped through vital components of cells like a tornado, causing extensive damage.

## Birth of a Free Radical

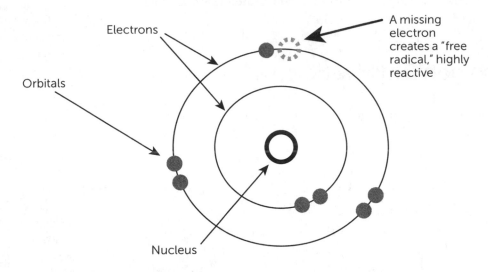

Electrons

Orbitals

A missing electron creates a "free radical," highly reactive

Nucleus

## Antioxidants

Our bodies are not helpless in the face of these oxidative assaults. We have several defenses against oxidative stress:

- Use the body's own antioxidant enzymes to contain free radicals within cells
- Consume plant-derived antioxidants that neutralize reactive forms of oxygen
- Consume antioxidants, such as vitamin C and vitamin E, that can "quench" free radicals by donating electrons to them and cutting off the chain reactions early in their course

# Neurotoxins

Damage to the brain and nervous system can lead to long-term reductions in our ability to think, move, and perform. Sometimes this damage can occur due to toxic compounds that react chemically with the cells of the nervous system. More to the point, they inflict damage on the DNA in our cells or the microscopic organelles, those components of the cell that create energy and manufacture essential proteins. In the case of Alzheimer's disease, free radical damage and perhaps environmental toxins can contribute to its development. If we are aiming to slow down the progression of aging-related neurological diseases, then we must strengthen our body's own systems for processing and neutralizing toxic compounds.

Toxins can develop in the body as bacteria or from exposure to insecticides, herbicides, and heavy metals. There are many other items from the environment — thousands of compounds, actually — that overwhelm the detoxification systems of many people, especially those with poor diets.

## Good and Bad Bacteria

The gastrointestinal (GI) tract is home to a whole universe of microorganisms. These include bacteria, fungi, yeasts, protozoa, and even a few viruses from time to time. At birth, our colon and the rest of the GI tract are sterile, but within a few minutes (longer if the baby is born by cesarean section), the microorganisms in the environment begin to colonize the gut. The breast milk or formula that the baby consumes provides a growth substance for these bacteria and other organisms. In fact, human breast milk contains natural prebiotics. These oligosaccharides (a fancy term for medium-length chains of sugars) act as a super-fuel for gut bacteria.

**Q** **How do toxins act in the gut?**

**A** These bacteria are not just along for the ride. They help to mature the immune system. They crowd out more aggressive bacteria and make the gut a kind of safe neighborhood. They produce some vitamins, such as vitamin K, and they make nutritional substances that help energize and heal the gut. They also reduce allergy and help the body to become less sensitized to allergens in the environment.

However, even the mighty figure of 100 trillion gut bacteria can be altered by the choices we make. Our diet can shift the species that we have in the gut — for instance, eating a lot of meat can cause one type of bacteria to predominate. More importantly, our use of antibiotics (which are necessary and helpful, even lifesaving in some instances) can drastically rearrange the world of microbes within our gut.

## Parkinson's Disease Toxins

Many patients with Parkinson's disease undergo toxic damage in the substantia nigra, that part of the basal ganglia in their brain that manufactures dopamine, a neurotransmitter essential to smooth, natural movements of the muscles. There is scientific investigation and debate about what ultimately destroys the dopamine-storing cells in the basal ganglia. One theory is that dopamine itself becomes oxidized and that it acts as a free radical that destroys dopamine-making or -storing cells. Another theory is that cell proteins are not broken down correctly and that they can accumulate and cause cell damage. Incidentally, the street drug ecstasy (MDMA) can destroy these cells, leading to a tremor condition much like Parkinson's disease. In other cases, specific toxins, such as the herbicide paraquat, can potentially damage these cells.

## CASE STUDY

### Parkinson's Disease (continued from page 32)

With a nudge from his partner, Ron recognized he should see his doctor for a checkup. At his first appointment, a nurse conducted a brief neurological examination, checked his reflexes, observed his gait, and tested his strength. She saw no problems. Despite her reassurances, the symptoms became worse and Ron insisted on being referred to a neurologist. As was his habit, Ron had researched various neurological conditions he might have. By the time he met with Dr. Davis, he had narrowed down the list, and when Dr. Davis finished a brief 3- or 4-minute examination, he asked Ron if he had any inkling what might be wrong. "I've narrowed it down to three choices," Ron said. "TIA, Parkinson's, or MS." Dr. Davis prompted, "Guess." Ron ventured, "Parkinson's?" Small consolation, he guessed right… (continued on page 108)

### Detoxification

If more aggressive organisms begin to gain dominance there, they may produce byproducts that our liver has to then detoxify. Recall that the liver is connected to the circulation of the gut. Overindulging in meat, sugar, and other rich foods can provide food for things like yeasts in the gut, which can lead to an abundance of unwanted compounds that we have to detoxify.

Some people are unaware that this is going on in their bodies, while others are very aware. Many sufferers of the skin condition psoriasis will notice that their skin condition worsens when they eat fast food, too much sugar, or too much animal protein. This can be directly connected to some of those gut byproducts (of bacteria, yeast, and fungi) entering the bloodstream and making the scaly, whitish lesions on their skin worse.

Having an active metabolism will lead to the development of intermediary compounds. For example, when we exercise or do any kind of repetitive workout or lifting, we get a "burn" in our muscles. This sensation is caused by lactic acid. Lactic acid is produced when our muscle cells break down a storage form of energy — called pyruvate — without the use of oxygen. This is known as anaerobic metabolism, the creation of cellular fuel without the use of oxygen. Note that our brains cannot do this, but our muscle cells can. This is only a short-term energy source, useful for bursts of activity. Lactic acid is an irritant and it causes a burning sensation in our muscles for several minutes or less. Athletes will often become acutely aware of this "burn" as they undergo rigorous training. It is a sign that the muscles exceeded their capacity to create energy from glucose and oxygen from the blood and had to switch to this alternative power source. Our body's cells produce all sorts of byproducts in the course of normal cell function, and many of these must be detoxified as intermediary metabolites (lactic acid, pyruvic acid, sulfuric acid, urea, homocysteine, nitric acid). That is to say, the cell creates a certain amount of refuse, just like a household, and that refuse has to be exported to the bloodstream and eventually broken down or neutralized.

## Detox Routes

When a toxin enters the body or is incidentally produced in the body, there is almost always a route of disposal. In our homes, we have ways to transport washing water, toilet water, food waste, and dry trash to other locations for disposal or processing. Our bodies work the same way. We dispose of toxic chemical compounds using several pathways in the body, and several organs are vital to this process, especially the liver and kidneys.

## Liver Detoxification

The liver is the master organ of detoxification. This vital organ contains a hearty blood supply, much of it derived from the intestine and other parts of the gastrointestinal tract. The liver is also loaded with enzymes, which are proteins capable of rearranging the structure of certain chemicals. Think of the liver as a very sophisticated chemical laboratory that can create, destroy, or alter an endless array of compounds.

## Phase I and II Detoxification

In the liver, there is a system of enzymes that render a toxic or foreign compound harmless before it is excreted into the urine, passed through the gut, expelled through the breath, or sweat through the skin. This process is called Phase I and Phase II detoxification.

**DID YOU KNOW?**

### Acetaminophen Poisoning

Many people use the drug acetaminophen (such as Tylenol) for pain or fever every day, and in most cases, it is safe. However, if too much of the drug is consumed, even just a tiny bit more than the maximum dose, the liver runs out of ways to detoxify it and it becomes harmful. This is because the rate at which that harmful byproduct of acetaminophen piles up is faster than the rate at which the liver's Phase II enzyme can get rid of it. There are thousands of cases of emergency room visits in North America for acetaminophen poisoning each year.

The colon is another detoxification battleground. The liver dumps many toxins into the gastrointestinal tract through the bile. Not only does bile help us digest fat, it is a kind of disposal route for end products of liver detoxification. It contains trillions of microflora. Some are beneficial and some form toxins.

**Meters of Skin**

The skin is a very large organ of elimination, the average adult having about 22 square feet (2 sq m) of skin, about 23 feet (2 m) long, that can excrete toxins. This is mostly done through perspiration. For example, the toxin urea is ultimately destined to be eliminated from our kidneys, but some urea circulating in the bloodstream can leave the body through perspiration.

Phase I enzymes make a toxin more reactive by oxidizing it. If the process ended there, the toxic products of Phase I might be stronger than free radicals. Fortunately, Phase II produces chemical compounds that attach to the Phase I product and neutralize or detoxify it. This creates a nonreactive, safe, water-soluble, and easily disposable product.

## Dietary Function

Typically, most people have sufficient Phase I activity; in fact, our livers can often produce more Phase I enzymes in response to having more drugs or toxins to break down. Sometimes, a person can have all the Phase I capacity they need to begin to transform a toxin, but they lack the Phase II compounds needed to truly finish the job of disposing of this toxin in a safe manner. Phase II is nutritionally powered — and our diet is often lacking in the compounds needed to support Phase II enzymes. The compounds needed to neutralize toxins require various nutrients, vitamins, minerals, and enzymes. There are limits as to how many of these Phase II compounds we can make, and the reason that we cannot make what we need may be genetic — or it may reflect our diet. Nutritional deficiencies or marginal deficiencies can also affect levels of detoxification enzymes.

The worst-case scenario is when a person has a large number of foreign and self-made compounds to detoxify and yet their Phase I enzyme system is very active and their Phase II detoxification enzymes are lacking. In this scenario, nasty free radicals and toxic compounds can build up in the liver and perhaps throughout the body.

## Kidneys

Although it is pivotal, the liver does not act alone in the detoxification process. The kidneys excrete many compounds that the liver has rendered water-soluble. Kidney circulation and filtering is so intense that an entire vascular compartment of fluids (all the fluid in our blood vessels) can be filtered more than 50 times daily. Support the kidneys by drinking plenty of water to avoid becoming dehydrated. A diet that overemphasizes protein can also put a strain on the kidneys.

## Breath

With each exhalation, we release $CO_2$ as well as volatile organic compounds into the air. Deep and effective breathing is beneficial for the proper flow of oxygen and for the disposal of toxins. If you want a demonstration, eat some raw garlic. Brush your teeth several times to make the odor go away. In a short while, your breath will be garlicky and sulfurous again. Why? Because the lungs are excreting the garlic compounds that end up on the breath.

---

**Q** **What is the lymphatic system and what role does it have in dementia?**

**A** The lymphatic system moves waste throughout the body, and with good blood circulation and lots of physical activity, it can drain itself properly. In poor health and immobility (common in older individuals with arthritis, heart problems, and — ironically — dementia), the lymph flow can stagnate and increase the impact of toxins. The lymph nodes provide small channels between cells, which connect to a drainage system that empties into a major vein. Lymph nodes can become repositories for toxins or infections.

---

## Organic Toxins

Molds and fungi can produce compounds that are poisonous to the human body; for instance, the black mold *Stachybotrys chartarum*, which loves to grow in damp basements, behind drywall in a home that has moisture build up behind it, and any structure with poor air circulation and high moisture. Perhaps because of the fact that children with asthma will suffer aggravations from spending the entire day in a classroom with mold issues, increasing attention has been brought to bear on mold contaminations of schools. Schools can accumulate moisture when not in use during the summer months, and some schools districts lag behind in their maintence schedules and some of their schools have water leakage and roofing/window issues. Portable classrooms seem to have a more severe issue. These mold toxins can do more than just cause severe lung problems and allergies. It can also cause toxicity in the brain and cause inflammation in the body. Overall, mold exposure can lead to a "tired and toxic" state, and the mental sluggishness that follows can be a major drain on the brain. This is not just a problem from the air; our food can also have fungal contamination. Peanuts, for instance, contain aflatoxin, which can be toxic to the liver. The U.S. Department of Agriculture (USDA) sets limits on how much aflatoxin can be allowed on peanuts, but it finds its way onto other foods, too.

> **DID YOU KNOW?**
>
> **Total Maximum Daily Load**
>
> Total maximum daily load (TMDL), a regulatory term used in the United States Clean Water Act, measures the maximum amount of a pollutant that a body of water can contain while still meeting water quality standards. TMDL has been extrapolated to measure the amount of a pollutant in the human body.

## Environmental Neurotoxins

There are numerous environmental toxins, or xenobiotics, that have emerged in our advanced industrial society, with thousands of compounds in common use that never existed 100 years ago. Some toxins are from natural sources. A good example would be the radioactive gas radon, which is a formed by the decay of radium and is found in some basements, especially in the American Midwest. Others are manufactured, such as dichlorodiphenyltrichloroethane (or DDT, a colorless, odorless insecticide) and 2,4-dichlorophenoxyacetic acid (or 2,4-D, a common pesticide/herbicide). Whatever the source, these toxins will age the brain if their cumulative effect, or the total maximum daily load of them in the body, becomes too great. Sometimes limited exposures over the course of many years can be a problem, and sometimes our body can adapt.

## Insecticides and Herbicides

These chemicals are widely used in agriculture, and when they were first developed, they were hailed as major breakthroughs. Pests were eating farmers' crops, sometimes to the point of creating famine and suffering. The development of chemicals that could protect these crops was an impressive feat. However, the shortcomings of introducing large-scale toxins, such as DDT, into the food chain soon became apparent. Birds, such as the bald eagle, were not able to tolerate the effects of the toxin in their system — specifically in their reproductive system. Some bird species began to approach extinction because their eggs would not form properly. The book *Silent Spring*, by Rachel Carson, introduced this fact to the public in 1962, and it's often credited with helping launch the creation of government agencies such as the U.S. Environmental Protection Agency (EPA).

Although organophosphates are more directly neurotoxic than herbicides, herbicides carry their own risks and also have nasty implications. The herbicide 2,4-D has been linked to cancer (it's banned in Canada). Recent research has also shown the ability of 2,4-D to induce brain cells to shut down and die — another reminder to eat more organic food and wash your food!

## Overstimulation

Most insecticides are, in fact, neurotoxins that poison the nervous system. Insects are more sensitive to them than we are, and the total amount that humans might ingest is much, much smaller per body weight than an insect dose (although many people who work in agriculture are exposed to much more). Neurotoxins cause many nerves in the body to be overstimulated, to the point that they are not able to shut themselves off, and interfere with the proper clearance of a neurotransmitter called acetylcholine, a crucial brain chemical.

## Food Additives

There are many food additives and they are used for a number of different reasons. Some are used to prevent mold and decay. Others are added to food to enhance flavor, and still others to add texture.

Some individuals are very sensitive to certain additives. Take sulfites as an example. These are added to fruitcakes and dried fruits — even dried instant potatoes. Their purpose is to prevent mold and decay. But some people do not detoxify sulfites very well. When they eat them, they experience headaches, a rush of blood to the head, and mental confusion. Not all food additives create such dramatic reactions, but they all need to be processed and disposed of by the body.

When we eat too much processed food, we are again increasing the burden of compounds that cause neurological degeneration — chemical compounds our body must detoxify. Vital enzymes and nutrients are used for this process, diverted from their inherent purpose of nourishing our bodies and optimizing health.

## Medications

One of the significant sources of chemicals that our body must detoxify is pharmaceutical medications. Our society uses these in great quantities. Without a doubt, the advent of modern pharmacology has done enormous good for countless people. A well-timed antibiotic, blood pressure medication, or antidepressant can have a healing impact on your life — but it also has a toxic effect. The average American uses 12 to 13 prescriptions per year, and the average Canadian uses approximately 14 per year. These pharmaceuticals introduce another substance into the body that must be broken down and excreted, competing for the natural detoxification pathways in the liver. Take acetaminophen as an example. For an adult, a daily 3-gram dosage (6 capsules of the strong dose) is safe, provided that the liver is healthy and the patient is properly nourished. Beyond that dose, the liver runs out of glutathione for dealing with the breakdown product of acetaminophen (N-acetyl-p-benzoquinone imine — NAPQI). The toxic NAPQI so derived from acetaminophen builds up and can cause very severe damage to the liver.

## Brain Medications

Some medications are toxic to the nervous system. Some drugs damage the dopamine-containing cells of the brain, which can lead to Parkinsonian movement disorders. Even the overuse of normally tolerable drugs like beta-blockers for high blood pressure, or benzodiazepines (Valium or Xanax) for treating anxiety, can begin to interfere with thinking. Consult with your pharmacist before using these drugs that may affect your brain.

## Common Medications with Neurological Side Effects

- Amphetamines
- Anticonvulsants
- Antidepressants
- Anti-psychotics
- Blood pressure medications
- Cardiac glycosides
- Diuretics
- Pain medications
- Sedatives

**DID YOU KNOW?**

**Detox Diet**

To keep your brain young, pay attention to the chemicals you are exposed to and reduce contact with them whenever possible. Eat foods that are detoxifying agents.

### Synthetics

We live in sea of synthetic compounds — clothing and carpets made from synthetic materials, food stored in plastic containers, the interiors of automobiles. They all produce toxins, called off-gassing, that must be handled by the liver. For example, at one time, chemical compounds known as phthalates were added to the composition of children's toys, bottles, and pacifiers to make these plastics flexible and able to withstand bending without fatiguing and cracking too soon (all plastics do eventually). As a side effect, these chemicals acted like synthetic estrogen. In time, they began to disrupt the endocrine system. Fortunately, phthalates are not used to make plastics anymore.

### Heavy Metals

Toxic heavy metals also influence brain health. These minerals are natural to the environment but can be toxic to humans when used in combination with other chemicals in industry and even in household cleaning products and paints.

### Lead and Arsenic

Combined or alone, lead and arsenic are notoriously neurotoxic and insidiously accumulate in the body and brain. Lead and arsenic are often combined as lead arsenate, a highly toxic pesticide. Children are particularly vulnerable, but lead content in adults can be high, too. Lead is able to not only damage the brain (especially the developing brain), but it can cause damage to nerves, leading to a loss of sensation, muscle function, and pain. Lead is still found in the paint on the walls of many older homes. Sanding or scraping must be done with great caution (it is sometimes best left to professionals who can mitigate the release of lead dust into the home). Lead pipes are still is use in some places, and lead pollution will remain in the environment for hundreds of years thanks to its use in automobile fuel until the 1980s. Blood tests can identify if your body contains dangerous levels of lead and arsenic.

## Mercury

Mercury is toxic to brain cells and can accumulate in the body for decades. It tends to be found in fatty tissues, such as the brain. Mercury was used in dental amalgams until recently. Mercury has contaminated many species of fish in our lakes, rivers, and oceans. This contamination puts pregnant women who eat fish at a high risk for having children with neurological conditions. Mercury poisoning can also contribute to the premature aging of the brain. Be sure to consult with your public health agency for lists of fish species that are safe to eat without neurological risk.

## Aluminum

This heavy metal is used in the fabrication of many products, from aircraft to cookware, due to its durability and lightweight quality. Aluminum is found in the plaques of individuals with Alzheimer's disease. This is not to say that exposure to aluminum causes dementia. However, given that the brain likes to concentrate aluminum and that it finds its way into the lesions found in the brains of patients with Alzheimer's, it seems prudent to keep our exposure down to a minimum. Our body requires trace amounts of aluminum, but this amount is easily provided by a normal diet.

Many detoxification systems require the same body proteins and enzymes to function well, and therefore the same nutrients to power them. When we allow these pathways to become overburdened or compromised, our capacity to deal effectively with all needs, including heavy metal detoxification, decreases.

# Glucose Damage

Eating contaminated foods is not the only dietary danger for developing aging-related diseases. If eaten in excess, glucose can contribute to these diseases, too. If glucose levels are high in

**DID YOU KNOW?**

**Methylation**
Removing heavy metals from the body is possible, but they tend to be resistant. One important detoxification step is methylation. In this procedure, nutrients are combined to create a chemical unit, or methyl group, that sticks to the heavy metal and makes it water-soluble so that it can leave the body. Folic acid and vitamin $B_{12}$ are commonly combined to make a methyl group. Sulfur-containing proteins are used to help drive the toxin out of the cells.

the diet, two things can happen slowly in the brain and nervous system. In the Schwann cells that protect the nerves, glucose can accumulate and be converted to a sugar called sorbitol. This new sugar crystallizes and damages those cells. In a broader sense, the high glucose can attach itself to proteins, making them dysfunctional. This targets the vascular system, and diabetes causes that critical vascular system to age very rapidly in some cases, especially when the diet is pro-inflammatory. The aim is to eat low-glycemic foods to control binging or the spiking of glucose levels.

**Q** **If the brain is dependent on glucose for fuel, how can glucose damage the brain?**

**A** The problem comes when glucose levels are too high in the brain for too long. It is the old example of having "too much of a good thing." A perfect example of this is the disease diabetes. Although there are many types of diabetes, the common symptoms include thirst, urination, and, above all, high levels of glucose in the blood — very high levels after meals and too high in between meals.

## Glycemic Index and Glycemic Load

When we consume a large amount of sugar, special cells in our pancreas secrete insulin in response. Insulin helps pull sugar from the blood and into the cells, where it can be used for immediate energy or stored for later use. However, certain foods, like white bread, turn into sugar so quickly that as far as the body's release of insulin is concerned, eating white bread, donuts, or similar foods is just like eating raw glucose. The glycemic index (GI) and glycemic load (GL) measure how quickly any food raises blood sugar levels after being ingested.

The glycemic index estimates how much each gram of available carbohydrate (total carbohydrate minus fiber) in a food raises a person's blood glucose level following consumption of the food, relative to the consumption of pure glucose. Glucose has a glycemic index of 100.

GI 0–55 = Low
GI 56–59 = Medium
GI 75+ = High
Glucose = 100

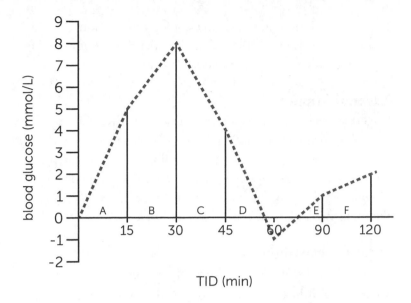

However, the glycemic index does not take into account the amount of carbohydrate actually consumed. The glycemic load accounts for this by multiplying the glycemic index of the food in question by the carbohydrate content of the actual serving.

Note that high-glycemic-index foods cause a rapid spike in blood sugar, followed by a an equally rapid lowering of blood sugar levels — in some patients this leads to symptoms of reactive hypogloycemia and is very unpleasant.

GL > 10 = Low
GL 11–19 = Medium
GL < 20 = High

## Sugar Roller Coaster

The North American diet is very high in high-glycemic-index foods, such as white rice, potatoes, white bread, and white noodles. Many people begin their day with a high-glucose breakfast of white foods (white bread, white cereal, white sugar) that causes blood sugar levels to rise sharply and prompts the pancreas to secrete insulin. When a person's blood sugar levels are high, they may have a temporary sense of energy, or may be overexcited, giddy, and impulsive. By midmorning, the burst of steam they experienced from their sugar-based breakfast has subsided and they can feel tired, anxious, shaky, surly, and confused. Why? Their blood sugar level has crashed due to their body's successful release of insulin. Now the blood sugar levels drop too low. The brain has trouble coping with plummeting blood sugar levels. If this up-and-down roller coaster reaction becomes extreme, hypoglycemia may result.

## Adrenal Support

The body will try to combat dangerously low levels of blood glucose by turning to the adrenal glands. These two glands are near the kidneys. In response to impending hypoglycemia, the adrenal glands release the hormone epinephrine, also known as adrenaline. This surge of adrenaline mobilizes any remaining blood sugar stored in the body (the liver, typically).

## Insulin Resistance

Chronic exposure to high insulin levels creates an environment where the body begins to ignore insulin. This effect is called insulin insensitivity or insulin resistance. In response to this condition, the pancreas will secrete even more insulin.

## Metabolic Syndrome

Some individuals go on to develop metabolic syndrome, which presents clinically as weight gain, high blood pressure,

**Q**
**A**

### What does "gluten-free" mean?

Some people are very sensitive to the proteins in wheat, known as gluten. For years, health professionals recommended eating whole grains because they are a stable source of slow-release energy in the body. And this is often true: a complex carbohydrate is better than purely refined food. (A complex carbohydrate is composed of many sugars bound together in a chain that needs to be broken up before the sugars can be burned in the body; a whole grain still has some fiber and some natural plant material in it — and has not been refined into a white powder). High-gluten grains, often from genetically modified or hybridized wheat, appear to really trigger the release of the hormone insulin in some people. The mechanisms are not entirely clear, but there is no doubt that modern wheat has been genetically manipulated to have a much higher gluten content than its ancestor that humans consumed traditionally. Insulin will cause blood sugar to drop and create cravings for more grains. Not everyone reacts this way, but it is clear that the whole-grain advice that was handed out for two decades simply does not work for many people.

There are plenty of people eating bagels, bread, and noodles all day long who have insulin levels higher than they ought to be. Some of these individuals eliminate wheat and gluten-containing foods from their diet and experience remarkable changes in their weight, cholesterol levels, energy levels, and food cravings.

high blood sugar, and problems with cholesterol. There is a high risk of developing atherosclerosis, which will eventually destroy the network of blood vessels upon which the brain is entirely dependent. The brain does not function well during the degradation of the blood supply or during injury from being awash in too much sugar.

## Diabetes Mellitus

The outcome of metabolic syndrome may be diabetes mellitus, a disease with a variety of causes and one that is defined by high blood sugar levels. To be diagnosed with diabetes, a person must have a high count of blood glucose when they are fasting (approximately 12 hours after their last meal).

## Hyperglycemia

The physician may also look at a form of hemoglobin called A1c (or glycated hemoglobin), a form of hemoglobin that has been modified by glucose in the blood; if there is too much of the A1c form, it is a telltale sign that blood sugar levels have been high for several weeks. This is known as hyperglycemia, which is caused by lack of insulin or a resistance of the body to insulin.

# Type 1 and Type 2 Diabetes

There are two common forms of diabetes, insulin-dependent diabetes mellitus (IDDM, or type 1) and non-insulin-dependent diabetes mellitus (NIDDM, or type 2).

**IDDM** is responsible for approximately 10% of cases of primary diabetes. The insulin-secreting cells of the pancreas, the beta cells, are destroyed by the body's own immune system. When these cells run out, or there are too few of them still functioning, the symptoms of the disease appear (frequent urination, thirst, hunger, and weight loss).

Not only will blood levels of glucose be high in the blood when diabetes mellitus occurs, but the levels of ketones are high, too. Ketones are the product of breaking down fatty acids and are used for energy when blood levels of glucose are too low for any length of time or when the muscles cannot use the glucose that is there (such as in the disease diabetes). High levels of ketones can lead to diabetic ketoacidosis, a very dangerous condition that can result in coma and death.

**NIDDM** is much more common than IDDM. It occurs mainly in adults but is becoming ever more common in adolescents and even children. These patients have a decreased sensitivity to insulin in the peripheral tissues. There may be a lack of insulin in the blood, or, in many cases, there is actually too much insulin.

# Protein Deposition

For reasons that are not always clear, abnormal proteins can be deposited in the brain. One of these proteins is tau protein, found in high amounts in Alzheimer's disease. These proteins may be the wreckage of some other phenomenon, such as hypoxia or free radical damage. There seem to be other triggers as well, including genetic ones.

Some amount of protein deposition in the brain is normal as we age, but it should not reach levels that begin to seriously interfere with our base function. At some point, we accrue damage to the brain from living long enough, but we compensate by developing skills and activating other areas, alternative pathways, that make us more efficient and better problem solvers. What we lack in brute thinking power, we make up for in higher-order thinking. In bona fide aging diseases of the brain (as opposed to normal aging), the protein deposition has reached a point that overwhelms the brain's compensatory mechanisms and there is a breakdown.

# Physiological Stress

Oxidative stress needs to be distinguished from physiological stress. Almost everybody feels under stress at some time or another. The term has become a synonym for the pressures of life, but in medical terminology, the word "stress" refers to a physiological state that can have a pronounced impact on aging-related diseases. Two hormones, adrenaline and cortisol, from the adrenal glands play the key roles in this process.

## Alarm Phase

Stress accounts for our ability to respond to an external threat or harsh condition. When we are first confronted with a dangerous condition, our body experiences an alarm reaction. Our adrenal glands expel a surge of adrenaline (epinephrine), and blood flow increases to the muscles. Our reflexes quicken and our alertness increases. This is the classic fight-or-flight response. We are ready to either outrun the saber-toothed tiger or confront it.

This biological response worked very well in a more primitive and nature-based existence, where survival was often a physical struggle. It can, of course, still serve us well. A near-miss collision on the highway will provoke the same response and might save our life if quick reflexes are required. A police officer who must corner and overpower a dangerous criminal will know this feeling, as will any firefighter who must penetrate a burning building to rescue someone. These alarm reactions are supposed to come and go. The whole thing is over quickly.

## Adaptation Phase

After the alarm phase, our body goes into the second phase of the stress response. This is the adaptation phase and the hormone cortisol is released into our bloodstream from adrenal glands. This survival hormone originates from a different part of the adrenals than adrenaline. Cortisol brings down inflammation and seems to help us survive some of the extremes of harsh conditions and trauma.

## Exhaustion Phase

What happens if the adaptation phase goes on for too long? Eventually, high levels of cortisol stop being the solution and become the problem, and the body enters the exhaustion phase. They wear the body down. The adrenals show the wear and tear of this state of stress, and the immune system becomes compromised.

**Q**
**A**

**What is the role of stress in brain health?**

Many things can provoke an alarm reaction in people. For example, a person finds out that the company they work for may go out of business. It comes as a shock. Or a parent learns their child has a medical issue and they have many bills to pay. As this plays out, they begin to feel the adaptation phase kick in, especially if it happens as a period of financial distress sets in. Eventually, and it depends on many factors (such as nutritional status, social support, and genes), that person may arrive at the exhaustion, or burnout, phase. They need antidepressant medication to carry on. They feel disengaged and powerless. They get very sick whenever a cold or flu comes along.

Long-term stress can even be caused by a long-term sense of urgency; many people have schedules that are just too full. Expectations of success are inflated (sometimes we compare our current situation to characters on television who have opulent lifestyles), and many of us are type A, or very competitive by nature.

## Chronic Stress

When we are in a state of chronic stress, our cortisol levels go up. This can damage the brain on some level. High cortisol levels depress the growth of new brain cells. This is particularly true in the hippocampus, that part of the brain that is responsible for learning and memory. The human brain is always capable of growth and it can sprout new connections. The hippocampus can become very active later in life if we keep our brain active, and this can offset a lot of the brain decline of aging. But if we are in a state of chronic and serious stress, we may lose this critical adaptive response of the brain. Our brain will age because it has lost its ability to replenish and grow.

# Determinants of Health

Our general day-to-day health is determined by a number of related functions, called determinants of health, including drinking an adequate volume of water to prevent dehydration and getting adequate sleep to refresh body and mind. The basic determinants of health have a significant impact, directly and indirectly, on cognitive function, brain aging, and several disease pathways.

Disturbances to the factors that determine our general health — those absolutely essential to health needs — eventually create a disturbance in the body and mind. For instance, if you do not drink enough water, your kidneys will struggle to remove toxins from the body. If you skimp on sleep, you can mask the symptoms with coffee or energy drinks, but eventually your body's ability to heal and your emotional well-being will be compromised. Over time, this disturbance becomes chronic. The person might experience symptoms — such as fatigue in the case of lack of sleep or headache in the case of mild dehydration.

Sometimes these symptoms are seen as a problem, but they are not the underlying problem — the real issue is the disturbance to this determinant of health. It doesn't get better — it gets worse.

## Determinants of Good Brain Health

- Sleep
- Hydration
- Exercise
- Exposure to nature

### Sleep Deficiency

Sleep deficiency is one of the greatest disturbances to our health today and has a direct impact on brain function. About 80% of sleep is non-REM (rapid eye movement), and REM sleep, which displays fast activity on the EEG (electroencephalogram), takes up the other 20%. Non-REM sleep ranges from levels 1 to 4 in "depth." Most night terrors, sleepwalking, and talking occur during the deeper levels (3 to 4) of this phase. During REM sleep, heart rate, respiration rate, and depth increase. Dreaming, including nightmares, occurs in REM.

### Causes of Poor Sleep

The causes of poor sleep are many. Some sleep issues are the outcome of an underlying medical issue, such as pain or fever. In other instances, it is almost all due to psychological well-being — be it a short-lived bout of anxiety or worry or a long-term psychological issue. Night sweats due to a chronic infection, or in some cases an undetected malignancy in the body, can lead to sleep disturbance, as can temperature shifts in the body associated with menopause. The easiest causes of poor sleep to address are the ones that occur because of choices we make: staying up too late, eating late at night, and excess caffeine intake.

## DID YOU KNOW?

**Brain Decay**

Without adequate sleep, the brain can decay. People differ in their requirement for sleep, but everyone must spend time in this state of unconscious rest.

# Social Interaction

The old adage "Use it or lose it" is apt for the human brain. When we are learning, our brain comes to life. In fact, learning new skills or simply processing new experiences causes our brain to physically sprout new connections. These new connections begin to wire themselves to other pathways of the brain, and more activity in one area leads to more activity in another. In this way, the brain is very much like a muscle — exercise it and it gets stronger; let it sit idle and it shrinks. This is structurally and functionally true for the brain. The brain has regenerative capabilities, but these are rare and limited. The right thing to do is to prevent damage.

### Retirement

Retirement can have very serious negative effects on the brain. No longer needed to solve problems at work, never called on for wisdom, many people withdraw from family and community life. Nothing could be more dangerous to the brain, short of trauma or loss of blood flow. However, you can redirect your brain to other activities to regenerate it. Volunteering is a great way to use talents gained through life for a good cause. Learning a new language is another.

# PART 2

## Smart Nutrients

# Nutrient Deficiencies

## CASE STUDY

### Alzheimer's Disease (continued from page 37)

As Elizabeth neared her 85st birthday, her symptoms intensified and it became more difficult for her to organize her thinking enough to take care of basic housework and some of her personal care. An occupational therapist was used to help organize the home and deal with potential safety issues. The strain of what was happening began to take its toll on Ben's health, and he was experiencing high blood pressure and what his doctor thought was mild depression. Elizabeth's daughter, Cindy, who lived a mile (1.5 km) away, had been helping out more and more with shopping, cooking, and banking, but she had two children of her own. One day Elizabeth began to shout at Ben and her daughter about how they had hidden her favorite necklace, which she herself had lost several months before. Cindy began to cry and went home. This was a wakeup call for the family to obtain some counseling about this situation.

In more lucid moments, Elizabeth was very anxious about what was happening, but it was clear that she was slowly losing her memory. It was discovered that insurance would not pay for a personal home support worker, but the family decided to keep Elizabeth in her home (they also had a son, Greg, about 50 miles/80 km away in a nearby city), and draw upon their pension money in order to have someone visit daily to help her shower and do other activities… (continued on page 94)

Nutrient deficiencies can lead to damage in our cognitive abilities. Sometimes this is simply due to a lack of support for cognitive functions. If we need a certain brain chemical to think and that chemical is lacking, we may suffer the consequences. Or a person can have a true deficiency of a nutrient. This can be due to problems absorbing the nutrient (for example, the failure to absorb vitamin $B_{12}$ in pernicious anemia) or the lack of it in the diet. Some people need a megadose of a specific nutrient to gain and maintain brain health. An average person might need a teaspoon (5 mL) of a specific nutrient, and other people might need a bucketful. The reasons for this dependency are usually genetic. In treating aging-related brain disease, we need to respect the biological individuality of each patient. One treatment does not fit all cases.

## Nutrient Supplements

Increasing the intake of the needed nutrients is an obvious solution, but the amount to ingest for preventive and therapeutic purposes depends upon the individual. In some cases, the amount of nutrient needed is preventive; that is, the minimum amount of the nutrient needed to prevent a disease condition is prescribed. In other cases, the dose is therapeutic; that is, a larger, or megadose, is prescribed to help heal an existing disease condition.

Practitioners of this field of medicine distinguish between nutrient deficiency and nutrient dependency. A nutrient deficiency is present when the body does not synthesize or consume a diet that prevents disease. A nutrient dependency is present when the needs of the body are so great that even the best diet cannot provide an adequate amount.

This practice of using nutrients not only preventively but also therapeutically was introduced to modern medicine in the 1950s by Dr. Abram Hoffer and Dr. Linus Pauling, and it is now known variously as orthomolecular medicine, clinical nutrition, or dietary therapy.

Nutrient deficiency can be addressed by eating food rich in the required nutrient, by taking supplements, or by combining food sources with supplements. Nutrient dependency requires megadoses of the nutrient that are larger than food sources alone can supply. In his book *Smart Nutrients: Prevent and Treat Alzheimer's and Senility, Enhance Brain Function and Longevity*, Dr. Hoffer presents the case for using megadoses of vitamin B3, vitamin C, chromium, and zinc for restoring brain function and quality of life.

# Dietary Reference Intakes

The amount of nutrient needed to gain and maintain good health has been established by the National Institutes of Health as the Dietary Reference Intakes (DRIs). The DRIs are divided into macronutrient and micronutrient values. These are reference values for healthy individuals eating a typical North American diet. An individual may have physiological, health, or lifestyle characteristics that may require a tailoring of specific nutrient values.

## Kinds and Functions of Macronutrients and Micronutrients

Macronutrients comprise carbohydrates, proteins, and fats. Carbohydrates comprise sugars and fiber, proteins comprise amino acids, and fats comprise fatty acids. Macronutrients provide the body with energy and fiber.

- Carbohydrates
- Proteins
- Fats

Micronutrients comprise vitamins, minerals (elements), and enzymes. Micronutrients enable the metabolism of macronutrients.

- Vitamins
- Elements (minerals)
- Enzymes

## Macronutrient Values

### Estimated Energy Requirement (EER)
An EER is defined as the average dietary energy intake that is predicted to maintain energy balance in healthy, normal-weight individuals of a defined age, gender, weight, height, and level of physical activity consistent with good health. In children and pregnant and lactating women, the EER includes the needs associated with growth or secretion of milk at rates consistent with good health.
- Relative weight (i.e., loss, stable, gain) is the preferred indicator of energy adequacy.

**Acceptable Macronutrient Distribution Range (AMDR)**

The AMDR is a range of intake for a particular energy source (protein, fat, or carbohydrate), expressed as a percentage of total energy (kcal), that is associated with reduced risk of chronic disease while providing adequate intakes of essential nutrients.

# Micronutrient Values

### Recommended Dietary Allowance (RDA)

The RDA is the average daily dietary intake level that is sufficient to meet the nutrient requirement of nearly all (97% to 98%) healthy individuals in a particular life-stage and gender group.

- The RDA is the goal for usual intake by an individual.

### Estimated Average Requirement (EAR)

- The EAR is the median daily intake value that is estimated to meet the requirement of half the healthy individuals in a life-stage and gender group. At this level of intake, the other half of the individuals in the specified group would not have their needs met. The EAR is based on a specific criterion of adequacy, derived from a careful review of the literature. Reduction of disease risk is considered along with many other health parameters in the selection of that criterion.
- The EAR is used to calculate the RDA. It is also used to assess the adequacy of nutrient intakes, and can be used to plan the intake of groups.

### Adequate Intake (AI)

- If sufficient scientific evidence is not available to establish an EAR on which to base an RDA, an AI is derived instead. The AI is the recommended average daily nutrient intake level based on observed or experimentally determined approximations or estimates of nutrient intake by a group (or groups) of apparently healthy people who are assumed to be maintaining an adequate nutritional state. The AI is expected to meet or exceed the needs of most individuals in a specific life-stage and gender group. When an RDA is not available for a nutrient, the AI can be used as the goal for usual intake by an individual. The AI is not equivalent to an RDA.

**Q**
**A**
**What is a calorie?**

A calorie is a unit for measuring energy. An average adult male needs about 2500 calories a day to remain healthy, while an adult female needs about 2000 calories.

## Neurological Disease Deficiencies and DRIs

The tables in the following section of this book provide a summary of common neurological disease micronutrient deficiencies, RDA targets for prevention of brain disease, and UL values for treating micronutrient dependency. They are divided into four populations:

|                          |                        |
|--------------------------|------------------------|
| Females 51–70 years      | Males 51–70 years      |
| Females > 70 years       | Males > 70 years       |

These population groups represent the onset period (51–70 years) and the degenerative period (> 70 years) for most cases of dementia. In addition, these tables refer to recipes at the back of the book that can be prepared as a good food source for the micronutrient discussed.

*Caution:* Before taking any nutrient, especially in a high dose beyond its Tolerable Upper Intake Level (UL), consult with a licensed naturopathic doctor, medical doctor, of doctor of osteopathy.

# Recommended Dietary Allowances: Vitamins

> **Q** What is a vitamin?
>
> **A** This is one of the questions most frequently asked by patients. Vitamins are organic compounds that are needed in small amounts for normal growth and activity. Most vitamins cannot be synthesized by the body; instead, they are derived from our food. Vitamins are either water-soluble or fat-soluble. Most water-soluble vitamins, such as the vitamin B complex, act as catalysts and coenzymes in metabolic processes involving energy transfer. They are excreted fairly rapidly. Fat-soluble vitamins, such as vitamins A, D, and E, are necessary for the function or structural integrity of specific body tissues and membranes. They are retained in the body.
>
> Although it has been known for thousands of years that certain diseases can be treated with specific foods, the scientific link between vitamins and good health wasn't made until the early 1900s by Casimir Funk. While studying beriberi, Funk discovered an organic compound in rice husks that prevents the illness. He named the compound vitamine, derived from the chemical name amine and the Latin word *vita*, "life." Funk's compound is now known as vitamin $B_1$, or thiamine. He espoused the vitamin hypothesis of deficiency, which states that certain diseases, such as scurvy or rickets, are caused by dietary deficiencies and can be avoided by taking vitamins. Vitamins are carbon-containing organic structures, and they are different from minerals, such as calcium, iron, and magnesium, which are simple elements.

## Vitamin $B_1$ (Thiamine)

*Neurological effect of deficiency*

If not provided in adequate amounts:

- Results in fatigue, irritability, headaches, and lethargy
- Interferes with metabolism in brain cells, leading to profound loss of thinking ability, memory, and the ability to walk

| Vitamin $B_1$ | RDA Female | UL Female | RDA Male | UL Male |
|---|---|---|---|---|
| 51–70 years | 1.1 mg | ND | 1.2 mg | ND |
| > 70 years | 1.1 mg | ND | 1.2 mg | ND |

*Note:* Due to a lack of suitable data, UL could not be established for thiamine. This does not mean there is no potential for adverse effects resulting from high intakes. ND means no data.

*Supplement form:* Usually found in B-complex supplements, sometimes in amounts up to 50 mg. Lower amounts are usually adequate to maintain health.

*Food sources:* Found in high amounts in brown rice, enriched white rice, enriched grains, pork, peas, almonds, and potatoes (baked). Easily destroyed by processing and heating. Up to 80% of the thiamine content in food can be lost to cooking. Thiamine is needed for the enzyme system, which is involved in creating usable energy for the body. People who consume large amounts of refined carbohydrates, especially white sugar, may not get enough $B_1$. These foods increase thiamine requirements, but do not supply the nutrient. And because they are high-calorie foods, they displace other, more nourishing foods from the diet.

*Recommended recipes:* Barbecued Lemongrass Pork (page 315), Mandarin Rice and Walnut–Stuffed Acorn Squash (page 333)

*Signs and symptoms:* Deficiency signs include loss of appetite, weakness, pins and needles sensations, low blood pressure, increased heart rate, low body temperature, and swelling of the legs.

*Toxicity:* Excessive thiamine has been reported to cause headache, irritability, insomnia, tachycardia, and weakness, but this would be an extreme intake. Normally, this water-soluble B vitamin will wash out of the body if taken in excess.

## Vitamin B$_2$ (Riboflavin)

*Neurological effects of deficiency*
If not provided in adequate amounts:
- In experimental models, animals experience difficulty walking
- Humans show a decrease in the production of the critical detoxification enzyme glutaionine

| Vitamin B$_2$ | RDA Female | UL Female | RDA Male | UL Male |
|---|---|---|---|---|
| 51–70 years | 1.1 g | ND | 1.3 g | ND |
| > 70 years | 1.1 g | ND | 1.3 g | ND |

*Note:* Due to a lack of suitable data, UL could not be established for riboflavin. This does not mean there is no potential for adverse effects resulting from high intakes.

*Supplement form:* Found in B-complex supplements, but only lower doses are typically needed to maintain health.

*Food sources:* Found in many foods, especially in leafy vegetables, meat, yeast, milk, egg whites, and fish. As much as 50% of riboflavin content of foods is lost if food is exposed to light when cooking.

*Recommended recipes:* Power Pitas with Eggs and Vegetables (page 185), Parmesan Herb Baked Fish Fillets (page 288)

*Signs and symptoms:* Vitamin $B_2$ is part of an enzyme that produces a usable form of glutathione. Riboflavin deficiency presents with soreness of lips, mouth, and tongue. Light sensitivity, tearing, burning, and itching of eyes can occur as well. Dermatitis and changes to the skin, as well as a type of anemia, may occur. Alcoholics and people receiving hemodialysis for kidney failure are at risk of deficiency. Some drugs can interfere with the body's use of $B_2$, such as the antidepressant drug imipramine.

*Toxicity:* There are no known bad effects from riboflavin toxicity.

## Vitamin $B_3$ (Niacin)

*Neurological effects of deficiency*
If not provided in adequate amounts:
- Leads to profound changes to thinking, perception, mood, and personality
- Causes sleep disturbances, anxiety, depression, and thought disorders
- Can be followed by hallucinations, seizures, and psychotic episodes

| Vitamin $B_3$ | RDA Female | UL Female | RDA Male | UL Male |
|---|---|---|---|---|
| 51–70 years | 14 mg | 35 mg | 16 mg | 35 mg |
| > 70 years | 14 mg | 35 mg | 16 mg | 35 mg |

*Supplement form:* In treating cholesterol, physicians prescribe 1 g of vitamin $B_3$ three times daily. At this level, a phenomenon called vasodilation will occur, along with the release of a substance called histamine, which is not harmful but can be very unpleasant. Individuals who have been prescribed high doses of niacin need to work their way up to the maximum dose gradually. They should also have a blood test performed periodically to ensure that their liver is not adversely affected by the high dose. Although uncommon, this does occur for some individuals.

*Food sources:* Nicotinic acid is found in most foods, with the exception of fats and oils (niacin is a term used for both nicotinic acid and nicotinamide). It is added to some enriched foods, because processing removes vitamin $B_3$. Nicotinic acid levels are high in meats, fish, and grain products. It is also found in corn in a form that is not absorbable. Some of the first cases of documented $B_3$ deficiency, also called pellagra, were reported in people who ate corn as a staple food.

*Recommended recipes:* Turkey Apple Meatloaf (page 314), Tuna Casserole (page 293)

*Signs and symptoms:* Your body can make its own $B_3$ from the aminio acid tryptophan. Vitamin $B_3$ deficiency can occur due to a deficiency of vitamin $B_6$, because $B_6$ is needed for the conversion of tryptophan to nicotinic acid. In pellagra, the skin starts to crack and form crusts. The person has a red, swollen, and painful tongue. The lining of the intestines may slough off, leading to diarrhea. In the southern United States in the early 20th century, pellagra was common. Corn was one of the primary grains consumed and this otherwise-nutritious food is not very high in tryptophan. Anorexia nervosa, an eating disorder that leads to starvation, is an example where extreme pellagra has been reported. People with low niacin levels and low tryptophan in the diet are at risk.

*Toxicity:* Nausea, vomiting, and arrythmias may occur. Glucose intolerance, hyperuricemia, and aggravation of the peptic ulcer may be seen. Anyone taking a lot of niacin should ask their doctor for a periodic check of their liver enzymes, which is inexpensive and easy to obtain via a blood test.

## Vitamin $B_5$ (Pantothenic Acid)
*Neurological effect of deficiency*
If not provided in adequate amounts:
- Weakens energy metabolism in the brain
- Causes an inability to produce important neurotransmitters, such as serotonin, dopamine, and norepinephrine, which

---

**DID YOU KNOW?**

**High Dose Niacin**

Orthomolecular medical practitioners believe that some individuals require megadoses of $B_3$ at the UL level and beyond to regain and maintain mental health.

---

are critical brain chemicals needed to process thinking and moving
- Causes impaired function of the adrenal glands, which are key components in our ability to handle stress

| Vitamin B$_5$ | AI Female | UL Female | AI Male | UL Male |
|---|---|---|---|---|
| 51–70 years | 5 mg | ND | 5 mg | ND |
| > 70 years | 5 mg | ND | 5 mg | ND |

*Note:* RDAs are not available; AIs are provided.

*Supplement form:* Found as part of B-complex supplements, but only lower doses are typically needed to maintain health.

*Food sources:* Widely distributed in food (the root word "pantothen" in the name pantothenic acid is from the Greek for "from everywhere"). If you eat a mixed diet, you are likely to get enough vitamin B$_5$, but avocados, whole grains, and broccoli are particularly good sources.

*Recommended recipes:* Peppery Meatloaf with Quinoa (page 322), Saucy Swiss Steak (page 316)

*Signs and symptoms:* Although it is hard to develop a vitamin B$_5$ defiency, crash dieting, starvation, ill health with poor appetite, or living on refined foods and sweets could lead to less-than-optimal intakes. People with vitamin B$_5$ deficiency develop malaise, abdominal discomfort, and pins and needles sensations. Due to wide distribution, deficiency is likely to occur in conjunction with other B-complex vitamins.

*Toxicity:* Vitamin B$_5$ does not have any reported toxicity.

## Vitamin B$_6$ (Pyridoxine)
*Neurological effect of deficiency*
If not provided in adequate amounts:
- Causes a breakdown in the manfacturing of amino acids, precursors to many important brain chemicals, such as dopamine
- Causes a possible impaired conversion of linoleic to arachidonic acid, an important brain cell fatty acid
- Causes a possible impaired production of vitamin B$_3$ from tryptophan (B$_3$ being an important brain nutrient)

| Vitamin B$_6$ | RDA Female | UL Female | RDA Male | UL Male |
|---|---|---|---|---|
| 51–70 years | 1.5 mg | 100 mg | 1.7 mg | 100 mg |
| > 70 years | 1.5 mg | 100 mg | 1.7 mg | 100 mg |

*Supplement form:* Supplements are often given at 50 or 100 mg doses but should not exceed this.

*Food sources:* Found in rice, meats, bananas, and potatoes, and in low concentration in many other foods. The heating and storage of these foods can cause a loss of B$_6$. Boiling broccoli for 5 minutes can cause a loss of up to 50% of the B$_6$ content. Likewise, the canning of vegetables can cause over half of the B$_6$ to be lost and the canning of fruits can cause about a third of the B$_6$ to disappear. Even freezing food can destroy about half of the B$_6$.

*Recommended recipes:* Shrimp Risotto with Artichoke Hearts and Parmesan (page 302), Beef with Broccoli (page 318)

*Signs and symptoms:* Patients who consume large amounts of dietary amino acids will have higher needs, so anyone who consumes a lot of whey protein shakes should make sure they have enough vitamin B$_6$. Individuals who consume a lot of heavily processed foods may not be meeting their requirement for vitamin B$_6$ if they do not also contain enough fresh, B$_6$-rich foods (due to the loss of B$_6$ in cooking, canning, and freezing). Vitamin B$_6$ deficiency leads to skin abnormalities and to thickening and redness around the eyes, nose, and mouth. Deficiency can also cause inflammation of the mouth and tongue. Extreme deficiency can lead to convulsions.

*Toxicity:* Doses of 2–6 g daily may cause nerve damage. This can also occur with lower doses (such as 500 mg) taken over a long period of time.

## Vitamin B$_9$ (Folic Acid)

*Neurological effect of deficiency*
If not provided in adequate amounts:
- Prevents formation of active DNA
- Impedes clearance of the toxic amino acid homocysteine
- Disturbs methylation reactions
- Darkens mood, leading to fatigue and depression

| Vitamin B$_9$ | RDA Female | UL Female | RDA Male | UL Male |
| --- | --- | --- | --- | --- |
| 51–70 years | 400 mcg | 1000 mcg | 400 mcg | 1000 mcg |
| > 70 years | 400 mcg | 1000 mcg | 400 mcg | 1000 mcg |

*Supplement form:* Typically, folic acid is supplemented at 1 mg daily. There is a fraction of the population that has real difficulty using folic acid in their body and they may need to take a form of it called methylfolate. The problem lies in the inability to convert folic acid into a form that is needed to be metabolically active once in the body.

*Food sources:* Good sources of folate (the naturally occuring form) are green leafy vegetables, asparagus, cauliflower, almonds, liver, eggs, dried beans, and oranges. It occurs in different forms and is bound to proteins in some foods. Low-availability forms of folate are found in oranges, lettuce, egg yolks, cabbage, soybeans, and wheat germ; the high-availability form is found in bananas, lima beans, liver, and yeast. Steaming and frying can lead to losses as high as 90%. Boiling vegetables for 8 minutes can destroy 89% of folate in vegetables.

*Recommended recipes:* Everyday Salad (page 240), Tabbouleh (page 251)

*Sign and symptoms:* Symptoms of folic acid deficiency include loss of appetite, nausea, diarrhea, mouth ulcers, and hair loss. Chronic deficiency leads to fatigue, a sore tongue, and anemia. People with very low folate status may begin to experience a type of anemia (hemoglobin deficiency). Deficiency might be an issue for people taking certain medications, such as methotrexate, commonly used to treat rheumatoid arthritis. Alcoholics may also be deficient, which can be due to poor nutrition as well as the effect of alcohol on the body. Smoking increases the need for folic acid.

*Toxicity:* Folic acid competes with the drug phenytoin for uptake, so individuals relying on this drug to prevent convulsions should not take large doses. At doses of 1 to 10 mg, rare cases of hypersensitivity (allergic-type reactions) have been seen, with fever, hives, itching, and respiratory distress. Folic acid can mask vitamin B$_{12}$ deficiency by temporarily reversing one of the telltale signs of B$_{12}$ deficiency: macrocytic anemia. This is problematic because the neurologic damage from B$_{12}$ deficiency will progress in this case, and can be irreversible.

## DID YOU KNOW?

### Genetic Test

Some people are not able to use folic acid efficiently due to a genetic characteristic. They actually ingest and absorb enough, but the normal biochemical pathway for folic acid in the body is disrupted. Although this is not deemed deficient by medical standards, these people may not be getting all the folic acid they need for optimal health because their individual need is extremely high compared to the average person. Consult with a clinical nutritionist, such as a dietitian skilled in nutrigenomic testing and the analysis of nutritional deficiencies.

# Vitamin B$_{12}$ (Cobalamin)

*Neurological effect of deficiency*

If not provided in adequate amounts:

- Causes difficulty conserving folic acid
- Creates risk for pernicious anemia
- May lead to problems with DNA synthesis
- Causes an overall decrease in proper neurologic function
- Causes a breakdown of myelin formation
- Eventually leads to degeneration of the spinal cord and extreme neurological problems

| Vitamin B$_{12}$ | RDA Female | UL Female | RDA Male | UL Male |
|---|---|---|---|---|
| 51–70 years | 2.4 mcg | ND | 2.4 mcg | ND |
| > 70 years | 2.4 mcg | ND | 2.4 mcg | ND |

*Note:* Due to a lack of suitable data, UL could not be established for vitamin B$_{12}$. This does not mean there is no potential for adverse effects resulting from high intakes.

*Supplement form:* Vitamin B$_{12}$ is often given in doses of 1 mg. Some people who cannot absorb it efficiently try the sublingual form (under the tongue). Others need a B$_{12}$ injection into their arm muscle because they cannot absorb it well.

*Food sources:* Microorganisms in the colon produce vitamin B$_{12}$, but it is not available for absorption. Vitamin B$_{12}$ is found in meat and milk. Strict vegetarians can develop a B$_{12}$ deficiency. Absorption is dependent on the production of intrinsic factor in the stomach. Vitamin B$_{12}$ is absorbed in the very last part of the small bowel in the ileum.

*Recommended Recipes:* Orange Ginger Beef (page 319), Beef and Quinoa Power Burgers (page 321)

*Signs and symptoms:* Deficiency may take up to 2 years to present symptoms. It is insidious in onset. Weakness, fatigue, and dyspnea are seen as a result of the anemia resulting from B$_{12}$ deficiency. Numbness and tingling in the feet and hands, diarrhea, hair loss, impotence, irritability, depression, and memory disturbances are also reported. Vitamin B$_{12}$ deficiency can mask folic acid deficiency, so folic acid should be given with vitamin B$_{12}$.

*Toxicity:* No toxic effects are reported.

# Vitamin C (Ascorbic Acid)

*Neurological effect of deficiency*

If not provided in adequate amounts:

- Interferes with the formation of norepinephrine, a key neurotransmitter in thinking, memory, and organ system function, and particularly important in dementia
- Impedes the production of serotonin, a key brain neurotransmitter associated with mood and also active in the human gut
- Weakens absorption of iron, especially iron from nutritional supplements
- Skin and soft tissue repair are defective
- Impairs immune function, bone formation, and adrenal gland function

| Vitamin C | RDA Female | UL Female | RDA Male | UL Male |
|-----------|-----------|-----------|----------|---------|
| 51–70 years | 75 mg | 2000 mg | 90 mg | 2000 mg |
| > 70 years | 75 mg | 2000 mg | 90 mg | 2000 mg |

*Supplement form:* Vitamin C can be supplemented at 100 mg daily, but many people take 500 mg. A naturopathic physician might prescribe higher amounts in many situations.

*Food sources:* Found in green vegetables, fruits (especially citrus, cantaloupe, strawberries), broccoli, cabbage, spinach, tomatoes, green bell peppers, and potatoes. Heat and oxygen can damage vitamin C. Prolonged exposure to iron, copper, and oxygen will destroy it. Vitamin C is lost in cooking water.

*Recommended recipes:* Orange Zinger (page 362), Cherry Juice (page 360)

*Signs and symptoms:* Presents as scurvy, with weakness, irritability, bleeding gums, inflammation of gums, and the loosening of teeth. There is also bleeding in the skin, conjunctiva (eye lining), nose, and genitourinary tract. Anemia can occur. People with a low intake of fresh fruits and vegetables are at risk. Alcoholics may present with scurvy. Individuals with increased oxidative stress, such as smokers, may have a greater requirement for ascorbic acid. Anyone with a high burden of chemicals to detoxify may escape the extremes of scurvy but will definitely need additional vitamin C.

*Toxicity:* There is a risk for kidney stones at large doses. Higher doses also cause diarrhea and may reduce semen production. Vitamin C can impact people with inherited blood conditions, such as sickle-cell anemia, thalassemia, and glucose-6-phosphate dehydrogenase deficiency. Very high doses of vitamin C may be problematic in kidney failure. Chewable vitamin C is not recommended for any length of time because it can cause dental erosion (it is a weak acid). Vitamin C may interfere with laboratory tests of liver function and blood sugar. It can also affect fecal occult blood measurements (a simple screening test for colorectal cancer) and urine glucose measurements. In spite of these considerations, vitamin C is a very safe vitamin, and it is frequently given in large doses with no observed toxicity.

## Vitamin D

*Neurological effect of deficiency*
If not provided in adequate amounts:
- Increases calcium and phosphate absorption, which can be a medical emergency because nerve, muscle, and heart function depend on these levels being very well controlled
- Impairs brain receptors for vitamin D in the areas that control body function and impact movement
- Diminishes vitamin D receptors in the hippocampus and in the progress of Alzheimer's disease

| Vitamin D | RDA Female | UL Female | RDA Male | UL Male |
|---|---|---|---|---|
| 51–70 years | 600 IU | 4000 IU | 600 IU | 4000 IU |
| > 70 years | 800 IU | 4000 IU | 800 IU | 4000 IU |

*Forms:* Vitamin D has three forms. Vitamin D2 is produced synthetically from ultraviolet (UV) irradiation of ergosterol. Vitamin D3, cholecalciferol, is formed from 7-dehydrocholesterol in the skin by UV exposure. In the liver, the active form of D is made — D3 becomes 25-hydroxyvitamin D3 and a similar product is made of D2. With more UV exposure, you can make more — but only to a limit (probably not above 150 IU daily). Dietary intake of vitamin D is important in individuals with normal absorption who live somewhere with limited exposure to sunlight. As a unit of measurement, 10 ug cholecalciferol equals 400 IU vitamin D.

*Supplement form:* Supplemental doses of D3 vary widely. Some formulations deliver 200 IU, but some regimens (which should only be recommended by physicians who focus on nutrition, and naturopathic physicians) will exceed 2000 IU daily.

*Food sources:* Fish liver oils and, to a lesser extent, fish meat oils provide vitamin D, as do egg yolks and beef liver. Some dairy products and margarines are fortified with vitamin D.

*Recommended recipes:* Cream of Broccoli Soup (page 219), Salmon Oasis (page 290)

*Signs and symptoms:* New research has shown that higher amounts of vitamin D are needed by a much larger portion of the population in order to maintain healthy plasma levels of vitamin D. The elderly do not always get the sun exposure they need to make sufficient vitamin D, and nutritional issues (both dietary deficiencies and inefficiencies digesting and absorbing food) can reduce vitamin D intake. Chronic vitamin D deficiency may be a factor in osteoporosis seen in the elderly.

*Toxicity:* The active form of vitamin D, 25 D3, can induce high blood calcium and too much calcium in the urine. High blood calcium levels leads to nausea, loss of appetite, itching, frequent urination, abdominal pain, constipation, bone pain, metallic taste in the mouth, and dehydration. Chronic use can lead to the calcification of the kidneys, calcium deposits in various tissues throughout the body, kidney stones, and even kidney failure. Weight loss, irritability, pancreatitis, light sensitivity, hypertension, cardiac arrhythmias, elevated blood urea nitrogen, cholesterol, liver enzymes (a sign of liver damage), and psychosis may also be seen. Although vitamin D deficiency is a real phenomenon, we stress again, you should not exceed the daily guidelines.

**DID YOU KNOW?**

**Suboptimal Vitamin D**

A large segment of the population, even those who are exposed to regular sunshine, have suboptimal levels of plasma vitamin D. The implications for bone health and cancer prevention are far-reaching.

## Vitamin E
*Neurological effect of deficiency*
If not provided in adequate amounts:
- Damages the brain, spinal cord, and nervous system in advanced deficiency
- Leads to walking difficulties as a result of damage to the nerves, causing pain or loss of sensation and clumsiness
- Leads to retinal damage

Vitamin E is also known as d-alpha-tocopherol. It is found in fatty foods and in nature, and it is there to protect these fats from oxidation. Remember that when fatty acids get oxidized, they are hazardous to our health — think about rancid butter or meat drippings left on a barbecue grill for a week.

Vitamin E is localized in the cell membranes and provides a defense against oxidative damage to the delicate fats in the cell membrane. This is certainly the case in the cells of the brain. Vitamin E works with selenium to help glutathione deal with a number of potentially damaging free radicals.

This essential fat-soluble antioxidant vitamin protects the components of cells (the membranes on the organs, or organelles, of human cells) from damage. These are the microscopic structures inside our cells that are in essence the organs of the cells — the machinery that runs them. Vitamin E can therefore act independently to mop up certain free radicals. If there is not enough of it, aging of the brain and changes to the spinal cord can occur.

| Vitamin E | RDA Female | UL Female | RDA Male | UL Male |
|---|---|---|---|---|
| 51–70 years | 15 mg | 1000 mg | 15 mg | 1000 mg |
| > 70 years | 15 mg | 1000 mg | 15 mg | 1000 mg |

*Supplement form:* D-alpha-tocopherol is the active human form, and about 400 IU daily is found in many supplement protocols. Approximately 1 mg of vitamin E is needed for each 0.6 g of polyunsaturated fatty acids (PUFAs) consumed.

*Food sources:* Vitamin E is found in lipids of leafy green plants, oils, and seeds. Animal sources include eggs, liver, and muscle meats. The vitamin E content is greatly affected by processing, storage, and preparation. Freezing does not prevent peroxide formation and the destruction of biologic activity. The median intake in the United States is less than the RDA. This may be due to the fact that many dietary recommendations to reduce fat steer us away from vitamin E–rich foods, and also because some oils that ought to be sources of vitamin E have been altered to the point of losing some of their tocopherols. Those who consume large amounts of PUFA without accompanying vitamin E may not be meeting their requirements, and those who eat too many undercooked grains may also be at risk.

*Recommended recipes:* Cranberry Mandarin Coleslaw with Walnuts and Raisins (page 249), Walnut Flax Waffles (page 197)

*Signs and symptoms:* Progressive nervous system symptoms are associated with low serum vitamin E in children with certain types of liver disease. Symptoms include lack of reflexes, difficulty or changes to walking, decreased sensation in the legs (especially where position of the legs or a sense of vibration are concerned), and weakness or paralysis of the eye muscles.

Vitamin E deficiency is seen in adult malabsorption syndromes where the person cannot properly absorb nutrients from the gastrointestinal tract. Malabsorption is reported in individuals with inflammatory bowel disease, such as Crohn's disease, with short bowel syndrome (surgical removal of part of the intestine), and in those who have had gastric bypass surgery. Individuals may present with red blood cell destruction, muscle destruction, unsteady gait, tremor, weakness, eye muscle weakness, damage to the retina, and impairment of the sense of limb/joint position.

There are serious questions about the efficacy of vitamin E supplementation, and research in the past 15 years has questioned its prevention value and, in some cases, its safety. In 2005, an editorial in the *Annals of Internal Medicine* warned the public not to use supplemental vitamin E, citing research that indicated it increased cardiovascular mortality and was useless in stopping cognitive decline in patients with Alzheimer's disease.

*Toxicity:* Vitamin E can interfere with the absorption of other fat-soluble vitamins. At very high doses, vitamin E can block the oxidation of vitamin K to its active form, and this can increase the tendency to bleed and bruise (vitamin K helps the blood to clot). This can be a big problem for those who are already on blood-thinning drugs, those who have a blood-clotting problem in general (easy bleeding), and those who are about to have surgery. In these scenarios, moderate and large doses of vitamin E should be avoided. Generally, intakes below 400 IU are safe.

## Vitamin K

*Neurological effect of deficiency*
If not provided in adequate amounts:
- Leads to issues with blood clotting
- Causes mineralization and the hardening of bone

---

### DID YOU KNOW?

**PUFA Paradox**

The requirements for vitamin E depend on the intake of polyunsaturated fatty acids (PUFAs). Requirement increases with PUFA intake. Foods that contain PUFAs should also have vitamin E, but some vitamin E may have been lost during processing. For example, a natural oil that has been extracted from a nut, seed, or olive in a gentle way (without chemical solvents) will have plenty of vitamin E. An oil that is extracted using heat, light, and chemicals, and is then processed to look clear, will be lacking the very vitamin E that is supposed to protect these fats in the human body.

- Does not seem to directly affect the brain and the central nervous system, but the production of vitamin K in the colon does demonstrate the importance that gut flora (friendly bacteria in the colon) can play in our health

| Vitamin K | AI Female | UL Female | AI Male | UL Male |
|---|---|---|---|---|
| 51–70 years | 90 mcg | ND | 120 mcg | ND |
| > 70 years | 90 mcg | ND | 120 mcg | ND |

*Note:* Due to a lack of suitable data, UL could not be established for vitamin K. This does not mean there is no potential for adverse effects resulting from high intakes.

*Supplement form:* Supplementation is uncommon.

*Food sources:* Vitamin K is found in green leafy vegetables and in some forms in bacteria and animals. Colonic bacteria provide some vitamin K.

*Recommended recipes:* Everyday Salad (page 240), Tabbouleh (page 251)

*Signs and symptoms:* Easy bleeding (especially for those already on blood thinners) might occur with deficiency. Many patients who have had multiple courses of antibiotics have had their colonic bacterial flora altered permanently, and unless they recolonize the gut with the right bacteria, they may have impaired vitamin K synthesis. This is more of an issue if they consume few leafy greens.

*Toxicity:* People taking anticoagulants should definitely not take vitamin K.

# Recommended Dietary Allowances: Minerals

Minerals include those that are present in the body in a larger amount, such as sodium, potassium, magnesium, and calcium, as well as phosphorus. There are also widespread minerals with multiple functions, and these include iron, zinc, copper, iodine, flouride, selenium, and chromium. Trace minerals are present in very small amounts, but often play vital roles. These include cobalt, molybdenum, vanadium, silicon, and nickel.

## Calcium

*Neurological effect of deficiency*
If not provided in adequate amounts:
- Impairs nerve conduction
- Leads to hypocalcemia, resulting in stiff or spastic muscles and heart arrhythmias

| Calcium | RDA Female | UL Female | RDA Male | UL Male |
|---|---|---|---|---|
| 51–70 years | 1200 mg | 2000 mg | 1000 mg | 2000 mg |
| > 70 years | 1200 mg | 2000 mg | 1200 mg | 2000 mg |

*Supplement form:* Calcium citrate can be given at 500 or 1000 mg daily. Recent scientific evidence suggests that lower amounts are more helpful and that higher amounts of supplemented calcium may not be helpful or may even be harmful.

*Food sources:* Sources include dairy products, meats, beet greens, spinach, almonds, kale, canned salmon, and collard greens. Calcium in vegetables is bound to phytate. In animal sources, it is bound to protein, which does get into the body more easily than some forms of plant calcium. Gastric acid is needed for calcium absorption. The eldery and people who take medications that reduce stomach acid are at risk of calcium deficiency.

*Recommended recipes:* Tofu Quinoa Scramble (page 187), Vegetable Cheese Loaf with Lemon Tomato Sauce (page 264)

*Signs and symptoms:* Chronic deficiency of calcium will force the body to pull calcium from the bones. Calcium is not very well absorbed and it is lost from the body quite easily. Vitamin D is needed to absorb and maintain an optimal plasma calcium level.

A deficiency of vitamin D will probably lead to abnormalities in calcium metabolism (under normal circumstances, high but not toxic doses of vitamin D should be taken with calcium in order to help feed calcium to the bones and to prevent a buildup of calcium in the arteries). Calcium absorption decreases with aging, resulting in suboptimal calcium status and a decrease in bone mass. Individuals with an intestinal mucosal disease (such as Crohn's disease), which causes malabsorption, and individuals with renal disease are at risk for calcium deficiency.

*Toxicity:* Too much calcium in the body can build up if individuals take extreme amounts of vitamin D. A buildup would lead to weak muscles, paralysis of the bowel muscles, and eventually brain issues, such as coma. Calcium in this case might deposit into soft tissues, and the kidney may start to form stones.

## Chromium

*Neurological effect of deficiency*

If not provided in adequate amounts:

- Increases likelihood of blood sugar issues (blood sugar is crucial for short-term brain energy requirements and long-term brain health; chromium is part of glucose tolerance factor, which works with insulin to allow glucose uptake into cells)

| Chromium | RDA Female | UL Female | RDA Male | UL Male |
|---|---|---|---|---|
| 51–70 years | 20 mcg | ND | 30 mcg | ND |
| > 70 years | 20 mcg | ND | 30 mcg | ND |

*Note:* Due to a lack of suitable data, UL could not be established for chromium. This does not mean there is no potential for adverse effects resulting from high intakes.

*Supplement form:* Supplements of chromium tend to deliver 50 to 200 mcg of chromium daily.

*Food sources:* Chromium is found in meat, dairy, eggs, spices, and brewer's yeast.

*Recommended recipes:* Three-Spice Chicken with Potatoes (page 305), Rosemary Chicken Breasts with Sweet Potatoes and Onions (page 304)

*Signs and symptoms:* Deficiency can lead to type 2 diabetes, weakness, confusion, and possibly nerve damage. Deficiency is seen in some individuals on prolonged total parenteral nutrition, where they are fed a nutrient solution through a port into a vein.

*Toxicity:* Not well described, but dietary chromium does not seem to be toxic. Industrial forms of chromium are not safe.

## Copper

*Neurological effect of deficiency*
If not provided in adequate amounts:
- Impairs antioxidant systems of the brain
- Results in serious neuropathies and myelopathies (pain and degeneration of nerves)

| Copper | RDA Female | UL Female | RDA Male | UL Male |
|---|---|---|---|---|
| 51–70 years | 900 mcg | 10000 mcg | 900 mcg | 10000 mcg |
| > 70 years | 900 mcg | 10000 mcg | 900 mcg | 10000 mcg |

*Supplement form:* Copper is not often supplemented. When it is prescribed, the goal may be to balance zinc supplementation, given at 1 part copper to 10 parts zinc. An example would be 5 mg of copper given with 50 mg of zinc.

*Food sources:* Copper is found in shellfish, organ meats, nuts, legumes, dried fruits, and cocoa.

*Recommended recipes:* Pasta with Shrimp and Peas (page 296), Perfect Chocolate Bundt (page 346)

*Signs and symptoms:* Deficiency can lead to anemia. Copper deficiency can be caused by an inability to absorb food due to disease or a surgical procedure in the small bowel. A deficiency has been reported in people who have had gastric bypass surgery or other forms of bariatric surgery to lose weight.

*Toxicity:* Excessive copper intake can produce nausea, vomiting, diarrhea, abdominal cramps, and damage to the mucosa of the gastrointestinal tract. Larger doses cause gastrointestinal bleeding, liver necrosis, hemolysis, and neurologic damage. Copper toxicity can occur in Wilson's disease, an inherited condition of excessive copper accumulation in the liver.

## Iodine

*Neurological effect of deficiency*
If not provided in adequate amounts:
- Metabolism may suffer because iodine is a key component of active thyroid hormone

*Supplement form:* Just a few micrograms a day is all that would be supplemented.

| Iodine | RDA Female | UL Female | RDA Male | UL Male |
|---|---|---|---|---|
| 51–70 years | 150 mcg | 1100 mcg | 150 mcg | 1100 mcg |
| > 70 years | 150 mcg | 1100 mcg | 150 mcg | 1100 mcg |

*Food sources:* Iodine is found in seafood. The iodine content of dairy products, eggs, and meat depends on the iodine content of the animal feed. In coastal regions, atmospheric iodine is an additional source.

*Recommended recipes:* Shrimp Risotto with Artichoke Hearts and Parmesan (page 302), Shrimp and Corn Bisque (page 234)

*Signs and symptoms:* Deficiency of iodine leads to hypothyroidism due to a lack of thyroid hormone production. Deficiency symptoms include decreased cellular activity, decreased basal metabolic rate, weakness, fatigue, slow thinking, slow heart rate, swelling of the lower legs, delayed return of ankle reflex, thinning eyebrows, constipation, and slow, deep tendon reflexes. Some soils are iodine poor and the foods grown on them are iodine deficient.

*Toxicity:* Taking more than 2000 mcg daily of iodine has a negative effect and can actually decrease thyroid gland activity.

## Iron

*Neurological effect of deficiency*
If not provided in adequate amounts:
- Impairs brain function because the brain will not have enough oxygen and energy. Iron is part of hemoglobin and myoglobin, oxygen-carrying proteins that maintain body energy and brain oxygenation

| Iron | RDA Female | UL Female | RDA Male | UL Male |
|---|---|---|---|---|
| 51–70 years | 8 mg | 45 mg | 8 mg | 45 mg |
| > 70 years | 8 mg | 45 mg | 8 mg | 45 mg |

*Supplement form:* Approximately 25 to 50 mg of actual iron is supplemented. This is delivered in a matrix or is bound to something else, such as citrate, fumarate, or sulphate. Iron from yeast is a good source, as are protein- or amino acid–bound iron (such as iron that is bound to the amino acid glycine, which is easier to absorb). Iron preparations contain only percentages of elemental iron. The sulfate form (anhydrous) contains 30% iron, fumarate form contains 33%, and gluconate form contains 11.6%.

*Food sources:* Iron is found in red meat, nuts, seeds, and egg yolks. Vegetable sources of iron vary with the growing conditions of the plant. Inorganic salts and vegetable iron need ascorbic acid present to help absorption. Heme iron (the type of iron found in red blood cells), which is found in animal sources, is better absorbed. Iron absorption increases when the total body pool is decreased. Gastric acid helps convert iron to a more absorbable form. Amino acids can bind to iron and make it easier to absorb. Absorption is decreased by phytates (found in many plant foods) and by inorganic zinc.

*Recommended recipes:* Beef and Quinoa Power Burgers (page 321), Beef with Broccoli (page 318)

*Signs and symptoms:* Iron deficiency presents as anemia, weakness, pallor, mouth sores, and increased susceptibility to infection. In children, decreased growth and effects on cognitive function are seen. Those at risk include vegetarians and individuals with low levels of stomach hydrochloric acid (from atrophic gastritis or hydrogen chloride–suppressing medications). Individuals with excessive blood loss due to chronic bleeding from the gastrointestinal tract, as well as females during menstruation, are at risk.

*Toxicity:* Excess iron ingestion leads to nausea, diarrhea, and abdominal pain, and extreme amounts can lead to shock, intestinal perforation, oliguria (low urine output), coagulopathy, acidosis, and lethargy. Iron can be stored in the body chronically, leading to iron overload and liver damage. Iron supplementation should be used with caution in those with cardiovascular disease because it can promote free radical reactions.

## Magnesium

*Neurological effect of deficiency*

If not provided in adequate amounts:

- Leads to problems with energy and nerve function
- Impairs neuromuscular transmission
- Affects bone matrix
- Affects nucleic acid synthesis
- Affects energy production in cells
- In severe deficiency, causes difficulty in the mobilization of calcium into the bloodstream (from storage in bone)

| Magnesium | RDA Female | UL Female | RDA Male | UL Male |
|---|---|---|---|---|
| 51–70 years | 320 mg | 350 mg | 420 mg | 350 mg |
| > 70 years | 320 mg | 350 mg | 420 mg | 350 mg |

*Supplement form:* Take 400 mg daily. Higher amounts are divided up to prevent diarrhea.

*Food sources:* Found in cereals, legumes, nuts, vegetables, fish, hard water, and meat.

*Recommended recipes:* Baked Risotto with Spinach (page 339), Mushroom Spinach Quiche (page 194)

*Signs and symptoms:* Signs of deficiency include muscular twitching, numbness, and tingling; in severe deficiency, muscle weakness, convulsions, apathy and depression, delirium, and heart problems. Those with long-standing dietary restrictions, malabsorption syndrome, and alcoholics are at risk. Alcoholics have decreased intake, as well as increased urinary excretion and magnesium loss from diarrhea and vomiting, so they are often in need of magnesium.

*Toxicity:* Hypermagnesemia is seen in renal failure as well as eclampsia, severe diabetic ketoacidosis, and Addison's disease. Excessive magnesium can cause serious problems, including stopping heart function. The patient may have drowsiness and muscular weakness prior to the most serious symptoms.

## DID YOU KNOW?

### RDA/UL Confusion

You're reading it right: the magnesium ULs for men over 51 are *lower* than the RDAs. This is because some people experience gastrointestinal symptoms when taking a magnesium dose as low as 350 mg. Even though the vast majority of people can tolerate much higher levels, the UL is set at the level where symptoms arise in *any* individual.

# Manganese

*Neurological effect of deficiency*

If not provided in adequate amounts:

- Impairs detoxification because manganese is part of several enzymes, including the detoxification enzyme superoxide dismutase

| Manganese | RDA Female | UL Female | RDA Male | UL Male |
|---|---|---|---|---|
| 51–70 years | 1.8 mg | 11 mg | 2.3 mg | 11 mg |
| > 70 years | 1.8 mg | 11 mg | 2.3 mg | 11 mg |

*Supplement form:* Dosage should be approximately 5 mg daily.

*Food sources:* Manganese is found in nuts, dried fruits, unrefined grains, tea, and prunes.

*Recommended recipes:* Couscous Salad with Basil and Pine Nuts (page 252), Cranberry Mandarin Coleslaw with Walnuts and Raisins (page 249)

*Signs and symptoms:* Retarded skeletal growth, weight loss, dementia, nausea, vomiting, and altered hair color can all occur if someone does not have enough manganese. Some people with epilepsy have been found to have low blood manganese levels.

*Toxicity:* Manganese is rarely toxic, but when inhaled as dust (by miners, for example), it can cause psychiatric disease and movement disorders, somewhat like Parkinson's disease.

# Selenium

*Neurological effect of deficiency*

If not provided in adequate amounts:

- Causes the detoxification systems to suffer; selenium is essential for the activity of the master detoxification enzyme glutathione peroxidase (this enzyme protects membranes from oxidative damage and is an important liver and brain/nervous system protector)

| Selenium | RDA Female | UL Female | RDA Male | UL Male |
|---|---|---|---|---|
| 51–70 years | 55 mcg | 400 mcg | 55 mcg | 400 mcg |
| > 70 years | 55 mcg | 400 mcg | 55 mcg | 400 mcg |

*Supplement form:* Dosage should be up to approximately 200 mcg daily.

*Food sources:* Selenium is found in foods as selenomethionine or selenocysteine. High levels are found in seafood, organ meats, muscle meats, and whole grains. Selenium in grains is lost in milling. Organic selenium is best assimilated.

*Recommended recipes:* Vegetable Quinoa Salad (page 254), Shrimp, Vegetables and Whole Wheat Pasta (page 297)

*Signs and symptoms:* A deficiency of selenium leads to Keshan disease, which is associated with the destruction of heart muscle. People eating foods derived from selenium-poor soils are at risk, as are individuals on highly refined diets with low selenium levels, and individuals who have high oxidative stress (from cigarette smoking and environmental factors).

*Toxicity:* Toxicity may present with nausea, vomiting, fatigue, hair loss, diarrhea, irritability, parasthesias (skin sensations), and abdominal cramps.

## Zinc

*Neurological effect of deficiency*
If not provided in adequate amounts:
- Declines many basic enzyme functions of the body and brain; zinc is crucial for many reactions in the body and it is involved in chemical reactions that support the healing and the life of body cells in general

| Zinc | RDA Female | UL Female | RDA Male | UL Male |
|---|---|---|---|---|
| 51–70 years | 8 mg | 40 mg | 11 mg | 40 mg |
| > 70 years | 8 mg | 40 mg | 11 mg | 40 mg |

*Supplement form:* Dosage should be up to 10 mg daily.

*Food sources:* The zinc content of foods can vary depending on the zinc content of the soil that the food was grown on. Muscle meats and seafoods have high levels. Vegetable sources have zinc-binding anions and phytates.

*Recommended recipes:* Beef with Broccoli (page 318), Salmon Chowder (page 238)

*Signs and symptoms:* Extreme deficiency is illustrated by acrodermatitis enteropathica, which is a childhood disease with zinc deficiency. There are oozing and crusty eruptions on the skin, diarrhea, and oral, anal, and genital ulcers. In children, delayed growth is the hallmark of zinc deficiency. Zinc deficiency leads to a loss of appetite and no desire to eat, which may compound the problem. Immune dysfunction occurs. Alcoholics may have low zinc status. People on total parenteral nutrition may not meet their zinc requirements. People who consume diets high in refined and processed foods, and those with eating disorders, such as anorexia nervosa, are at risk.

*Toxicity:* Shaking and chills as well as copper imbalances can occur.

# PART 3

# Standard Care
# for Dementia

# Medications

## CASE STUDY

### Alzheimer's Disease (continued from page 64)

That winter, things took a turn for the worse. Getting out of the car at church, Elizabeth slipped on the ice and broke her hip. The recovery was slow, and, in Ben's words, "She was never really the same." Although she recognized immediate family, at times she slipped into reminiscences about days long gone by and it was impossible to get her to focus on the moment. Eventually, the house was sold and Ben moved to a seniors residence. Elizabeth was moved to a nearby long-term care facility — and although Ben visits her daily and they can still eat together and celebrate important times together, there is no doubt that she needs to be there.

## DID YOU KNOW?

### Choice of Care

Consider the effectiveness of standard therapies, including pharmaceutical medications and botanical medicine. Drug treatment is the mainstay of Western medicine in the treatment of dementia, while herbal treatments of brain disease underpin Eastern approaches through traditional Chinese medicine and Ayurvedic medicine.

Most types of dementia can be prevented but cannot be cured. However, doctors can help to slow down the progression of symptoms and improve quality of life using a variety of therapies

Most of the medicines that help with neurological or aging-related brain diseases are drugs that target the central nervous system. They usually have an affinity for a particular region or receptor in the brain. A receptor is a protein that is embedded on the surface (usually) of a brain cell, and this acts as a docking station for various agents. The most common agent that latches on or binds to a receptor in the brain is a neurotransmitter. In fact, this is how the brain cells communicate with each other. The neurotransmitters cause changes in a brain cell that lead to changes in electrical activity, or the firing of the neuron. This triggers activity in other neurons. The arrival of the neurotransmitter (or several such inputs) might make the brain neuron more active or less active.

Most drugs that impact the central nervous system attach themselves to some receptor in the brain. They might also have a secondary effect, such as making that brain cell's response to neurotransmitters more pronounced, or they may have their own direct effect. Consult with your doctor about the efficacy and safety of the medications mentioned in this book.

# Alzheimer's Disease

The U.S. Food and Drug Administration (FDA) has approved two kinds of medications for treating the symptoms of Alzheimer's disease. These drugs are not curative, but they are working beyond the level of prevention to offer improvement to those who already have active Alzheimer's disease. Both kinds of drugs are used to treat the cognitive symptoms of Alzheimer's disease (memory loss, confusion, and problems with thinking and reasoning).

## Cholinesterase Inhibitors (Aricept, Exelon, Razadyne, Cognex)

These drugs work by raising the levels of the neurotransmitter acetylcholine in the brain. This neurotransmitter is involved in memory and learning. Its levels start to drop in the brain of an Alzheimer's patient.

## Antidepressants

Alzheimer's disease patients may also suffer from symptoms beyond troubled thinking and memory. The disease affects multiple areas across the brain, including those that regulate mood. Antidepressants are used not only for depression, but also for the simple lowering of mood and irritability (common occurrences in Alzheimer's disease). Some medications commonly used to treat behavioral and psychiatric symptoms of Alzheimer's disease are listed here in alphabetical order by generic name:

- citalopram (Celexa)
- fluoxetine (Prozac)
- paroxetine (Paxil)
- sertraline (Zoloft)
- trazodone (Desyrel)

## Anxiolytics

These drugs are given to relieve anxiety and restlessness. As the disease progresses, patients may express verbally disruptive behavior and resist efforts of assistance from caregivers.

- lorazepam (Ativan)
- oxazepam (Serax)

**DID YOU KNOW?**

**Brain Cell Death**
An FDA-approved drug, memantine (Namenda), regulates the neurotransmitter glutamate in the brain. If glutamate is too active, it can lead to an increased level of calcium entering brain cells and to brain cell death.

**DID YOU KNOW?**

**Drug Authorities**
The Mayo Clinic and Johns Hopkins University provide authoritative information on drug treatments for aging-related conditions. Consult their websites, which elaborate on the information provided here.

## Antipsychotics

Some drugs are used to alleviate hallucinations, delusions, aggression, agitation, hostility, and uncooperativeness. Although these medications are not specifically approved as Alzheimer's memory drugs, they are considered standard treatment.

- aripiprazole (Abilify)
- clozapine (Clozaril)
- haloperidol (Haldol)
- olanzapine (Zyprexa)
- quetiapine (Seroquel)
- risperidone (Risperdal)
- ziprasidone (Geodon)

# Lewy Body Dementia

The treatments for Lewy body dementia are similar to Alzheimer's disease, although the way they might be used and the way such cases are managed will have differences. There may be more focus on symptoms of rigidity, as well as the dysfunctions across the nervous system, such as the autonomic nervous system that controls body functions.

# Vascular Dementia

The FDA has not approved any drugs to specifically treat changes in judgment, planning, memory, and other affected thought processes caused by vascular dementia. However, certain medications approved by the FDA to treat these symptoms in Alzheimer's disease may also help people with vascular dementia to the same modest extent they help those with Alzheimer's.

Most causes of dementia associated with cerebrovascular changes result from damage due to atherosclerosis, which may, in time, lead to small blot clots or infarcts, hemorrhage, or transient ischemic attacks. The actual dementia caused by this might be treated with the cognitive enhancers used in Alzheimer's disease, but efforts to slow down the progression of atherosclerosis are employed as well.

## Controlling Risk Factors

Controlling the conditions underlying the health of your heart and blood vessels can slow the rate of degeneration. Depending on your individual situation, your doctor may prescribe medications to:

- Lower your blood pressure
- Help control your blood sugar if you have diabetes

- Lower your cholesterol (statin drugs or niacin)
- Treat atherosclerosis-associated conditions, such as diabetes or obesity

Changes to diet and other lifestyle modifications (such as smoking cessation) may also be recommended.

# Parkinson's Disease

Parkinson's disease results from a lack of the neurotransmitter dopamine and affects movement, which is seen as stiffness with rigid muscles and tremor in many cases. This will ultimately impact walking and movement in general. The loss of dopamine action in the brain and the tremor issues are the primary targets for treatment. Medications can help with movement and tremor by increasing the supply of dopamine. Because it cannot enter the brain, dopamine cannot be given directly.

## Carbidopa-Levodopa (Parcopa)

Levodopa (L-dopa) has been shown to be the most effective Parkinson's disease medication. It is typically combined with carbidopa, which allows more of it to penetrate into the brain. It can work very well, but dosage is progressive, with higher doses typically needed year by year, and the effect tends to wax and wane. At high doses, tardive dyskinesia can result, where uncontrolled movements happen as a reaction to the drug. Doctors may lessen the dose or adjust the times of doses to control tardive dyskinesia.

## Dopamine Agonists

Another approach is to administer drugs that stimulate the dopamine-sensitive areas of the brain directly. These so-called dopamine agonists that act like dopamine tend not to work quite as well as carbidopa-levodopa, but they can give extra assistance.

The side effects of dopamine agonists are similar to those for carbidopa-levodopa, but the list also includes hallucinations, swelling, sleepiness, and compulsive behaviors, such as hypersexuality, gambling, and eating. If you are taking these medications and you start behaving in a way that is out of character for you, talk to your doctor.

# Dopamine Agonists Versus Levodopa

Unlike levodopa, dopamine agonists don't change into dopamine. Instead, they mimic dopamine effects in your brain. They aren't as effective in treating your symptoms as levodopa. However, they last longer and may be used with levodopa to smooth out the sometimes off-and-on effect of levodopa. Here are three examples:

- pramipexole (Mirapex)
- ropinirole (Requip)
- apomorphine (Apokyn), a short-acting injectable dopamine agonist, is used for quick relief

## Anti-tremor Medications

Anti-tremor medicines are used to treat Parkinson's disease, specifically anticholinergic drugs, but these can have unpleasant side effects. Individuals may experience a significant improvement of symptoms after beginning Parkinson's disease treatment. Over time, however, the benefits of drugs frequently diminish or become less consistent, although symptoms usually can continue to be fairly well controlled.

## Monoamine Oxidase B (MAO-B) Inhibitors

These medications include selegiline (Eldepryl, Zelapar) and rasagiline (Azilect). They help prevent the breakdown of brain dopamine by inhibiting the brain enzyme monoamine oxidase B (MAO-B). When added to carbidopa-levodopa, these medications can increase the risk of hallucinations. These medications cannot be used in combination with most antidepressants or with certain narcotics due to potentially serious reactions. Check with your doctor before taking any additional medications with an MAO-B inhibitor.

## Catechol-O-Methyltransferase (COMT) Inhibitors

Entacapone (Comtan) is the primary medication from this class of drugs. This medication mildly prolongs the effect of levodopa therapy by blocking an enzyme that breaks down levodopa. The side effects are primarily those due to an enhanced levodopa effect, including an increased risk of involuntary movements (dyskinesias). Tolcapone (Tasmar) is another COMT inhibitor, but it is rarely prescribed due to a risk of serious liver damage and liver failure.

## Anticholinergics

These medications were used for many years to help control the tremor associated with Parkinson's disease. Several anticholinergic medications are available, including benztropine (Cogentin) and trihexyphenidyl. However, their modest benefits are often offset by side effects, such as impaired memory, confusion, hallucinations, constipation, dry mouth, and impaired urination.

## Amantadine

Doctors may prescribe amantadine alone to provide short-term relief of the symptoms of mild, early-stage Parkinson's disease. It also may be added to carbidopa-levodopa therapy for people in the later stages of Parkinson's disease, to help control involuntary movements (dyskinesia) induced by carbidopa-levodopa. Side effects may include a purple mottling of the skin, ankle swelling, and hallucinations.

# Motor Neuron Disease

There are a number of motor neuron diseases. Amyotrophic lateral sclerosis (ALS) is one of the most common diseases of the nerves that control muscles or motor neurons. Medications are used to relieve muscle cramps and to reduce any accumulation of saliva and phlegm in the mouth and throat due to weakness of the mouth and throat muscles.

# Peripheral Neuropathy

Symptoms of peripheral neuropathies include sensory loss, muscle weakness, muscle, and pain. Treatment might include various pain medicines, both nonsteroidal anti-inflammatory drugs (NSAIDs, such as ibuprofen) as well as opioid drugs to suppress the pain. Some antiseizure medicines seem to help with peripheral neuropathy. Some antidepressants, such as the tricyclic antidepressants, seem to decrease pain as well.

> ## DID YOU KNOW?
> ### Sole Drug Approved
> Riluzole (Rilutek) is the sole drug approved by the FDA for slowing ALS. It seems to regulate glutamate in the brain, and excess glutamate activity can lead to cell death in the parts of the nervous system that control muscle movement.

Topical treatments include capsaicin (from hot chile peppers) and lidocaine (which deadens nerve sensation). Lidocaine might be applied in a patch for longer action. Therapies that dampen pain signals — such as transcutaneous electrical nerve stimulation (TENS) therapy, where small electrical currents block pain signals from reaching the brain — are commonly used.

# Sleep Disorders

The classic prescription for sleep disorders for many years was benzodiazepines, such as alprazolam, which cause relaxation and deeper sleep (but they often also cause a morning hangover and grogginess and have a potential for dependency). Newer drugs bind to what is known as the gamma-aminobutyric acid (GABA) receptor in the brain. Drugs in this category include Ambien and Lunesta.

# Diabetes

The management of diabetes with medications is complex. Some diabetics require insulin, and there are many forms, release times, and delivery methods (needle or pump) to choose from. Medications can both increase the body's own secretion of insulin (which brings blood sugar levels down) and make the body and muscles more sensitive to insulin (which they often are not in diabetes, thus exacerbating the disease). Weight loss and diet change are a big part of standard care.

# Botanical Medicines

**B**otanical medicines can have a profound effect on the brain and nervous system. However, the evidence does not support using them as stand-alone treatments for Parkinson's disease, Alzheimer's disease, or any of the other aging-related diseases of the brain and nervous system. This does not mean that they cannot have beneficial effects. We ought to do all that we reasonably can to support the normal function of our brains and nervous systems. Our aim is to minimize the forces that age our brain. In this light, some botanicals have beneficial properties.

*Caution*: Because botanical extracts can deliver a large dose of certain compounds, it is possible to experience vigorous effects and unwanted effects. Occasionally, an herb can have negative or dangerous effects, and it can certainly interact with medications. We advise consulting with a medical practitioner trained in both pharmaceutical approaches and naturopathic approaches and consulting with your family physician about any herbs you choose to use.

## Evidence-Based Effects

Herbal medicine products have been used in the treatment of the behavioral and psychological symptoms of dementia, but with various responses. A systematic review of the use of herbal medicine in Alzheimer's disease was conducted in 2006 and published in the journal *Evidence-Based Complementary and Alternative Medicine*. The treatments of choice in Alzheimer's disease were identified as cholinesterase inhibitors and NMDA-receptor antagonists (NMDA stands for N-methyl-D-aspartate excitotoxic amino acid). Several sources remain skeptical about the therapeutic effectiveness of these drugs. The objective of this article was to review evidence from controlled studies in order to determine whether herbs can be useful in the treatment of cognitive disorders in the elderly. Randomized controlled studies assessing Alzheimer's disease in individuals older than 65 years were identified through searches of MEDLINE, LILACS, Cochrane Library, Dissertation Abstract (USA), ADEAR (Alzheimer's Disease Clinical Trials Database), National Research Register, Current Controlled Trials, Centerwatch Trials Database, and PsycINFO journal articles. The search combined the terms "Alzheimer disease," "dementia," "cognition disorders," "herbal," and "phytotherapy." The crossover results were evaluated by the Jadad scale.

The review identified two herbs and two herbal formulations with therapeutic effects for the treatment of Alzheimer's disease: *Melissa officinalis* (lemon balm), *Salvia officinalis* (common sage), yi-gan san (YGS), and ba wei di huang wan (BDW). Another herb, *ginkgo biloba,* was identified in a related meta-analysis study. All five are useful for treating the cognitive impairment of Alzheimer's disease. *Melissa officinalis* and yi-gan san are also useful in treating agitation, for they have sedative effects. Further large multicenter studies should be conducted to test the cost-effectiveness of these herbs for Alzheimer's disease and the impact on the control of cognitive deterioration.

## Herbs Effective in Treating Alzheimer's Disease

- *Ginkgo biloba*
- *Melissa officinalis*
- Ba wei di huang wan (BDW)
- *Salvia officinalis*

- Yi-gan san (YGS)
- *Bacopa monnieri*
- Huperzine A

## Ginkgo Biloba

*Gingko biloba*, also known as just gingko or the maidenhair tree, is a very hardy, pollution-resistant tree once thought to be extinct but kept in Oriental gardens. It is widely used today for circulatory disorders and contains antioxidants useful in treating dementia. It seems to help open up medium-sized arteries, such as those in the brain. Ginkgo also seems to protect the brain tissues from brief episodes of oxygen deprivation, something that can take its toll on the brain. It does seem to improve memory in some older adults.

However, large trials with Alzheimer's patients have not shown a reversal of dementia, although some studies have shown small improvements in daily functioning. Frankly, once the damage has been done to the brain, the effects of ginkgo, although useful, are not enough to reverse it. However, any person who wants to take care of their circulation to the brain and also "pretreat" themselves against limited and mild circulation issues to the brain should consider taking it.

*Standard Dose:* 80 mg two or three times daily of an extract standardized to 24% ginkgoflavonglycosides.

## Bacopa Monnieri

Also known as bacopa or brahmi, this herb has been used in India for centuries, perhaps millennia. Its traditional usage was to improve concentration and thinking — people have sought to do this for a long time across different eras and cultures. Recent research shows that it may, in fact, be a memory booster, and for this reason, it could be a useful adjunct (an extra treatment).

*Standard dose:* Bacopa extract, 300 mg daily.

## Huperzine A

Derived from the Chinese herb *Huperzia serrata*, this herb is a cholinesterase inhibitor that is currently being investigated in clinical trials. It is available as a dietary supplement and may prove useful in augmenting acetylcholine activity (acetylcholine is a crucial brain chemical). Pharmaceutical treatments are also available to boost acetylcholine and can help maintain mental function, and these have been much better researched. Recent research casts doubt on huperzine A's value as a stand-alone treatment for established Alzheimer's disease. It may make an impact on some individuals with less advanced dementia. This is best used under the supervision of a physician familiar with the interactions between botanical medicine and pharmaceuticals.

*Standard dose:* 50 to 200 mg twice daily.

## Acupuncture

Acupuncture is a part of the system of traditional Chinese medicine and is used in other systems of traditional medicine

**DID YOU KNOW?**

**Ginkgo Caution**

Consult with your physician before taking ginkgo. Ginkgo thins the blood, and it can interact with many medications. Anyone taking blood thinners, even aspirin, can develop easy bleeding from using this herb. You should never take ginkgo within 2 weeks of surgery because it can make the bleeding from surgery more dangerous. If you are on a heavy-duty clot buster drug, such as warfarin, do not take ginkgo. There are other options for circulatory support.

(there are Korean, Japanese, and other systems of acupuncture). The traditional system of diagnosis of neurological conditions is different from a biomedical-based diagnosis. For example, tremor in traditional Chinese medicine is attributed to "interior wind," the etiology of which may be quite complex. There is a very long and very large clinical experience with using acupuncture for neurologic issues and a fair number of contemporary clinical trials, some of which demonstrate efficacy. While we would not advocate completely substituting acupuncture for the best of what conventional approaches can offer, it can make a very powerful and helpful adjunctive therapy. In some conditions, there are few conventional options for treatment, which makes the need for relief from acupuncture even more relevant.

# Deep-Brain Stimulation

Deep-brain stimulation (DBS) is an option for treating patients with advanced Parkinson's disease who have unstable levodopa responses. DBS can help stabilize medication fluctuations, reduce or eliminate involuntary movements (dyskinesia), reduce tremor, reduce rigidity, and improve the slowing of movement. However, DBS is not helpful for treating problems that don't respond to levodopa therapy — except for tremor.

## Procedure

In DBS, surgeons implant electrodes into the specific part of the brain related to the patient's condition. The electrodes are connected to a generator implanted into the chest. The generator sends electrical pulses to the brain and may help improve many of the symptoms in Parkinson's disease. The doctor may adjust the settings, as necessary, to treat specific conditions. Surgery involves risks, including infections, stroke, and brain hemorrhage.

# Physical and Occupational Therapies

Physical therapies can be targeted at the deficits created by the neurological condition. For instance, loss of muscle strength in one leg due to a brain or spinal cord degenerative issue may necessitate therapy and exercises to strengthen other muscles (such as the opposite leg) and training in gait (how to walk

## Deep-Brain Stimulation

An implanted pulse generator sends mild electrical signals that may help with tremor and other neurological issues.

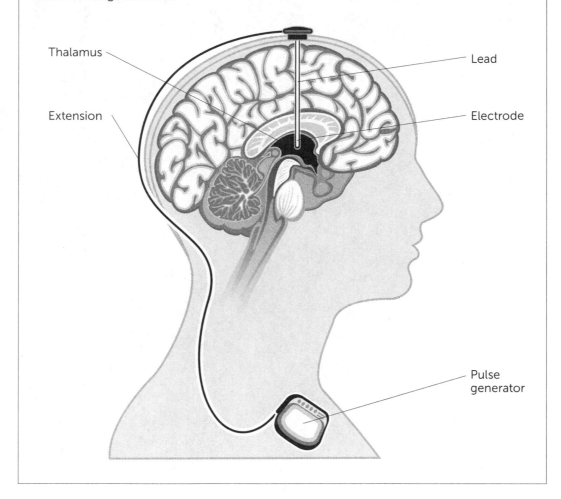

Thalamus

Extension

Lead

Electrode

Pulse generator

efficiently in a new way). Sometimes physical therapy is aimed at reducing pain and spasm, especially when the brain's control of muscles is interrupted or diminished and the muscles contract involuntarily and become stiff and painful.

An occupational therapist can help with retraining in the daily activities of life. As a neurological or brain disease takes its toll, the patient needs help to relearn certain skills (such as using the supplies and appliances in their kitchen) or they need to learn to do things in a different way. An occupational therapist can also do a risk assessment and safety plan for the home; all of the good natural and conventional therapies in the world won't help a person if they are at risk for falls or other sources of harm in their own home.

**PART 4**

# The 12-Step Healthy Brain Diet Program

# Program Goals

## Parkinson's Disease (continued from page 46)

Ron's diagnosis of Parkinson's disease did not sink in for a few days, but after thinking things through and reading more about treatments for Parkinson's, Ron set out to "draft" his Parkinson's team, to use the sports metaphors he was fond of. Ron had played sports all his life and had often observed how a team could achieve more than the individual "star" — there is no "I" in team, the cliché reads. He set out to draft a team of neurological experts to manage his Parkinson's symptoms. First, he asked his family doctor to take charge. That he was trained in traditional Chinese medicine in Hong Kong and traditional Western medicine at Cambridge University in England was a distinct advantage. Dr. Chung brought acupuncture and herbal formulas to the examination table, along with a healthy respect for the use of medications — the levadopa and the dopamine agonists that Ron's neurologist prescribed. Dr. Gio invited Ron to participate in several studies involving balance at the local teaching hospital. Rounding out the team was Dr. Elash, a naturopathic doctor and professor of clinical nutrition who recommended large doses of antioxidants, especially coenzyme Q10.

Keeping Ron informed at every stage was his partner Irene, a medical research associate, and his daughter, Jayne, who decided to study motor control disorders at McGill University (MSc) and the University of Toronto (PhD). Not surprisingly, discussions at the dinner table revolved around new research in Parkinson's disease. The value of patterned exercise, such as swimming and skating, for alleviating symptoms proved to be true. Ron swam most days and played hockey twice a week. The neurology department at the university hospital found it remarkable that he could maintain his balance while playing hockey. It was challenging at times, but Ron did score the odd goal and no longer "froze up." Not everything came up roses, though… (continued on page 162).

The Healthy Brain Diet Program is designed to provide an optimal physical and mental environment for your brain and nervous system to function at their best. On the one hand, this program is designed to help slow down the brain's aging process by reducing — or, in some cases, preventing — the common causes of aging in the brain. On the other hand, it is meant to support the cognitive functions of the brain by incorporating nutrients that boost the brain's abilities, such as omega-3 fatty acids, and addressing lifestyle factors that determine good health. In many cases, the preventive and enhancing factors are one and the same.

# No Cure

We are not advocating or claiming that any one of these recommendations is a single, stand-alone cure for dementia. In some cases, the recommendations may improve dementia, depending on the severity, but even so, it takes a range of supportive lifestyle and nutritional factors to make a difference there. Any change to diet and lifestyle can have unpredictable effects.

# Holistic Approach

For example, exercise is a powerful tonic to the brain, helping it to sprout new connections, but this benefit is limited if the arteries that carry blood and oxygen to the brain are compromised. So although we are presenting this plan in actionable steps, the way to experience the most success is to take an holistic approach to health, including brain health. From the perspective of nutritional support, we are providing the substances needed for the best structure and function of the brain. We are also trying to provide a diet that minimizes the risks for premature brain wear and tear, based on what we know about the relationship at this time. From a lifestyle perspective, understanding how certain choices can negatively impact the brain helps to make sense of the necessity of certain good habits and practices.

## Characteristics of the Healthy Brain Diet

- High-energy
- Low-glycemic
- Low-fat
- Anti-inflammatory
- Antioxidant
- Omega-3-rich
- Detoxifying
- Neuroplastic

# Rules of Thumb

The first rule of thumb with this plan is that steady progress is better than overdoing change and then not being able to sustain that change. So if you find that aspects of the diet plan are too difficult to carry out for a few days (you are traveling, your work has become extra busy for a few days, you are ill and cannot cook), don't give up! Continue to apply the principles we are talking about. Aging and damage to the brain are accumulations of little events, gradual influences that span decades. Likewise, small adjustments and daily decisions over time can improve your health. You do not have to be perfect — just persevering.

# Conscious Eating

Conscious, or mindful, eating is the second rule of thumb. As we become more conscious of what we eat, we start making better choices and become healthier in body and brain. It is easier to think of a positive than a negative. It's easier to eat a delicious corn and quinoa pasta within a savory recipe than it is to dwell on the fact that you are not choosing the typical wheat-based spaghetti that you've eaten since childhood.. And there is nothing wrong with the more traditional foods. In our menu plan, there is still spaghetti and there is still cake. But we are encouraging you to use the many opportunities throughout the day to eat something that will improve your cognitive function or simply put you in a healthier state. Look at good food as health maintenance and brain therapy.

# Program Steps

## Lay a Good Nutritional Foundation

Step 1

One sure way to keep dementia at bay is to cultivate general good health, eating the right foods in the right amounts. Start the program by following the guidelines for general good health established by the U.S. Department of Agriculture (USDA) and Health Canada.

### Food Guides

Perhaps the two best guides to eating well for optimal health are the United States Department of Agriculture Choose MyPlate diet program (ChooseMyPlate.gov) and Health Canada's Eating Well with Canada's Food Guide (www.hc-sc.gc.ca). Both programs break the three macronutrients — carbohydrate, protein, and fat — into four food groups and seek to strike a balance in their consumption.

### Balanced Food Groups

The food guides recommend eating a balanced or proportioned diet of macronutrients, deriving 45% to 65% of your total calories for the day from carbohydrates, 10% to 30% from proteins, and 20% to 35% from fats.

**Carbohydrates:** 45% to 65% of your total daily calories
**Proteins:** 10% to 30% of your total daily calories
**Fats:** 20% to 35% of your total daily calories

## Macronutrients

- Carbohydrates
- Proteins
- Fats

## Food Groups

- Fruit and vegetables
- Grains and legumes
- Meat and alternatives
- Dairy and alternatives

**Q**
**A**

**What does it mean to "burn calories"?**

Calories are a unit of measure for counting the energy required to maintain basal metabolic rate (breathing, sleeping, and digesting) and to enable physical activity (walking, talking, and writing). Calories are expended, or "burned," during these unconscious and conscious metabolic activities, including brain activity. Food analysis calculators have been developed to determine the calorie content of most food items. These are available in print from a dietitian and on the Internet.

# Energy Rules

### Healthy Energy Rule

When the amount of energy from the food we eat is balanced exactly with the amount of energy the body needs to stay alive and carry out activity, our body will maintain the same amount of stored body fat.

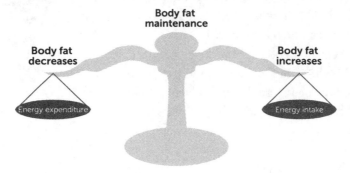

### Positive Energy Rule

When the amount of energy from the food we eat is more than the amount of energy the body needs to stay alive and carry out activity, our body will store the extra energy as fat.

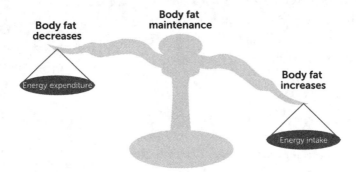

### Negative Energy Rule

When the amount of energy our body needs to stay alive and carry out activity is more than the amount of energy we get from the food we eat, our body simply uses up stored fat as its energy source.

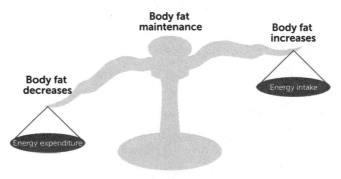

## Energy Balance and Weight Maintenance

If you consume more calories than your body "burns" from basal metabolism and physical activity, you will likely gain weight because the excess calories are stored in the body as fat. This is a state of energy excess. If you burn more calories than you consume, an energy deficit can occur and you will likely lose weight as your body burns those calories stored in body fat. Once you achieve your desired weight, you can maintain that weight by balancing the calories you consume with the calories you burn.

## Energy Reserves

At one time, fats were considered a form of energy. They can be burned as fuel and stored in a stable way. Anyone who has tried to lose weight can attest that the storage form of fatty acids can be very stable. Fats are deposited into a triple fatty acid form called a triglyceride (tri meaning "three," and glyceride meaning stuck to a molecule of glycerol — which acts as a kind of "coat hanger" to put the fatty acids on).

We now know that fats are not simply fuel for the fire. They are involved in many metabolic processes in the body. No less important is the fact that our cells are coated in them. All human cells have a membrane, and although complex, the basic ingredient is made of fatty acids.

## Good Fats, Bad Fats

Several kinds of fat have been isolated. Some are considered to be healthy — in fact, they are essential to our well-being. Others threaten our health.

---

## Kinds of Fats

1. Saturated fats
2. Unsaturated fats
   *Monounsaturated fats*
   *Polyunsaturated fats*
3. Trans fats
4. Omega-3 fatty acids
   *Alpha-linolenic acid (ALA)*
   *Docosahexaenoic acid (DHA)*
   *Eicosapentaenoic acid (EPA)*
5. Omega-6 fatty acids

Adapted from Kim Arrey, *The Complete Arthritis Health, Diet Guide and Cookbook.* Toronto, ON: Robert Rose Inc., 2012

---

**DID YOU KNOW?**

### Calorie Measurements

There are two ways to measure calories:

**1. Small calorie (symbol: cal):** 1 cal is the amount of energy required to raise 1 gram of water by 1 degree Celsius.

**2. Large calorie (symbol: Cal, kcal):** 1 Cal is the amount of energy required to raise 1 kilogram of water by 1 degree Celsius.

---

**DID YOU KNOW?**

### Neuron Cell Membranes

The neurotransmitter, or electrical signal, that makes up a nerve impulse is carried along the membrane of the cell. Think of the brain as an electrical system and a chemical system. Sometimes impulses are sent as an electrical signal along cell membranes. To jump from neuron to neuron, however, the signal requires a chemical messenger across a super-small space.

**Q**
**A**

**Which fats are good to eat and which ones should be avoided?**

Trans fats should be avoided and saturated fats should be limited. Fats affect the cholesterol levels in the body. The saturated and trans fats raise LDL ("bad") cholesterol levels in your blood. Monounsaturated fats may decrease the total cholesterol as well as the LDL ("bad") cholesterol. Polyunsaturated fats can not only decrease the total and LDL ("bad") cholesterol, but certain types of polyunsaturated fats may protect against heart disease and sudden death, and they have beneficial effects on the nervous system. Eating the foods high in beneficial omega-3 fats may help to raise HDL ("good") cholesterol — which is usually beneficial.

## Energy as Therapy

Food guides specify the number and size of servings needed to receive adequate calories, which vary according to a person's gender, age, and activity level. For example, on average, a moderately active 50- to 70-year-old adult should take in about 2000 calories per day. But this can be increased with a larger body mass, and with more physical activity. For individuals with aging-related brain diseases, their specific issue may decrease caloric needs (if they are sedentary because of advanced dementia). On the other hand, some people may need to avoid caloric restrictions, as they become sensitive to fluctuations in blood sugar or if they need to maintain muscle mass due to aging and the effects of a neurological disorder such as Parkinson's disease or motor neuron disease. In this case, restricting calories may simply mean that dietary protein gets consumed as energy instead of being used to fabricate tissues of the body or, even worse, some of the amino acids from the body's own muscle tissue are broken down to be used as energy in a person who lacks dietary caloric intake.

## How to Eat for Energy

The USDA not only offers practical guidelines on what to eat but also provides tips on how to eat, which are outlined here:

1. Determine your ideal daily calorie intake. Use a calorie calculator on the Internet or consult with a dietitian.
2. Balance your calorie sources. Derive your sources of energy proportionately from carbohydrates, proteins, and fats.
3. Eat more fresh vegetables and fruits. Fill half your plate with fruits and vegetables.

4. Use whole grains. Limit processed carbohydrates.
5. Reduce the amount of meat containing saturated and trans fats. Try substituting with beans and legumes as sources of good protein.
6. Switch to fat-free or low-fat milk. Look for other ways to reduce fat in your diet.
7. Cut back on foods that are high in solid fats, added sugars, and salt.
8. Select low-sodium or no-salt-added products. Sodium is not healthy for the heart or arteries.
9. Drink water instead of sugary drinks, juice drinks, and sodas. Excessive blood sugar is not diabetes-friendly.
10. Enjoy your food but eat less. Reduce oversized portions to prevent unnecessary weight gain.
11. Eat therapeutically. Select the foods that can support general good health, but also foods that can help you heal.

Adapted from the USDA MyPlate food guide

# Restore the Determinants of Good Health

Step 2

Good nutrition is the cornerstone of the determinants of general good health. Sleeping well, drinking adequate amounts of water, exposing yourself to sunlight, exercising regularly, lowering stress, and maintaining social interactions — these are the determinants of good health that apply to dementia. Neurodegenerative diseases typically disturb the determinants of good health. Addressing these factors will help prevent the onset of brain disease, promote mental wellness, and help improve the quality of life in full-blown cases of dementia.

## Determinants of Good Health

- Exposure to nature
- Fresh air
- Love
- Movement (exercise)
- Posture
- Recreation

- Sleep
- Sunlight
- Water (hydration)
- Wholesome food
- Stress solutions

## Sleep Health

Although not directly influenced by diet, sleep allows the growth hormone level to rise and helps heal the nervous system. Sleep also reduces stress and the hormone cortisol, which can have a deteriorating influence on the brain. Without sleep, our muscles do not heal and our brains do not learn. Any program for boosting brain power or keeping the nervous system in working order must include healthy sleep.

## Cognitive Function

Lack of sleep has been linked to decreased cognitive function in the elderly, so one sure way to support brain health and the memory system is to sleep. If you are serious about keeping your brain and nervous system in tip-top shape, you must address your sleep habits.

## Growth

During deep sleep (meaning stages 3, 4, and REM sleep), energy is restored and growth hormone is released. Growth hormone is essential for growth and development, including muscle development.

## Stress

Stress can disturb sleep. Emotions of anger, worry, and excitement make it difficult to fall asleep and stay asleep. The person who said, "I worked all night and didn't make a buck," after worrying about her job had it right. This type of sleep disturbance robs us of our strength and decreases our learning skills and adaptability. Sleep apnea, sinusitis, cough, restless legs syndrome, pain, and muscle tension can all impede sleep.

## Sleep Solutions

Sleep habits can be improved by trying these healthy sleep strategies:

### 1. Improve Your Sleep Environment

Review your sleep environment, including noise levels, light, temperature, and bedding. Try to avoid light pollution and don't let stuffy, overheated rooms sabotage your sleep. Choose bedding that is not too soft, too hard, or too small. Keep the space dark and quiet. A relaxing bedtime routine — a bath, light conversation, soothing music — can pave the way for sound sleep.

### 2. Do Not Eat Late

Having a late-night dessert at a wedding reception or ordering a midnight pizza on special occasions can be fun, but habitual

**Q** **Is it true or just a legend that caffeine disturbs sleep?**

**A** Yes, caffeine can make sleep elusive, but caffeine is also an active component of certain antioxidants. Caffeine activates the adenosine system, which is a chemical system in the body that fights fatigue. The aftermath of a caffeine "buzz" is a secondary and reactive sense of being tired. When this occurs at 2 a.m., it is a bit too late to have a sound night's sleep. Most people who have overindulged in caffeinated beverages will know that this leads to waking up groggy. However, caffeine is often a component of powerful antioxidants like chocolate, cocoa, and other compounds that support vascular health and act as brain-friendly foods. Cocoa, for example, contains caffeine, theophylline, and theobromine (these compounds activate the nervous system), as well as a compound called phenethylamine (a natural amphetamine). What do we advise? Eat and drink caffeine foods well before bedtime so that the adenosine system is not triggered while you are sleeping.

late-evening eating is not a good idea. Not only does it provoke insulin release in the body and feed us calories we often don't need, but the late-night lump of food in our GI track diverts blood flow and can cause simple indigestion or acid reflux symptoms that can impede sleep, especially as we age.

## 3. Change Your Attitude

In our busy world, we tend to neglect sleep and to disparage it. We have no time for sleep; sleep is a lazy behavior. Instead, respect sleep and take time to sleep until you feel refreshed. A lack of sleep is a perfect example of diminishing returns. It gradually decreases our learning skills and memory. It accelerates aging and may increase the risk for certain cancers. Without a doubt, lack of sleep lowers our emotional health. We do our best work when we are cheerful and feel that we have a reserve of emotional energy at our disposal. Why would we think we can get away with feeling drained and groggy and still be productive?

## 4. Close Down Social Media

Staying up late, sleeping at irregular hours, watching television (especially emotionally disturbing shows), playing video games, and surfing the Internet can all throw us off our sleep schedule. Although brain activity can be a good thing for dementia, brain activity before bedtime causes a level of arousal that postpones sleep. Visiting your favorite Internet sites, checking your social networks, writing replies to emails — these activities can divert you from settling into the presleep mode.

## 5. Set a Schedule

It's important to set regular times for going to bed and waking up. Not only babies and toddlers need to follow a sleep schedule. Most of us need at least 8 hours, but there are individual differences. At all costs, we must go into REM and stage 3 and 4 sleep if we are to be healthy and mentally fit.

## 6. Turn Off Your Brain

Do not perform any serious or lively mental activity at bedtime. If you must do nighttime work, try not to make a nightly habit of it.

# Adequate Hydration

Sleep is not the only determinant of health that has a positive impact on dementia. Being dehydrated can impair performance in tasks that require attention, psychomotor skills, and immediate memory skills. Many aspects of brain function are improved with optimal hydration.

Water is the medium of life. We can survive for days or even, in some cases, weeks without food — but without water, we perish. Water acts as a medium for chemical reactions, and it enables the cohesion of our cells. We need water to excrete toxic substances, including the byproducts of our metabolism. We need water to digest food and carry nutrients throughout the body.

## Diuretics

Some people take diuretics to control their blood pressure, but they should watch carefully to ensure that they are not dehydrated. These diuretics take sodium, which is a substance that can exacerbate high blood pressure, out of their system. Sodium that occurs naturally in food or is added to food is another problem, because the body must spend water to get rid of excess sodium. Many processed foods are loaded with sodium. According to the Centers for Disease Control, our bodies can function on 500 mg of sodium per day, but the average sodium intake of Americans age 2 and up is 3436 mg of sodium — far in excess of the needed or tolerable upper intake.

## Central Nervous System Disturbance

Dehydration occurs when water output exceeds water intake. The body wants to keep the blood levels of sodium, potassium, and other electrolytes balanced, so it will draw water from cells to perform this function. This can happen automatically, via osmosis. The cells begin to shrink. Eventually, if this process becomes chronic or more severe, dehydration begins to have an impact on brain cells. Waste products can accumulate in the spaces between cells and cause disturbance or damage to the central nervous system.

As a person dehydrates, the body tries to compensate for a lack of water. For instance, if not enough water is consumed in a day, urine becomes more concentrated. The body is conserving water. If this state continues, a disturbance of function occurs. The body may try to rectify the situation with some kind of "push back" — for example, in the form of a fever, illness, or pronounced symptoms of fatigue.

If the disturbance continues, new imbalances appear. Eventually these become a chronic problem and can lead to serious wear and tear on some parts of the body, including the brain.

## Water Intoxication

Water can also be intoxicating to the body and brain if the water between the cells becomes too diluted. This can be caused by overdrinking water, which is something that people with more advanced dementia might do. This dilutes the ions in the bloodstream and creates an environment that the brain does not like. Water enters cells too quickly — and cells swell. Muscle contractions, convulsions, confusion, and coma can occur. These individuals need emergency care with sodium-containing fluids.

## Water Contamination

Even when we drink the right amount of water, we may cause harm to ourselves by drinking water from a source that is contaminated by bacteria or heavy metals, which can influence brain health.

**DID YOU KNOW?**

**Thirst Mechanism**

Some patients with dementia, including Alzheimer's disease, do not drink enough. This can be part of a general decline in self-care or it can be due to a difficulty in remembering to do this specific task. The thirst mechanism in the elderly is also somewhat unreliable. In perfect health, we thirst for just enough water to replace what we have lost. In the elderly, thirst is more easily satisfied and this demographic may not completely fill up.

# Healthy Water Sources

**Tap water:** In North America, tap water is generally free enough from bacteria and other microbial contaminants to be safe to drink.

**Well water:** There is no guarantee that well water is safe.

**Groundwater:** Agricultural and mining practices can contaminate groundwater, making it unsafe. Regular testing is advised.

**Springwater:** Springwater, which can be purchased in large containers with dispensing setups for the home, is usually pure but might have been sourced near contaminants and may contain bacteria. Most commercial providers will screen for this, however. The plastic that contains the water is another concern, and the leaching of the plastic's phthalates can exert estrogen effects on the body and may be linked to an increased risk of breast cancer and other problems.

## DID YOU KNOW?

### Distilled Water

Distilled water is missing electrolytes (small amounts of sodium, potassium, and magnesium) and should not be consumed. Drinking distilled water every day is like diluting your body's fluids. Some people choose to drink it because it is more likely to be free of impurities and heavy metals, but other sources of clean water are preferable (such as properly tested springwater).

## How to Stay Hydrated

1. Avoid diuretics, including excessive amounts of caffeine.
2. Don't overeat protein, because it creates the need to excrete urea, the breakdown product of ammonia, which is the byproduct of proteins. These nutrients are valuable, but many people consume too many (eating a 12-oz/375 g cut of meat when a 4-oz/125 g cut would be more than sufficient).
3. Aim for water balance. Drink the RDA for fluids: at least 10 cups (2.5 L) daily of springwater or better-quality tap water. Closer to 12 cups (3 L) daily is best — more if you are active.
4. Drink beyond thirst to create a reserve of water if needed.
5. Drink evenly. Do not cram drinking into a short timeframe.

## Exposure to Nature

There seem to be cognitive benefits in communing with nature. Natural environments have a distinct look, feel, and aroma that activate good feelings and seem to stimulate the brain in a powerful way. Exercising in natural settings has been found to create positive feelings.

Take time to explore nature several times a week. Note that this may include gardening in a lush backyard or walking along a heavily tree-lined street that is not too laden with traffic. Some is better than none, and the exposure to nature helps meet this requirement. Sitting at home, in front of the television, does not, and if we really want to keep our brains young, we must act young in the best sense — play outdoors!

## Circadian Rhythms

This may be a surprising recommendation. For years, we have been encouraged to reduce our exposure to the sun to prevent skin diseases and possibly cancer, but we do need a small amount of sunlight for the production of vitamin D in our body and for nervous system health.

When we are in the sun, our retina (the receptor-rich area at the back of our eyes) is stimulated. This sends a message down a very crucial pathway in the brain that connects with the pineal gland. This gland will produce melatonin, which helps set our daily 24-hour life rhythm, also known as the circadian rhythm.

## Exercise

Exercise makes us feel good. Take a fast walk or go for a run and you have s a feeling of well-being. Many people have heard of endorphins, which are released in the brain and cause this feeling of well-being, called the runner's high. We now know that the positive effect of exercise on the brain goes way beyond this. In numerous studies, exercise has been shown to increase brain growth and increase learning and memory. If you are aiming to keep your brain young, there is every reason to exercise within the safe limits of your current health.

### Brain-Derived Neurotrophic Factor

Exercise potentiates insulin-like growth factors 1 (IGF-1), vascular endothelial growth factor (VEGF), and fibroblast growth factor (FGF-2). Together they affect brain-derived neurotrophic factor (BDNF), which is responsible for causing growth and the regeneration of neurons within the brain. Some of this growth is in the hippocampus itself. This structure is "memory central," because it writes the experiences and lessons of the day into the long-term circuits of the brain.

### Rewiring

Evidence suggests that movement with intention enables the brain to rewire itself to be more powerful and that growth occurs after movement. A senior doing tai chi in the park would get the same type of positive results as the 30-year-old doing a spin class at the health club.

## Stress Solutions

People with dementia often experience worse symptoms — such as impaired memory — when they are frustrated or anxious. Exercise is one means of reducing stress, as is relaxation.

**Q** **A** **What is the best exercise for managing dementia?**

There is a great variety of sports and fitness machines that you can try, but some of the old exercises are equally effective.

- Walking
- Dancing
- Yoga
- Pilates
- Tai chi
- Jogging
- Qigong
- Gardening
- Cycling

Alternating exercise routines with relaxation strategies will help people with dementia better manage their behavior.

## Relaxation Therapies

*Music therapy*: involves listening to soothing music

*Pet therapy*: involves use of animals, such as visits from dogs, to promote improved moods and behaviors

*Aromatherapy*: involves the use of essential plant oils

*Massage therapy*: involves touch techniques

## Meditation and Mindfulness

Meditation centers the mind on something positive and often something universal. Mindfulness is a meditative practice that has a more specific function, which is to develop self-awareness and objectivity about what our subjective experiences are. Many people enroll in mindfulness training; it reduces their stress and they feel better.

**Q** **A** **Does meditation work?**

Contemporary research in this area confirms that meditative practices, including mindfulness, can improve thinking ability. There is some evidence that these practices can even slow down aging in the brain by altering the fundamental mechanisms of aging. Meditation may be linked to a religious practice for some; for others, it is a self-directed practice that is non-religious and non-denominational in nature.

If you can encourage your brain into a meditative state for a set period every day, you will slow down the aging of the brain and help harness its power. You do not need fancy equipment or an electrocardiograph (EKG) from your physician to do this. It is a self-directed activity and the effects are turning out to be profound.

## Social Interaction

"All you need is love," sang the Beatles. Well, we need a bit more than love, but we certainly do not thrive without it. In fact, seniors who are socially isolated or who have lost a spouse are at greater risk for cognitive decline. The fact that children may live far away or that a spouse has passed away does not make this inevitable, but it does necessitate finding other social connections and support that will continue to be nurturing. Social engagements with neighbors, new friends, old friends, and relatives, as well as a membership in a place of worship or health club, are all ways to make these connections.

In addition to nurturing our brains, we also learn strategies and resources for dealing with health issues and life issues. Social support also lowers our stress levels. "A problem shared is a problem halved" is one old adage, but there seems to be a great benefit from getting things off your chest. Just the fact that someone else listens and cares will cause biochemical changes that reduce your anxiety and help activate your adaptive mechanisms, such as problem solving, creative thinking, and self-efficacy — our sense of being able to meet challenges.

### DID YOU KNOW?

**Maintaining Relationships**

When we maintain or create relationships, our brains respond by keeping vital connections internally alive. When we are socially isolated, the shrinkage that is part of the normal aging process is likely to accelerate.

## How to Address the Determinants of Health

In addressing these determinants of good health, you start to change your lifestyle and lay the foundation for various therapies. In themselves, these activities help the brain sprout new connections. We can replace brain cells now, and we can rebuild the internal wiring of the brain. The energizing power of these activities helps harness this power. In the next section, we will explore the sources of energy needed to prevent and treat neurodegenerative diseases.

- Make an inventory of your determinants of health and your lifestyle.
- Identify what needs to be addressed and improved.
- Make a plan to change behaviors, and start with the "doable" ones.
- Reward steps and gain confidence as you continue to successfully make changes.

# Energize the Brain

The brain is the hungriest kind of tissue in the body. Eat an energy-rich, low-glycemic-index diet that fuels the brain steadily without spikes in blood sugar levels. Spiking blood sugar damages neurons moment by moment.

## Blood Sugar Regulation

Steady is the word. The brain cannot store energy for long, and if the supply is interrupted for even a few minutes, the brain can be damaged. Just as a car would count on some kind of steady and reliable fuel injection, the brain is counting on a fairly consistent range of blood sugar levels. They may rise after a meal and drop several hours later, before the next meal, but if they stay within a certain range, the brain is not affected adversely.

But this is not the case for many people. Some people's blood sugar levels tend to swing wildly; at some times of the day, they can be very high, and then at other times, they are close to normal or even low. Diabetes mellitus can cause this, but this condition tends to swing from near normal to high blood sugar in patients with the non-insulin-dependent type of diabetes. Many more individuals have swings of blood sugar because their mechanism for regulating it has been overly stressed. These swings in blood sugar level can be reduced by avoiding high-glycemic carbohydrates and by eating a rotation diet of low-glycemic foods.

## Low-Glycemic Diet

To spare the brain glucose fluctuations, consider limiting or even avoiding grains altogether — or, at the least, all processed grains that contain gluten. If the grain has been processed, there is little food value left. The germ (the most nutritious part) has been taken out, along with its natural fiber, and the endosperm is milled into white flour, alkalinized, baked, and often stored for long periods. Keep a food diary to see how often you eat grain products in a day — many people find that they eat wheat products seven to 10 times a day!

Avoiding grains is not a hard-and-fast rule for everyone. Some individuals will find that they can tolerate more grain intake without any ill effects. If an individual has been riding the blood sugar roller coaster for a long time, or the individual knows from experience that grains either charge them up or put them to sleep, then they should eat accordingly.

## DID YOU KNOW?

### Rotation Diet

Many people find that they can avoid the worst swings in their blood sugar levels if they rotate the food they eat, especially grains. For instance, if they avoid eating grains on Tuesday, consuming proteins, vegetables, and fruits instead, then on Wednesday, they can have some whole wheat pasta. This allows them to avoid an insulin surge and a blood sugar crash. However, unless they continue to rotate foods steadily, their blood sugar levels will not stabilize in the long term.

## Conquer Cravings

Eating grains makes you hungrier for grains. It is almost as if the brain becomes addicted. When you gorge on grains, the neurotransmitter dopamine is released, switching on a pleasurable feeling and providing a sense of reward. If you receive a compliment at work, a dopamine surge tells you all is well with the world. Sink your teeth into that chocolate cake — it happens again. Just thinking about a reward can start to arouse this system. One good dopamine surge deserves another. Grains are very effective at creating this surge. An ice cream sundae is not just a feast for the taste buds — it is a feast for the brain. When the reward chemicals wear off, we feel "blah" — we have a hole that needs to be filled. The answer is simple: eat some more! Although reducing grain intake sounds easy in theory, it is challenging. One effective solution is to eat low-glycemic-index carbohydrates.

**Q**
**A**
### What are good sources of energy?

Besides the adequacy and consistency of the glucose source is the question of what foods are effective and safe for energizing the brain. Certain fats and proteins are good long-term sources of energy, but a variety of low-glycemic-index carbohydrates, mostly in their natural form, feed the brain most effectively. Carbohydrates are an important form of energy, but we have to consider their source and their form.

## Low-Glycemic-Index and Low-Glycemic-Load Foods

To maintain a steady supply of glucose, without spiking blood sugar levels, eat low-glycemic-index or low-glycemic-load foods. The lower a food's glycemic index or glycemic load, the less it affects blood sugar and insulin levels.

Following is a list of the glycemic index and glycemic load for more than 100 common foods, available at the Harvard Health website. You will also find most of these foods and ingredients in the menu plan and recipe section later in this book. The complete list of the glycemic index and glycemic load for more than 1000 foods can be found as an appendix to the article "International Tables of Glycemic Index and Glycemic Load Values: 2008" by Fiona S. Atkinson, Kaye Foster-Powell, and Jennie C. Brand-Miller in the December 2008 issue of *Diabetes Care*, 31(12), pages 2281–83.

| Food | Glycemic index (glucose = 100) | Serving size | Glycemic load per serving |
|---|---|---|---|
| **BAKERY PRODUCTS AND BREADS** | | | |
| Banana cake, made with sugar | 47 | 2 oz (60 g) | 14 |
| Banana cake, made without sugar | 55 | 2 oz (60 g) | 12 |
| Sponge cake, plain | 46 | 2 oz (60 g) | 17 |
| Vanilla cake made from packet mix with vanilla frosting (Betty Crocker) | 42 | 3½ oz (111 g) | 24 |
| Apple cake, made with sugar | 44 | 2 oz (60 g) | 13 |
| Apple cake, made without sugar | 48 | 2 oz (60 g) | 9 |
| Waffles, Aunt Jemima (Quaker Oats) | 76 | 1¼ oz (35 g) | 10 |
| Bagel, white, frozen | 72 | 2¼ oz (70 g) | 25 |
| Baguette, white, plain | 95 | 1 oz (30 g) | 15 |
| Coarse barley bread, 75–80% kernels, average | 34 | 1 oz (30 g) | 7 |
| Hamburger bun | 61 | 1 oz (30 g) | 9 |
| Kaiser roll | 73 | 1 oz (30 g) | 12 |
| Pumpernickel bread | 56 | 1 oz (30 g) | 7 |
| 50% cracked wheat bread | 58 | 1 oz (30 g) | 12 |
| White wheat flour bread | 71 | 1 oz (30 g) | 10 |
| Wonder bread, average | 73 | 1 oz (30 g) | 10 |
| Whole wheat bread, average | 71 | 1 oz (30 g) | 9 |
| 100% Whole Grain bread (Natural Ovens) | 51 | 1 oz (30 g) | 7 |
| Pita bread, white | 68 | 1 oz (30 g) | 10 |
| Corn tortilla | 52 | 1¾ oz (50 g) | 12 |
| Wheat tortilla | 30 | 1¾ oz (50 g) | 8 |
| **BEVERAGES** | | | |
| Coca-Cola, average | 63 | 1 cup (250 mL) | 16 |
| Fanta, orange soft drink | 68 | 1 cup (250 mL) | 23 |
| Lucozade, original (sparkling glucose drink) | 95±10 | 1 cup (250 mL) | 40 |

| Food | Glycemic index (glucose = 100) | Serving size | Glycemic load per serving |
|---|---|---|---|
| Apple juice, unsweetened, average | 44 | 1 cup (250 mL) | 30 |
| Cranberry juice cocktail (Ocean Spray) | 68 | 1 cup (250 mL) | 24 |
| Gatorade | 78 | 1 cup (250 mL) | 12 |
| Orange juice, unsweetened | 50 | 1 cup (250 mL) | 12 |
| Tomato juice, canned | 38 | 1 cup (250 mL) | 4 |
| **BREAKFAST CEREALS AND RELATED PRODUCTS** | | | |
| All-Bran, average | 55 | 1 oz (30 g) | 12 |
| Coco Pops, average | 77 | 1 oz (30 g) | 20 |
| Cornflakes, average | 93 | 1 oz (30 g) | 23 |
| Cream of Wheat (Nabisco) | 66 | 8 oz (250 g) | 17 |
| Cream of Wheat, Instant (Nabisco) | 74 | 8 oz (250 g) | 22 |
| Grapenuts, average | 75 | 1 oz (30 g) | 16 |
| Muesli, average | 66 | 1 oz (30 g) | 16 |
| Oatmeal, average | 55 | 8 oz (250 g) | 13 |
| Instant oatmeal, average | 83 | 8 oz (250 g) | 30 |
| Puffed wheat, average | 80 | 1 oz (30 g) | 17 |
| Raisin Bran (Kellogg's) | 61 | 1 oz (30 g) | 12 |
| Special K (Kellogg's) | 69 | 1 oz (30 g) | 14 |
| **GRAINS (COOKED)** | | | |
| Pearled barley, average | 28 | 5 oz (150 g) | 12 |
| Sweet corn on the cob, average | 60 | 5 oz (150 g) | 20 |
| Couscous, average | 65 | 5 oz (150 g) | 9 |
| Quinoa | 53 | 5 oz (150 g) | 13 |
| White rice, average | 89 | 5 oz (150 g) | 43 |
| Quick-cooking white basmati rice | 67 | 5 oz (150 g) | 28 |
| Brown rice, average | 50 | 5 oz (150 g) | 16 |
| Converted, white rice (Uncle Ben's) | 38 | 5 oz (150 g) | 14 |
| Whole wheat kernels, average | 30 | 1¾ oz (50 g) | 11 |
| Bulgur, average | 48 | 5 oz (150 g) | 12 |

| Food | Glycemic index (glucose = 100) | Serving size | Glycemic load per serving |
|------|------|------|------|
| **COOKIES AND CRACKERS** | | | |
| Graham crackers | 74 | 1 oz (25 g) | 14 |
| Vanilla wafers | 77 | 1 oz (25 g) | 14 |
| Shortbread | 64 | 1 oz (25 g) | 10 |
| Rice cakes, average | 82 | 1 oz (25 g) | 17 |
| Rye crisps, average | 64 | 1 oz (25 g) | 11 |
| Soda crackers | 74 | 1 oz (25 g) | 12 |
| **DAIRY PRODUCTS AND ALTERNATIVES** | | | |
| Ice cream, regular | 57 | 1¾ oz (50 g) | 6 |
| Ice cream, premium | 38 | 1¾ oz (50 g) | 3 |
| Milk, full fat | 41 | 1 cup (250 mL) | 5 |
| Milk, skim | 32 | 1 cup (250 mL) | 4 |
| Reduced-fat yogurt with fruit, average | 33 | 7 oz (200 g) | 11 |
| **FRUITS** | | | |
| Apple, average | 39 | 4 oz (120 g) | 6 |
| Banana, ripe | 62 | 4 oz (120 g) | 16 |
| Dates, dried | 42 | 2 oz (60 g) | 18 |
| Grapefruit | 25 | 4 oz (120 g) | 3 |
| Grapes, average | 59 | 4 oz (120 g) | 11 |
| Orange, average | 40 | 4 oz (120 g) | 4 |
| Peach, average | 42 | 4 oz (120 g) | 5 |
| Peach, canned in light syrup | 52 | 4 oz (120 g) | 9 |
| Pear, average | 38 | 4 oz (120 g) | 4 |
| Pear, canned in pear juice | 43 | 4 oz (120 g) | 5 |
| Prunes, pitted | 29 | 2 oz (60 g) | 10 |
| Raisins | 64 | 2 oz (60 g) | 28 |
| Watermelon | 72 | 4 oz (120 g) | 4 |

| Food | Glycemic index (glucose = 100) | Serving size | Glycemic load per serving |
|---|---|---|---|
| **BEANS AND NUTS** | | | |
| Baked beans, average | 40 | 5 oz (150 g) | 6 |
| Blackeye peas, average | 33 | 5 oz (150 g) | 10 |
| Black beans | 30 | 5 oz (150 g) | 7 |
| Chickpeas, average | 10 | 5 oz (150 g) | 3 |
| Chickpeas, canned in brine | 38 | 5 oz (150 g) | 9 |
| Navy beans, average | 31 | 5 oz (150 g) | 9 |
| Kidney beans, average | 29 | 5 oz (150 g) | 7 |
| Lentils, average | 29 | 5 oz (150 g) | 5 |
| Soy beans, average | 15 | 5 oz (150 g) | 1 |
| Cashews, salted | 27 | 1¾ oz (50 g) | 3 |
| Peanuts, average | 7 | 1¾ oz (50 g) | 0 |
| **PASTA AND NOODLES (COOKED)** | | | |
| Fettucini, average | 32 | 6 oz (180 g) | 15 |
| Macaroni, average | 47 | 6 oz (180 g) | 23 |
| Macaroni and Cheese (Kraft) | 64 | 6 oz (180 g) | 32 |
| Spaghetti, white, boiled, average | 46 | 6 oz (180 g) | 22 |
| Spaghetti, white, boiled 20 min, average | 58 | 6 oz (180 g) | 26 |
| Spaghetti, whole-grain, boiled, average | 42 | 6 oz (180 g) | 17 |
| **SNACK FOODS** | | | |
| Corn chips, plain, salted, average | 42 | 1¾ oz (50 g) | 11 |
| Fruit Roll-Ups | 99 | 1 oz (30 g) | 24 |
| M & M's, peanut | 33 | 1 oz (30 g) | 6 |
| Microwave popcorn, plain, average | 55 | ¾ oz (20 g) | 6 |
| Potato chips, average | 51 | 1¾ oz (50 g) | 12 |
| Pretzels, oven-baked | 83 | 1 oz (30 g) | 16 |
| Snickers Bar | 51 | 2 oz (60 g) | 18 |

| Food | Glycemic index (glucose = 100) | Serving size | Glycemic load per serving |
|---|---|---|---|
| **VEGETABLES** | | | |
| Green peas, average | 51 | 2¾ oz (80 g) | 4 |
| Carrots, average | 35 | 2¾ oz (80 g) | 2 |
| Parsnips | 52 | 2¾ oz (80 g) | 4 |
| Baked russet potato, average | 111 | 5 oz (150 g) | 33 |
| Boiled white potato, average | 82 | 5 oz (150 g) | 21 |
| Instant mashed potato, average | 87 | 5 oz (150 g) | 17 |
| Sweet potato, average | 70 | 5 oz (150 g) | 22 |
| Yam, average | 54 | 5 oz (150 g) | 20 |
| **MISCELLANEOUS** | | | |
| Hummus (chickpea salad dip) | 6 | 1 oz (30 g) | 0 |
| Chicken nuggets, frozen, reheated in microwave oven 5 min | 46 | 3½ oz (100 g) | 7 |
| Pizza, plain baked dough, served with Parmesan cheese and tomato sauce | 80 | 3½ oz (100 g) | 22 |
| Pizza, Super Supreme (Pizza Hut) | 30 | 3½ oz (100 g) | 9 |
| Honey, average | 61 | 1 oz (25 g) | 12 |

Adapted from www.health.harvard.edu/newsweek/Glycemic_index_and_glycemic_load_for_100_foods.htm

### How to Use the Glycemic Index (GI)

For quick reference in shopping for these foods, post a list on your refrigerator door or smartphone.

1. Aim to eat five to 10 different whole fresh fruits, vegetables, and legumes each day. If you fill up on low-GI foods, you will naturally tend to eat less bread, simple sugars, and processed foods, which not only have a higher glycemic value but also contain less fiber, fewer nutrients, and (often) poorer-quality fats.

2. Avoid a diet that consists predominantly of the foods highest on the glycemic index (sugar, bread, rice, potatoes), especially at the exclusion of low-GI fresh fruits and vegetables.

3. Substitute foods high on the glycemic index with foods lower on the GI. For example, eat raw carrots (GI 35) instead of boiled potatoes (GI 82) for dinner.

4. Increase your fiber intake. Fiber helps slow the digestion of carbohydrates and improves insulin resistance. If you love a food high on the glycemic index, take care to not consume it often and aim to eat only a small portion of it combined with high-fiber foods that reduce the glycemic load.

5. Eat legumes to lower the high-GI foods in your meals. Legumes are low on the GI and contain an impressive amount of fiber and good-quality protein, which can serve to blunt the glycemic load.

6. With the glycemic index in hand, see how the ingredients in the recipes in this book are generally low on the GI and how cooking foods high on the index can reduce their GI. Evaluate the whole meal, rather than individual food items, to see if there is a glycemic problem.

Adapted from J. Stansbury, *The PCOS Health & Nutrtion Guide*. Toronto, ON: Robert Rose Inc., 2012.

## Cooking

Cooking methods will affect a food's glycemic index ranking. Cooked carrots have a much higher glycemic index than raw carrots (40 versus 20) because cooking breaks down the fiber and the glucose can be absorbed much more quickly compared to eating raw carrots with all the fiber intact. Cooking grains, beans, and vegetables for a long time will increase the glycemic index as fiber, which otherwise slows the digestion of starches and sugars, is broken down. Cooking with a bit of salt or vinegar may lower the glycemic index of many vegetables because this causes many molecules, not just the sugars, to be broken down, which results in trapping some of starches in complex structures that are digested more slowly.

## Calculation Variations

Due to the various ways that the glycemic index can be calculated, different glycemic index figures for a given food appear in the literature. Part of this also has to do with the test subjects chosen to gauge blood sugar responses, and when in the day a certain food is tested. For some people, a food consumed in the morning on an empty stomach will spike the blood sugar more than the same food eaten later in the day, after breakfast has already been digested. Those with good blood sugar control in general will show less of a spike in blood sugar than someone with poor blood sugar control.

### How to Eat Low-Glycemic-Index Foods

Changing eating habits to create a steady flow of glucose is challenging. To reverse the tide of insulin insensitivity and keep off the blood sugar roller coaster, try these dietary strategies:

1. Keep your blood sugar levels steady by eating low-glycemic-index foods.
2. Rotate your carbohydrates to maintain a steady blood sugar level from day to day.
3. Stabilize your body's energy systems as a whole, so that when you miss a meal or are under extra stress, you have the capacity to respond.
4. Get rid of the foods in your pantry that will spike your insulin levels.
5. Save a few high-sugar foods for treats or for when you are stuck with nothing else on the menu and you are ravenous (they will taste more like starch gruel in your mouth the more you become accustomed to healthier foods).
6. Stock up on good wholesome grains, like quinoa and brown rice.
7. Between meals, eat healthy snacks that don't send blood sugar through the roof: nuts, seeds, fruits, vegetables, and natural cheeses.
8. Plan your eating schedule so that you do not feel hungry.

**Step 4**

# Prevent Plaques

Keep the arteries, capillaries, and blood supply to the brain free of plaques and LDL ("bad") cholesterol by eating heart-healthy foods. Plaques can reduce oxygen supply to the brain and eventually cause ischemia and stroke.

## Heart Smart Diets

As go the arteries, so goes the brain. A heart-healthy diet aims to lower LDL ("bad") cholesterol in the blood by reducing the intake of saturated fats and increasing the intake of fiber. Eating more vegetables and fruit instead of meat and dairy foods will help lower LDL cholesterol. Lots of fiber in the diet naturally helps to lower cholesterol by absorbing some dietary cholesterol in the gut, especially if that fiber is of the soluble kind, like oat bran or the pectin naturally found in apples. There are many versions of a heart-healthy diet, but the American Heart Association endorses the popular Mediterranean diet. This diet is also healthy for the brain.

## Mediterranean Diet

In the late 20th century, epidemiologists noticed that people in the Greek Islands and other areas of the Mediterranean region had a lower incidence of cardiovascular disease. This prompted a study of their lifestyle and diet. In addition to a less frenetic pace of living, ample sunlight, and strong family ties, a specific way of eating seemed to be unify these populations. This diet included an emphasis on consuming fish, locally grown fruits and vegetables, olive oil, and red wine, with less intake of red meat, sugar, and saturated fats (certainly less than the average North American).

Recent study of this diet at the Mayo Clinic and elsewhere has borne out its value. The Mediterranean diet now signifies a way of eating that draws on this traditional diet. Since the 1990s, the emphasis has moved away from eating whole grains to vegetables, olive oil, and fish.

---

## Key Components of the Mediterranean Diet

- Plant-based foods, such as fruits and vegetables, whole grains, legumes, and nuts
- Olive oil (not butter)
- Herbs and spices (instead of salt) to flavor foods
- Red meat no more than a few times monthly
- Fish and poultry at least twice weekly
- Red wine (optional)
- The Mediterranean diet also recognizes the importance of being physically active and enjoying meals with family and friends.

---

### Whole Grains

The grains in the Mediterranean diet are whole grains, and whole-grain breads are dipped in olive oil. Use grains for energy, but do not overemphasize them in order to get the most benefit from this way of eating. Nuts and seeds contain powerful nutrients, including omega-3 fatty acids, and these can be enjoyed throughout the diet. Not only are they beneficial snacks, but lightly toasted nuts and seeds (unsalted) add lots of flavor to salads and rice dishes. Cheeses from goat's and sheep's milk, as well as cow's milk, add variety. Red wine is not required in the Mediterranean diet, but it provides powerful plant-derived antioxidants.

## DID YOU KNOW?

### Lifestyle

The other components of this diet are important, too: a relaxed atmosphere, the good company of family members or friends, and time enough to digest the food properly. The Mediterranean diet is not just a nutrient or calorie count diet; it is a way of life.

# Mediterranean Diet Pyramid

Meats & sweets

Poultry, eggs, cheese & yogurt

Fish & seafood

Fruits, vegetables, olive oil, grains (mostly whole), beans, nuts, legumes, seeds, herbs & spices

| Food Groups | Guidance |
| --- | --- |
| Meats and sweets | Less often |
| Poultry, eggs, cheese and yogurt | Moderate portions, daily to weekly |
| Fish and seafood | Often, at least two times a week |
| Fruits, vegetables, oilve oil, grains (mostly whole), beans, nuts, legumes, seeds, herbs and spices | Base every meal on these foods |

Adapted from Oldways Preservation & Exchange Trust, 2009

Step 5

# Reduce Inflammation

Control inflammation by avoiding pro-inflammatory foods and consuming anti-inflammatory foods instead. By limiting pro-inflammatory foods in your diet and substituting them for anti-inflammatory foods, the risk of atherosclerosis and brain damage can be reduced because plaque is less likely to form or rupture.

## Anti-inflammatory Diet

The foremost principle of an anti-inflammatory diet is to eat whole foods that are close to their natural state — not synthetic or processed foods. Eat corn on the cob rather than canned corn. Eat whole-grain brown rice rather than refined white rice. Processed foods (with their dozens of additives) are difficult to process by the body. The difference between a fresh fish fillet and a processed, salted fish stick battered in salty bread crumbs is plain for anyone to see, but it takes a deliberate effort to eat this way.

## Pro-Inflammatory Foods to Limit or Avoid

- Saturated fats from animal sources
- Hydrogenated fats or trans fats
- Deep-fried anything (the extreme heat of deep-frying damages fats and makes them pro-inflammatory)
- Excess omega-6 fatty acids from vegetable oils

### Anti-Inflammatory Diet Components

Omega-3 essential fatty acids and monounsaturated fats can help reduce inflammation. They are easy to use and bring great taste to your plate, not to mention a host of other nutrients. For example, nuts contain magnesium and fiber if you eat the skin. These foods also contain phytonutrients that are potent antioxidants. Try to eat these foods every day.

1. **Increase servings of vegetables and fruits:** To consume all the nutrients necessary to control inflammation, you need to eat seven to 10 portions of vegetables and fruit daily.
2. **Replace red meat with beans, legumes, and nuts:** To reduce LDL ("bad") cholesterol and inflammation, you need to increase brain-healthy phytonutrients and antioxidants.
3. **Increase omega-3 fatty acids:** To adjust the balance of omega-3 to omega-6 fatty acids, eat more flax seeds, flaxseed products, and fish.
4. **Moderate use of dairy products and eggs:** To maintain calcium levels without introducing excessive saturated fats, eat these foods in moderation.

### Cholesterol Moderation

Dairy foods and especially eggs include saturated fats that are considered to be pro-inflammatory. Some people are more susceptible to having their blood cholesterol go up when they

**DID YOU KNOW?**

**Pro-Inflammatory Foods**

Some degree of inflammation in the body is necessary to ward off infection and to remodel body tissues after injury. However, in the standard Western diet, some pro-inflammatory foods are eaten in excess. Simply avoiding a lot of processed foods will help, since vegetable oils are added to so many of these products.

**DID YOU KNOW?**

**Minimizing AGEs**

Do not cook meats at a high temperature without liquids, such as barbecuing. If you do, this will cause the formation of advanced glycation end products (AGEs), which increase inflammation. Cook meats at lower temperatures (medium-high and lower) to make stews, soups, braised dinners, or casseroles. Marinating meats in vinegar or lemon juice also reduces AGEs.

consume more cholesterol in food. Unfortunately, at this time, we have no way of determining if you are sensitive to the cholesterol that is in food, so if you have high cholesterol levels, it is best to moderate your consumption of dairy foods and eggs, consuming only 3 egg yolks weekly, for example. Discuss with your doctor or dietitian how many eggs you should eat.

Eggs are an amazing source of choline, an anti-inflammatory agent. They also contain lutein and other carotenoids, which have an antioxidant effect. They are one of the few dietary sources of vitamin D. Eggs that contain a significant amount of omega-3 fatty acids are also available.

## How to Add Healthy Fats to Your Diet

- Use olive oil and canola oil in cooking. If you want a buttery flavor, add a small amount of butter to the canola oil.
- Dip bread in olive oil instead of spreading butter on it.
- Use olive oil or other oils in salad dressings.
- Add ground flax seeds to recipes (such as cereal, muffins, and quick breads).
- Include slices of avocado in sandwiches, or use it as a spread.
- Use more spices and herbs, along with garlic and onions.

## Culinary Herbal Help

Herbs and spices can add a significant amount of powerful antioxidants and anti-inflammatory phytochemicals to our diets. Most herbs retain their phytochemicals if they are dried, so use dried herbs if you do not have access to fresh. However, you can keep a window box of fresh herbs in your home. They will add a wonderful fragrance to your kitchen. Keep dried herbs and spices away from the heat. Garlic and other members of the garlic family (onions, leeks, shallots, and green onions) can impart benefits when they are raw or cooked. Enjoy them any way you like.

**Q**
**A**

**Are sweet desserts and snacks inflammatory?**

One of the chief reasons to avoid desserts has nothing to do with their pro-inflammatory property. When we fill up on these treats, we may not have enough "room" for foods that we need to ensure good health. Desserts are also usually high in calories. Eating large amounts of high-calorie foods will ultimately result in weight gain. Gaining weight causes inflammation. Sweet desserts may be addictive. Some studies suggest that the more sweet treats and desserts you eat, the more you want to eat them. If you must consume sweets, consider following the Mediterranean diet, where desserts are reserved for special occasions.

# Protect Your Brain against Free Radicals

Damage to the brain tissues and cells by oxidative stress and free radicals can be mitigated through a diet rich in antioxidant foods, chiefly plant foods known as phytonutrients.

## ORAC Antioxidant Diet

The National Institutes of Health has developed the oxygen radical absorbance capacity (ORAC) unit of measure for the antioxidant capacity of various foods and spices. The higher the antioxidant count, the better. High-antioxidant foods greatly help to lower the risks of brain degeneration and disease.

## ORAC Value List
### Top 100 Antioxidant Foods

Have a look at the following list of foods and spices, with the information sourced from the U.S. Department of Agriculture (USDA), and consider making a conscious effort to obtain and consume more of them in your everyday diet. (The USDA led efforts to consolidate this information but no longer publishes it.) The ORAC values do not tell us exactly how a food or substance will behave in the body (versus the test tube), and the beneficial polyphenols themselves are not completely absorbed. Furthermore, the use of ORAC values on the labels of nutritional supplements can be misleading, and Health Canada, for instance, states that manufacturers should not include this data.

   We offer this table to help you gain some insight into the likelihood that a food contains many free radical–quenching molecules, but with the knowledge that this list does not necessarily represent a true ranking of these foods. We do, however, know that foods rich in polyphenols can provide strong health benefits. As we gain a better understanding of how these foods are absorbed and metabolized by the body, and what their ultimate function is, we'll know better which foods are best suited to protect our brains, and our bodies.

*Note:* ORAC values of a certain food can differ due to growing conditions, processing conditions, and variety. ORAC values are listed as µmol TE/100 g (micromol trolox equivalent per 100 grams).

| | | |
|---|---|---|
| 1 | Cloves, ground | 314,446 |
| 2 | Sumac bran | 312,400 |
| 3 | Cinnamon, ground | 267,536 |
| 4 | Sorghum, bran | 240,000 |
| 5 | Oregano, dried | 200,129 |
| 6 | Turmeric, ground | 159,277 |
| 7 | Acai berry, freeze-dried | 102,700 |
| 8 | Sorghum, bran, black | 100,800 |
| 9 | Sumac, grain, raw | 86,800 |
| 10 | Cocoa powder, unsweetened | 80,933 |
| 11 | Cumin seeds | 76,800 |
| 12 | Maqui berry, powder | 75,000 |
| 13 | Parsley, dried | 74,349 |
| 14 | Sorghum, bran, red | 71,000 |
| 15 | Basil, dried | 67,553 |
| 16 | Baking chocolate, unsweetened | 49,926 |
| 17 | Curry powder | 48,504 |
| 18 | Sorghum, grain, high-tannin | 45,400 |
| 19 | Cocoa powder, Dutch process | 40,200 |
| 20 | Maqui berry, juice | 40,000 |
| 21 | Sage | 32,004 |
| 22 | Mustard seeds, yellow | 29,257 |
| 23 | Ginger, ground | 28,811 |
| 24 | Pepper, black | 27,618 |
| 25 | Thyme, fresh | 27,426 |
| 26 | Marjoram, fresh | 27,297 |
| 27 | Goji berries | 25,300 |
| 28 | Rice bran | 24,287 |
| 29 | Chili powder | 23,636 |
| 30 | Sorghum, grain, black | 21,900 |
| 31 | Chocolate, dark | 20,823 |
| 32 | Flax hull lignans | 19,600 |
| 33 | Chocolate, semisweet | 18,053 |
| 34 | Pecans | 17,940 |

| 35 | Paprika | 17,919 |
|---|---|---|
| 36 | Chokeberry, raw | 16,062 |
| 37 | Tarragon, fresh | 15,542 |
| 38 | Gingerroot, raw | 14,840 |
| 39 | Elderberries, raw | 14,697 |
| 40 | Sorghum, grain, red | 14,000 |
| 41 | Peppermint, fresh | 13,978 |
| 42 | Oregano, fresh | 13,978 |
| 43 | Walnuts | 13,541 |
| 44 | Hazelnuts | 9,645 |
| 45 | Cranberries, raw | 9,584 |
| 46 | Pears, dried | 9,496 |
| 47 | Savory, fresh | 9,465 |
| 48 | Artichokes | 9,416 |
| 49 | Kidney beans, red | 8,459 |
| 50 | Pink beans | 8,320 |
| 51 | Black beans | 8,040 |
| 52 | Pistachios | 7,983 |
| 53 | Currants | 7,960 |
| 54 | Pinto beans | 7,779 |
| 55 | Plums | 7,581 |
| 56 | Chocolate, milk chocolate | 7,528 |
| 57 | Lentils | 7,282 |
| 58 | Agave, dried | 7,274 |
| 59 | Apples, dried | 6,681 |
| 60 | Garlic powder | 6,665 |
| 61 | Blueberries, fresh | 6,552 |
| 62 | Prunes | 6,552 |
| 63 | Sorghum, bran, white | 6,400 |
| 64 | Lemon balm, leaves | 5,997 |
| 65 | Soybeans | 5,764 |
| 66 | Onion powder | 5,735 |
| 67 | Blackberries | 5,347 |
| 68 | Garlic, raw | 5,346 |

| 69 | Cilantro leaves, fresh | 5,141 |
|---|---|---|
| 70 | Wine, white | 5,034 |
| 71 | Raspberries | 4,882 |
| 72 | Basil, fresh | 4,805 |
| 73 | Almonds | 4,454 |
| 74 | Dillweed | 4,392 |
| 75 | Cowpeas | 4,343 |
| 76 | Apples, Red Delicious | 4,275 |
| 77 | Peaches, dried | 4,222 |
| 78 | Raisins, white | 4,188 |
| 79 | Apples, Granny Smith | 3,898 |
| 80 | Dates | 3,895 |
| 81 | Wine, red | 3,873 |
| 82 | Strawberries | 3,577 |
| 83 | Peanut butter, smooth | 3,432 |
| 84 | Currants, red | 3,387 |
| 85 | Figs | 3,383 |
| 86 | Cherries | 3,365 |
| 87 | Gooseberries | 3,277 |
| 88 | Apricots, dried | 3,234 |
| 89 | Peanuts, all types | 3,166 |
| 90 | Cabbage, red | 3,145 |
| 91 | Broccoli | 3,083 |
| 92 | Apples | 3,082 |
| 93 | Raisins | 3,037 |
| 94 | Pears, fresh | 2,941 |
| 95 | Agave nectar | 2,938 |
| 96 | Blueberry juice | 2,906 |
| 97 | Cardamom | 2,764 |
| 98 | Guava | 2,550 |
| 99 | Lettuce, red leaf | 2,380 |
| 100 | Concord grape juice | 2,347 |

# Phytonutrient Food Sources

The Healthy Brain Diet Program is designed to deliver phytonutrients, such as lutein from peppers or lycopene from tomatoes, steadily to the brain. Phytonutrients are required for powering up the protective mechanisms within our cells. These nutrients include vitamins C, E, and D, as well as minerals such as zinc and selenium. Phytonutrients are compounds other than macronutrients and micronutrients that have antioxidant, anti-inflammatory, antiviral, and antibacterial properties. They tend to be found in highly colored vegetables from the carotenoid family, but tea, chocolate, nuts, flax seeds, and olive oil are also good sources.

None of these molecules is a surefire cure or absolute prevention for a neurological disease, but this fact does not negate their usefulness as part of a program of total health. This is important to know because often, when any one plant extract or nutrient is studied in isolation on a large population, the results are unclear or even sometimes negative in terms of benefit (in this case, retaining memory and staving off dementia). But in real life, these plant compounds are consumed together and there are variations in the manner in which different individuals respond.

| Q A | **Should we supplement antioxidant foods with phytonutrients?** |
| --- | --- |
| | As Dr. Louise Edwards of Durango, Colorado, says, "Supplements are just that — they are meant to supplement." They are not meant to take the place of actual food. Still, we may need to supplement in cases where some biochemical pathway is under extra stress due to diet, environment, or genetic makeup. Consider someone who smokes. That person has a much higher requirement for vitamin C to "quench" free radicals. |

## Carotenoids

Here are some of the major food-derived antioxidants — or if you like, plantoxidants. Carotenoids are found in more than just carrots, and they are much more than just beta-carotene. These helpful compounds give fruits and vegetables their distinct colors. The carotenoid beta-carotene can be converted in the body to vitamin A.

**Alpha-carotene:** Found in carrots, winter squash, tomatoes, green beans, fresh cilantro, and Swiss chard. This nutrient has been found to be higher in people who live longer. This is not surprising, because it is a potent antioxidant.

**Beta-carotene:** Found in high concentration in butternut squash, carrots, orange bell peppers, pumpkins, kale, peaches, apricots, mangos, turnip greens, broccoli, spinach, and sweet potatoes. This is also a very important antioxidant. Although some research has indicated that taking pure beta-carotene that is isolated from other carotenoids might be harmful, at least in some individuals (smokers), in the diet we recommend, it is embedded in healthy plant foods.

**Lutein and zeaxanthin:** Both these carotenoids, the two main carotenoids that are able to cross the barrier into the retina, accumulate there. The retina is the delicate tissue at the back of the eye, where blood vessels, special light receptors, and nerve cells come together to form our visual sense signal. These two carotenoids are the ones that tend to accumulate in the brain as well. There is some evidence that they can improve cognitive function. Lutein is found in high concentration in spinach, kale, Swiss chard, collard greens, beet and mustard greens, endive, red bell pepper, and okra. Zeaxanthin is found in kale, collard greens, spinach, turnip greens, Swiss chard, mustard and beet greens, corn, and broccoli.

**Q**
**A**
**What is meant by the phrase "French paradox"?**

One way to stay young is to consume lots of proanthocyanidins, found in berries and grapes. These compounds absorb the stress from oxidants. Ellagic acid is a smaller, shorter version of a proanthocyanidin and it is found in high concentration in raspberries and strawberries and in red wine tannins. Along with resveratrol, these proanthocyanidins are thought to be partially responsible for the "French paradox." Although cardiovascular mortality in France is lower than in North America, the average French citizen consumes more saturated fat from cheese and red meats and consumes more alcohol than the average American. There are other reasons for this paradox. For example, the French take it easy on portion sizes and eat foods that are lower on the glycemic index. The French also tend to eat more fresh food and less processed food.

**Cinnamic acid:** Found in cinnamon, brown rice, whole wheat, and oats, as well as in coffee, apples, artichokes, peanuts, oranges, and pineapples.

**Resveratrol:** Found in the skin of grapes but also widely distributed in plant foods. This potent antioxidant is also gaining more recognition in the prevention of cancer and cardiovascular disease. This is another suspected nutrient behind the French paradox. Red wine does contain resveratrol.

**Rosmarinic acid:** Found in high concentration in rosemary, oregano, lemon balm, sage, and marjoram. Rosemary itself has the ability to somewhat slow down the first phase of detoxification (Phase 1 detoxification), which involves oxidizing toxins. This makes them more chemically reactive and more likely to be able to bind to another molecule and then be whisked out of the body in some harmless form. It can happen that the rate of toxins that enter the detoxification "factory" is so high, so fast, that the Phase II part of detoxification — the part that renders the toxins water-soluble, safe, and easy to whisk out of the body — simply cannot keep up. The beauty of substances such as rosemary (in cooked food or in detoxification supplements) is that they help balance Phase I and II detoxification.

## Synergy

When eaten in consistent, generous quantities, from a variety of foods, the aggregate action of phytonutrients is greater than a single one may accomplish working in isolation. These foods and compounds slow down and protect brain tissue against aging. The medical model that looks for a single treatment for single diseases in a hypothetical patient is very useful for discovering drugs that target specific illness patterns. But this is not the way to think about nutritional therapy. In this case, it is more about creating an optimal environment for the cells of the nervous system to regenerate.

## Cooking Up Free Radicals

Some antioxidant compounds can be damaged during cooking. The reason is simple — heat plus light plus oxygen will form free radicals. Cooking, especially boiling, can deplete antioxidant foods of more than 50% of their nutrient value. This is why we do not recommend deep-frying as a cooking method; the oils and fats in the fryer become damaged and free radicals accumulate.

Likewise, an antioxidant can absorb a free radical (a molecule with a loose, or dangerous, electron), but once spent, it needs to be regenerated (a kind of reset). Vitamin C is useful in this regard. It can be used to recharge other antioxidants in the body. But some plant molecules are useful only once, and we need to eat more of them the next day.

### Raw Foods Diet

Many vegetables need heat and some kind of preparation to be appetizing to most people — think of squash, for example. But many vegetables are just fine in their raw form. Green, red, and yellow peppers can simply be washed, seeded, sliced up, and eaten as is or with a nutritious dip. Other vegetables, such as broccoli, can be consumed in the same way. Carrot sticks are easy, and organic baby carrots that are already prewashed are ready-made snacks. In the menu and recipe parts of this book, we recommend these as snacks.

### Superoxide Dismutases and Catalase

Superoxide dismutases (SODs) are enzymes that provide antioxidant defense in nearly all cells exposed to oxygen. Catalase is another common enzyme found in nearly all living organisms exposed to oxygen, and it protects the cell from oxidative damage by reactive oxygen species (ROS), which are chemically reactive molecules containing oxygen. One catalase molecule can convert millions of molecules of hydrogen peroxide to water and oxygen each second.

## How to Prepare and Eat Antioxidant-Rich Foods

1. Eat foods from high on the ORAC list.
2. Eat foods raw or cooked over medium heat to prevent the formation of free radicals.
3. Eat phytonutrients that quench free radicals.
4. Eat mineral-rich foods that support SOD and catalase enzymes in reacting to oxidation.

**Step 7** — ## Detoxify Your Body

Support the body's detoxification mechanisms by eating foods that lower the toxic load throughout the body. When detoxification is weak, harmful compounds accumulate in the body — compounds that can sometimes damage the nervous system. In Parkinson's disease, an oxidative process destroys nerve cells. When the body's detoxification system is working properly, we have more protection from disease processes that lead to neurologic aging.

## Detoxifying Dietary Agents

To combat toxins, the body has an array of weapons: enzymes, amino acids, and vitamins ready to take action. When combined with the detoxifying systems of the liver, kidneys, breath, and skin, this cleansing force is formidable.

> **Q** **Is this detoxification program the same as doing a fast or a cleansing diet?**
>
> **A** No, this is quite different. Cleansing diets and various types of fasting can support the body's efforts to dispel harmful substances, but we are speaking here of a specific biochemical process that happens at the cellular level. Detoxification involves making a compound less harmful and preparing it for disposal. Supporting our body's ability to navigate through a sea of chemical compounds is crucial. If we can perform this function, our physical and mental energy will improve — if we cannot, we are more likely to be fatigued and listless, and we may have problems with concentration and mental focus. Some of the compounds that we need to neutralize are indirectly damaging to the brain.

## Glutathione Action

Made from three amino acids, glutathione has the ability to quench free radicals (it gives up a proton to an unpaired "lonely" electron and renders that electron harmless), but it is best known as a master detoxification compound. It is produced in the liver (it is needed there to absorb the compounds that are being detoxified). The first step of detoxification, as we have discussed, is to oxidize toxic compounds so that they can be "stuck" to something else and excreted from the body. Glutathione is one of the major protective shields that help whisk toxic compounds from the body. Some of the glutathione produced in the liver goes into the body's circulation and helps suppress free radicals elsewhere.

## Fish Contamination

Fish that eat other fish, such as tuna, tend to build up toxins in their bodies. Although we recommend consuming fish in our menu plan, tuna, salmon, and other fatty fish should be consumed in moderation. The American Pregnancy Association rates the amount of mercury in various species of fish and advises against eating fish with a high mercury content. What's good for pregnant women should be good for all.

# Mercury Levels in Fish

### Highest Mercury Levels in Fish
- Mackerel (king)
- Marlin
- Orange roughy
- Shark
- Swordfish
- Tilefish
- Tuna (bigeye, ahi)

### High Mercury Levels in Fish
- Bluefish
- Grouper
- Mackerel (Spanish, Gulf)
- Sea bass (Chilean)
- Tuna (canned, white albacore)
- Tuna (yellowfin)

### Lower Mercury Levels in Fish
- Bass (striped, black)
- Carp
- Cod (Alaskan)
- Croaker (white Pacific)
- Halibut (Pacific and Atlantic)
- Jacksmelt (Silverside)
- Lobster
- Mahi mahi
- Monkfish
- Perch (freshwater)
- Sablefish
- Skate
- Snapper
- Sea trout (weakfish)
- Tuna (canned, chunk light)
- Tuna (skipjack)

### Lowest Mercury Levels in Fish
- Anchovies
- Butterfish
- Catfish
- Clams
- Crab (domestic)
- Crawfish (crayfish)
- Croaker
- Flounder
- Haddock
- Hake
- Herring
- Mackerel (North Atlantic, chub)
- Mullet
- Oysters
- Perch (ocean)
- Plaice
- Salmon (canned and fresh)
- Sardines
- Scallops
- Shad (American)
- Shrimp
- Sole
- Squid (calamari)
- Tilapia
- Trout (freshwater)
- Whitefish
- Whiting

**Q** **I've heard that glutathione can be injected intravenously. Is this effective?**

**A** Some physicians do use intravenous therapy, injecting a high dose of glutathione in sterile solution into a vein. The glutathione goes right into the bloodstream. There are also inhalation forms of glutathione. Intravenous administration of glutathione can rapidly raise the level of glutathione in the bloodstream. But these methods of delivering glutathione are usually not needed, because a plant-rich diet with fresh foods can provide the body with all of the starting ingredients it needs to make lots of glutathione.

Glutathione protects your nervous system as it finds its way into the circulation system. When it has done its job, it has to be regenerated into a useful form again. Vitamin E (d-alpha-tocopherol) helps to protect the cell membranes and to spare or conserve glutathione. Vitamin C can recharge glutathione back to a useful state. In chemical terms, it "reduces" glutathione so that it can once again give a proton to a dangerous free radical. When vitamin C is oxidized, it is a very weak radical but is not a menace to the body. It does need to be replaced, which is why we recommend several servings of vitamin C–rich foods daily.

## How to Avoid Free Radicals

1. Avoid rancid and hydrogenated fats.
2. Buy your produce fresh daily, preferably organic.
3. Don't overcook vegetables, to avoid nutrient loss and free radical formation.
4. Eat many different colors of food: orange, green, red, yellow. (Be sure the coloring comes from plant molecules, not from food coloring.)
5. Be mindful of contaminated food sources, including fish and foods susceptible to fungal contamination.
6. Drink green tea (preferably organic) at least once daily to support detoxification enzymes.
7. Drink enough water to support detoxification processes in the liver, kidneys, skin, and colon.
8. Move! Exercise not only directly stimulates the brain, but our lymphatic system, a major detoxification drainage route, needs muscle contraction to excrete toxins.

**Q** **What can I do to support detoxification at the cellular level?**

**A** Start by ensuring that the proper nutritional elements are readily available in your diet. Two kinds of detoxifying compounds are needed:

- Compounds that act as the required ingredients in the body's own detoxification systems (for example, selenium or vitamin $B_{12}$).
- Compounds that are direct "scavengers" of free radicals and toxic compounds (for example, lycopene from tomatoes and vitamin C. Vitamin C supports our body's own detoxification pathways (it recharges them), but it is also a great free-floating scavenger of free radicals.

**Q** **How should I manage pesticide and herbicide exposure?**

**A** To be clear, the small amounts of organophosphates on our food are not enough to cause poisoning, but if you are going to consider a plan to reduce all of the factors that can harm the nervous system, limit your exposure in the following ways:

1. Thoroughly wash fruits and vegetables, keeping in mind that this does not remove all the organophosphates.
2. Peel fruits and vegetables to reduce the amount of exposure.
3. Buy organic food, which should solve the problem of exposure.

**Step 8**

# Eat More Omega-3 Essential Fatty Acids

Surround the brain with essential fatty acids (EFAs) by consuming more fish oil and flaxseed oil. Omega-3 fatty acids protect the meninges surrounding the brain from damage and modulate inflammation in the nervous system. Increase your intake of omega-3 fatty acids but reduce omega-6 fatty acids in your diet. North American diets are already too saturated with omega-6 fatty acids. Saturate the brain with the optimal balance of these fats.

## Omega-3 EFAs

Omega-3 fatty acids are particularly important for the function of brain cells. They are the actual "conduit" through which electrical signals travel. They help neurons connect better. Our brains are meant to be rich in omega-3 EFAs.

EFAs are essential nutrients: they cannot be made in the body, so they must be consumed through diet or supplementation. Omega-3 EFAs are most commonly found in fish and fish oil and in flax seeds and flaxseed oil. Eating these foods in higher-than-average amounts has been shown to reduce symptoms of dementia.

---

## Kinds of Omega-3 EFAs

- Docosahexaenoic acid (DHA)
- Eicosapentaenoic acid (EPA)
- Linolenic acid

Generally, DHA and EPA are considered superior sources.

---

## Brain Growth

Our brains develop from a small node of starter neurons arising from stem cells, and they grow fantastically into a multibillion neuronal network at birth. It is no less wondrous than a galaxy's worth of stars emerging from a supernova! During this process, we have an absolute need for omega-3 fatty acids. This need continues after birth as the brain mass continues to grow at an explosive pace. Nature's perfect baby food — breast milk — is rich in omega-3 fatty acids.

### Q / A — What is IQ?

An IQ, or intelligence quotient, is a score derived from one of several standardized tests designed to assess intelligence. The normal score on these tests is 100. Approximately 95% of the North American population scores an IQ between 70 and 130. It has been shown that IQ scores are associated with such factors as morbidity and mortality, parental social status, and, to a substantial degree, biological parental IQ. These IQ scores are used as predictors of educational achievement, special needs, job performance, and income.

## DHA, Eyesight and Learning Ability

There is overwhelming evidence that babies are better off with abundant docosahexaenoic acid (DHA) in their nutritional supply before they are born and in that critical period of infancy. In fact, DHA seems to improve eyesight and increase learning ability as well. This is why infant formula is now fortified with DHA — to once again try to mimic what nature does perfectly in breast milk.

---

**Q**
**A**

**Does omega-3 improve brain function in adults?**

The answer is a resounding yes. Various types of studies on adults have confirmed that omega-3 fatty acids can improve brain function. In fact, physical increases in gray matter (brain cells) in key learning areas, like the hippocampus region, have been seen with increases in omega-3 fatty acids.

---

## Inflammation Connection

The DHA in your diet can decrease inflammation in many neurodegenerative diseases. Likewise, arterial health is better with omega-3 fatty acids. It decreases the propensity to clot and quells the inflammation in the lining of the arteries that leads to degenerative change. Eating these fatty acids not only encourages a better-functioning brain, it also helps maintain the healthy blood supply that the brain is absolutely dependent on.

## Executive Functions

The evidence for treating dementia with omega-3 EFAs is substantial. In one case, 65 healthy subjects (50 to 75 years old, 30 females and 35 males) completed 26 weeks of supplementing with either fish oil (about 2.2 grams a day of a potent omega-3 — just shy of a tablespoon/15 mL daily) or a placebo. Before and after the intervention period, the researchers looked at important signs of change, such as cognitive performance, changes to brain structure, and changes to blood and blood vessels. The focus was on the executive functions, which involve higher thinking — decision making, making choices, reasoning — and are a herald of increased brain capacity. The individuals treated with omega-3 supplementation showed an increase in brain power and displayed benefits in the integrity of the small connections of white matter (the connections between brain cells) as well as in the volume of gray matter in frontal, temporal, parietal, and limbic areas of the brain, primarily of the left hemisphere. The frontal, temporal, and parietal areas are all involved in thinking and reasoning. The scientists also observed good changes to the lining of the carotid arteries (the two arteries in the neck that bring much of the brain's blood supply to the head) as well as to diastolic blood pressure.

**Q** How much omega-3 and omega-6 EFAs should I include in my diet?

**A** The modern Western diet is dominated by omega-6 EFAs at the expense of omega-3 EFAs. The current ratio is approximately 10:1 omega-6 to omega-3 EFAs. This imbalance is pro-inflammatory and can promote symptoms of dementia. The recommended ratio is 4:1. An attempt to reach this recommended ratio is shown in the meal plans and recipe sections of this book. Simply stated, eat much more omega-3-rich foods than omega-6 foods.

## Omega-3 EFA Sources

Food sources include fatty fish and fish oils (bluefish, salmon, sardines, trout, and tuna, plus their fish oils). Fish are high in EPA due to the algae they consume, and algae-based products are available as vegetarian sources of EPA. Infants thrive on EPA, and human breast milk also contains EPA.

## Omega-6 EFA Sources

Olive, canola, corn, sesame, sunflower, soybean, and walnut oils, as well as most nuts, seeds, and whole grains, contain omega-6 EFAs. Omega-6 fatty acids are commercially available as evening primrose, flaxseed, borage, and currant oils. These oils can be used to prepare salad dressings, and in some cases of deficiency, omega-6 EFA oils are prescribed as nutritional supplements. Omega-6 fatty acids are not heat stable and should not be used to fry foods.

Linoleic acid is the most common omega-6 fatty acid in our diet. It has been shown to help prevent heart disease. However, omega-6 fatty acids are the precursor to inflammatory compounds in the body that can disturb the brain.

## Caution

Omega-3 EFAs do decrease blood clotting. If you have a blood-clotting disorder, easy bleeding, or easy bruising, or especially if you are on blood-thinning medications, you should not supplement with omega-3 fatty acids. Usually, adding more fish to the diet poses no problem, but if you are taking some of the more powerful anticlotting drugs (such as warfarin), you will want to be careful. Consult with your doctor before taking more omerga-3 EFAs.

**DID YOU KNOW?**

**Diminished Effects**

Omega-3 fatty acids are known to help balance the inflammatory effects of omega-6 fatty acids. When omega-3 fatty acids are deficient, the beneficial effects of omega-6 EFA oils may be diminished. Because corn, canola, and soybean oils are used widely in the production of commercial and processed foods, many people consume excessive amounts of omega-6 and insufficient amount of omega-3 EFA oils.

## How to Balance EFAs

**1.** Eat more omega-3 EFA foods:
- Fish and shellfish (seafood)
- Flax seeds
- Omega-3-enriched eggs and milk
- Walnuts

**2.** Reduce excessive intake of omega-6 EFA foods:
- Deep-fried foods
- Processed foods high in vegetable oils
- Snack foods

Step 9

# Enhance Brain Function with Special Nutrients

Several foods and supplements can be considered brain tonics that support circulation in the brain and protect against the aging effects of oxidation. Add these superfoods to your shopping list to protect yourself against the onset of a neurodegenerative disease or to treat a brain disease.

## Brain Tonics

Some foods enhance brain function by enabling the nerve cells of the brain to function optimally by resisting oxidative stress and by improving the function of key neurotransmitters.

### Superfoods and Nutrients

- Strawberries
- Sage
- Walnuts
- Acetyl-L-carnitine

### Strawberries

The botanical name of this fruit is *Fragaria ananassa*. Strawberries are packed with vitamin C and other nutrients, such as the mineral manganese. Strawberries contain compounds called anthocyanins. These molecules are excellent at absorbing free radicals that can damage tissue, and they have a strengthening effect on some body tissues. Recently, it has been found that the anthocyanins from strawberries can protect the mitochondria from oxidative stress damage. The mitochondria are the "power plants" of our cells, where food energy and oxygen combine to create a form of energy the body can readily use.

## DID YOU KNOW?

**Anthocyanin Therapy**

Damage to the mitochondria, especially oxygen-derived damage, is found in some neurodegenerative diseases. The anthocyanins from strawberries have been found to negate the effects of the oxygen damage. It is worth paying a few cents more to buy organic strawberries, because this food is often sprayed with pesticides.

Naturally, the effect of oxygen in the mitochondria has to be kept under control.

## Sage

Sage is an herb used in savory dishes. *Salvia officinalis* and *Salvia lavandulifolia* are the two species of sage used most commonly. Sage contains compounds called monoterpenes that boost the levels of acetylcholine in the brain. Acetylcholine is a neurotransmitter required for sending signals among brain cells. Raising the levels of this neurotransmitter in some brain regions can enhance memory. In fact, the medications prescribed for Alzheimer's disease are often aimed at raising acetylcholine levels.

The compounds from sage, monoterpenes (which are found in many foods and provide a distinct aroma and flavor), actually stop the brain from breaking down acetylcholine too quickly, and this stimulates more acetylcholine activity in the synapses of the brain.

## Walnuts

These nuts can serve as another cognitive powerhouse. They are packed with essential fatty acids, which are required for optimal brain function. Walnuts also contain melatonin, vitamin E, ellagic acid, and flavonoids that have antioxidant properties. In animal studies, walnuts have been found to improve learning, memory, and motor coordination in mice that had a genetic trait that caused brain damage similar to the damage found in Alzheimer's disease.

## Acetyl-L-Carnitine

Acetyl-L-carnitine (ALC) is an ester form of an amino acid called carnitine. Carnitine is essential for fatty acids entering the mitochondria and for the formation of acetylcholine, one of the brain's most important neurotransmitters. Acetylcholine is crucial for learning and memory. Decreased acetylcholine activity is one of the biochemical changes found in the brains of Alzheimer's patients.

ALC crosses the blood-brain barrier, which means it delivers acetyl groups directly to their receptors in the brain. The result is a decrease in free radicals and in lipofuscin deposits (lipofuscin is a sign of aging brain cells). Clinical studies have also shown improvements in behavioral and emotional measurements. ALC can be taken as a supplement at a recommended dose of 1 to 3 grams daily. Patients seem to tolerate ALC well.

---

### DID YOU KNOW?

**Sage Advice**

In clinical studies, sage ingestion led to improvements in memory. In healthy adults, there also seems to be an improvement in thinking ability and mood, and in people with dementia, some improvement in memory was shown. Although the weight of evidence of these studies is only beginning to accumulate, these are positive signs.

---

### DID YOU KNOW?

**Chocolate Therapy**

Cocoa, the main ingredient in chocolate, protects the vascular system and enhances cognitive function. Cocoa has been found to increase learning ability in animal studies and to enhance cognitive function in humans. Some chocolate preparations deliver plenty of cocoa, and some, like so-called "white chocolate," deliver little or none.

## How to Enhance Brain Function

- Eat strawberries several times per week.
- Incorporate sage into your diet.
- Add walnuts to salads or eat them as a snack.
- Supplement your diet with acetyl-L-carnitine (ALC).
- Keep eating chocolate — preferably dark and not loaded with sugar.

**Step 10**

# Regenerate the Brain

A healthy part of the brain will sometimes take over functions once held by damaged areas. This regenerative function is known as neuroplasticity. It is never too late to support the nervous system as best we can. Keep mentally active and perform specific brain and movement exercises that tone the nervous system. Tap into the regenerative potential of the brain.

## Mind Mapping

Neurologists once believed that the development of the brain ended during adolescence and that, once injured, the brain could not recover. Research has shown that, to the contrary, the brain keeps growing into old age and can recover, in part, from damage, such as from dementia and stroke. In addition, the brain can regenerate itself, moving a function of a damaged or diseased part to another that is healthy. This regenerative trait is called brain mapping, mind mapping, or neuroplasticity.

This "relearning" is facilitated by mechanisms such as axonal sprouting, in which undamaged axons grow new nerve endings to reconnect neurons whose links were injured or severed. Undamaged axons can also sprout new nerve endings and connect with other undamaged nerve cells, forming new neural pathways to accomplish a needed function.

## Types of Brain Plasticity

- *Functional plasticity:* Refers to the brain's ability to move functions from a damaged area of the brain to an undamaged area.
- *Structural plasticity:* Refers to the brain's ability to change its physical structure as a result of learning.

## Neuroplasticity Limits

Cognitive skills can be relearned through neuroplasticity. Learning certain skills and an overall stimulation to the brain that involves thinking, decision making, and reasoning seems to spur the same kind of transfer of function. The stimulation that prompts the activation of learning pathways can be a novel (new or fresh) experience or the challenge of learning a new skill, language, or group of people. However, in a disease like Alzheimer's or vascular dementia, there are limits as to what the brain can do to heal itself. This is especially true in aggressive forms of dementia. The physical damage to the brain tissue and vascular system can be so extensive that it really is a whole-brain problem.

When enough of the brain has been damaged by Alzheimer's disease or vascular dementia, it is as if the brain has run out of the healthy tissue to "remap" things. Through mechanisms that are not quite clear yet, when the brain starts to heavily compensate for loss of function, the compensation may backfire eventually and cause more function loss.

## Computer Analogy

Let's use the computer as an analogy. When a computer does not have enough short-term memory to run software, it sometimes swaps out the data stored in the short-term memory with very-short-term storage in its longer-term memory (the hard drive or internal drive). If this becomes too great, the computer becomes tied up with activating the hard drive and does not process instructions. Anyone who had a 486 computer in the 1990s and tried to run a program that had too many system requirements will remember what that was like. The principle here is that there are limits to what the brain can do to compensate for damage.

However, we must come back to the fact that the brain is composed of between 80 and 100 billion neurons. Not only does each of these neurons interact with thousands of other neurons, but chains of neurons can become involved in relays, and some of these relays can impact other relays. The number of possible neural circuits, or relays, that the brain can establish is a number so great that it has been estimated to exceed the known number of particles of matter in the universe. Although limited by oxygen, nutrition, blood flow, and time and space, the brain is a mysterious part of the body that has a vast potential to reassert its function, even if it does take time. Neuroplasticity is something that we can harness to maximize our brain potential. The Healthy Brain Diet Program promotes neuroplasticity.

**Q** **How about brain games? Are they effective in preventing symptoms of dementia?**

**A** Want to get strong? Do heavy work! If you want to strengthen the brain, exercise it. There are a growing number of products and websites developed to increase the brain's efficiency. One example is Lumosity (www.lumosity.com), which offers web-based activities to enhance brain function. These "brain games" can be done daily and purposefully in order to activate (prevent) or reactivate (treat) the learning process in the brain. Learning is the key. But there are other ways to increase cognitive reserve. Learning a new language strikes open the same vault of potential intelligence. It brings us back to a mode of brain growth and development that is similar to the one experienced in infancy.

Likewise, learning a new skill that does not just involve repeating skills we already have cracks open the brain's potential. Although proprietary products (some of which are created by people with great knowledge about neuroplasticity and other scientific brain issues) are wonderful, we are not limited to them. Our brains are meant to be used, doing challenging things in the world. We can seek out those activities that get us to "stretch" our thought powers, and we can invest our time in them.

## Learning to Learn

When we learn something entirely new, it activates the learning centers of the brain. Take the example of someone who wants to experience a new type of ethnic cuisine that they have never tried before. They could eat at the restaurant in their city or town that offers this type of cuisine or they could take a cooking class that focuses on that ethnic cuisine. At the restaurant, the menu is exciting and the food provides a new taste experience, but otherwise the overall experience of eating at a restaurant has not changed (there are interesting decorations, the wait staff takes your order, and you pay a check). But at the cooking class, you learn a new cuisine that combines ingredients that you have never tasted or even heard of. You ask questions, follow directions. You are reaching out to understand. All this time, your brain is making — literally, physically, chemically — new connections that never existed before. This active learning in the hippocampus takes us back to that super-learning state we lived in when we were children. So in this case, although there is some benefit in the novelty of just going to the restaurant for a new experience, the cooking class in this brand-new (to this person) cuisine is a more powerful activator of learning pathways in the brain.

Or consider the neurological implications of learning a new language in later life, even after accumulated damage has occurred in the brain due to dementia. Just like the days when you were learning your first language as a baby, your brain begins storing auditory information from spoken words, and it starts developing corresponding speech and eventually writing skills. The various regions of the brain involved in learning literally "light up" on brain scans when you start to learn something complex, such as a language. The brain goes into a growth mode, regardless of age.

For physical and mental health, the brain needs to be exercised at all stages of life. "Use it or lose it" is an apt expression of this principle of good health. When we simply repeat neural patterns that we have used for years, we are not causing those new connections in the brain to sprout. We actually become less effective at learning. This is accepted as normal aging by many people, but it is truly unhealthy, maladaptive, and strikingly unnecessary.

## How to Activate Brain Reserves

- Learn new things and have new experiences.
- Engage in specific cognitive exercises or tasks that stretch your intelligence.
- Move! Movement stimulates the brain and nervous system as a whole.
- Withdraw for rest and reflection. Meditation can take many forms, but it is definitely important to "unplug" and allow ourselves to mentally rest and disengage from our busy and driven lives.

# Create a Care Team

Invite medical professionals, family members, and friends to help you maintain a high quality of life. People with dementia and their caregivers experience a mixture of emotions — from confusion, frustration, anger, fear, uncertainty, depression, and grief — which tend to progress with the disease. At first, it appears as if there is nothing to be done other than to wait for the inevitable. On reflection, there is so much that can be done to improve the patient's quality of life and perhaps show signs of recovery. Scientists in this field make a discovery every day, it seems. Don't give up. For patients, there are rewards to be had in just trying; for caregivers, there are rewards in actively caring.

## Lifestyle Modifications

### Early Stages

Early dementia symptoms and behavior problems may be addressed by modifying lifestyle:

- **Modify the environment.** Reducing clutter and distracting noise can make it easier for someone with dementia to focus and function. It may also reduce confusion and frustration.
- **Modify responses.** A caregiver's response to a behavior can make agitation and fear even worse. It's best to avoid correcting and quizzing a person with dementia. Reassuring them by validating their concerns can defuse most situations.
- **Modify tasks.** Break tasks into easier steps and focus on success, not failure. Structure and routine also help reduce confusion in people with dementia.

### Later Stages

During the later stages of dementia, more significant steps may need to be taken:

- **Seek out support.** Many people with dementia and their families benefit from counseling and local support services. Contact your local Alzheimer's or Parkinson's association to connect with support groups, resources, referrals, home-care agencies, residential care facilities, a telephone help line, and educational seminars.
- **Give encouragement.** Caregivers can help a person cope with dementia by being there to listen, reassuring the person

that life can still be enjoyed, providing encouragement, and doing their best to help the person retain their dignity and self-respect.

- **Provide a calm environment.** A calm and predictable environment can help reduce worry and agitation.
- **Be predictable.** Establish a daily routine that includes enjoyable activities well within the comfort zone of the person with dementia. New situations, excess noise, large groups of people, being rushed or pressed to remember, or being asked to do complicated tasks can cause anxiety. As a person with dementia becomes upset, the ability to think clearly declines even more.

## Care for the Caregiver

Providing care for a person with dementia is physically and emotionally demanding. Feelings of anger and guilt, frustration and discouragement, worry and grief, and social isolation are common. But paying attention to your own needs and well-being is one of the most important things you can do for yourself and for the person in your care. If you're a caregiver:

- Learn as much about the disease as you can. Ask your primary-care doctor or neurologist about good sources of information. Your local librarian can also help you find good resources.
- Counseling and therapy for both the patient and caregivers can help with the frustration and the sense of loss as dementia progresses.
- Support groups for patients, caregivers, and families exist, and these can provide emotional support as well as the sharing of practical strategies and resources.
- Ask questions of doctors, social workers, and others involved in the care of your loved one.
- Call on friends and family members for help when you need it.
- Take a break every day.
- Take care of your health by seeing your own doctor.
- Make time for friends, and consider joining a support group.
- Get plenty of exercise.
- Eat brain-healthy meals using the menu plans and recipes in the next sections of this book.

# Prepare to Make Changes

Changing eating habits is one of the most difficult things we face in life. How do we substitute the addictive sweetness of a strawberry tart that contributes to plaque formation in our brain with the juicy texture and explosive flavor of a fresh organic strawberry that prevents free radicals? Although we have become accustomed to a daily diet that lacks nutrition, we can retrain our brain to want healthy foods.

## Implementing a Menu Plan

The key is to incorporate healthy food into our meals day by day. The nutty flavor of a quinoa salad soon becomes more enticing than a plate of fries. We still hear the siren call of a favorite take-out food, but we soon find the satisfaction of healthy foods instead. There are some barriers to changing our menu selections from "3 squares a day" to something more exciting. That's what the menu plans and recipes in this book are designed to do — present food that is new and nutritious without sacrificing flavor and texture. A tall order, yes, but it has been proven to change our eating habits.

The nutrition information detailed in the Healthy Brain Diet Program is the foundation for planning each meal, from compiling a shopping list to selecting ingredients, from cooking methods to preparation tips. Used preventively or therapeutically, menu planning is another way of supporting brain function.

## Stages of Change

There are proven techniques for making changes that last. How we make changes in our lives has been studied at length, most notably in the "Stages of Change" model proposed by James Prochaska and Carlo DiClemente. They identify five stages that a person goes through when wanting to change a behavior: precontemplation, contemplation, preparation, action, and maintenance. The process of change is ongoing. Having a strong support network to help you consolidate each stage of changes is important. Call on family and friends for support.

### Stage 1: Precontemplation or Denial Stage

In this stage, you have not yet identified an issue or challenge. Nothing needs to be changed, from your point of view, but others may have made comments or told you that there may be a problem. This is news to you; you do not agree.

## Stage 2: Contemplation or Acceptance Stage

In this stage, you now realize there is a problem, but you are not ready to address it. You begin to think about what is wrong, but you may not want to commit to making it better.

## Stage 3: Preparation or Planning Stage

In this stage, you intend to take action. You begin making plans to change.

## Stage 4: Action Stage

In this stage, you modify your behavior, experience, or environment in order to overcome your problem. This is the stage where you see what works for you and what does not. You gain access to resources to aid in your quest for change.

## Stage 5: Maintenance Stage

In this stage, you work on sustaining the change. You may backslide, but you quickly get back on course to change.

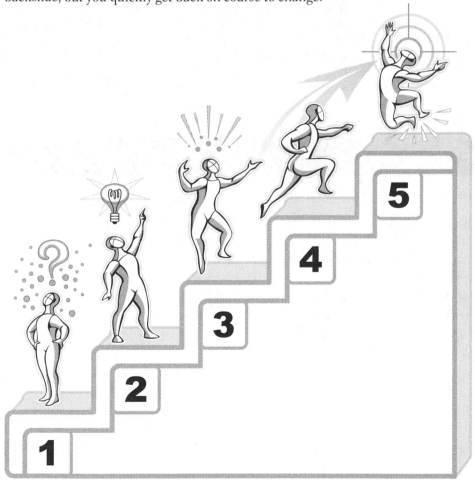

# Characteristics of Change

| Stage | Characteristics |
|---|---|
| **Precontemplation** | • "Ignorance is bliss"<br>• Not considering change |
| **Contemplation** | • "Sitting on the fence"<br>• Ambivalent about change<br>• Weighing the pros and cons of change<br>• Not going to make change in the next month |
| **Preparation** | • "Testing the water"<br>• Planning to act within the next month |
| **Action** | • "Giving it a try"<br>• Practicing new behavior for 3 to 6 months |
| **Maintenance** | • "Staying on course"<br>• Commitment to sustained behavior<br>• After 6 months to 5 years |
| **Relapse** | • "Fall from grace"<br>• Resumption of old behavior |

Adapted from S. Ekserci, *The Complete Weight-Loss Surgery Guide & Diet Program.* Toronto: Robert Rose Inc., 2011.

## CASE STUDY

### Parkinson's Disease (continued from page 108)

Ron thought his team had his symptoms under control, but there were some things that didn't work right. From time to time, he experienced what he called "Parkie" days when he forgot details, directions, and names — when he ran into anything that was fixed to the ground or loose on the floor — when he couldn't drive more than an hour before he started to nod off, and his eyes began to spin. Most problematic was his progressive loss of his voice. Everyone asked him to speak up; people referred to him as "soft spoken." The truth was that his speech volume was well below average — he just couldn't speak louder no matter how hard he tried. Thankfully, there was a speech therapist in town who specialized in Parkinson's cases. There would be many more Parkie adventures, Ron recognized, but he was ready for the challenge.

**PART 5**

# Menu Plans and Recipes for a Healthy Brain

# About the Menu Plans

These menu plan are for a month (28 days), plus a bonus detoxification week, but we are really looking at a way to eat all year round. The menu plans are a guidepost, and they offer a way to eat healthfully — most of the time — while supporting your nervous system.

# Strive for Balance

We are stressing balance in these menu plans, and sometimes balance means not trying to be too perfect. Most individuals find that the more healthy they eat, the more their body and taste buds begin to recognize real food as desirable, and to reject processed or fake food that is over-salted, over-stimulating, over-sedating, and generally unhealthy and unpleasant. This is not to say that it does not take an effort to keep choosing nourishing foods and to sometimes say no to the wrong foods, but in a surprising way, your brain and appetite become reprogrammed, or, one might say, we return to nature and start wanting real food and not a chemical buffet of fake foods. In time, you will be able to make substitutions and create your own plan based on the principles of this diet. Depending on how much you cook, you will also learn some new culinary skills here.

**Q**
**A**
**So how exactly do the menu plans work?**

Each week a specific preventive or therapeutic set of recipes is emphasized. Week 1 focuses on meals that are low on the glycemic index; Week 2 on antioxidant meals; Week 3 on meals that provide healthy dietary fats; and week 4 on meals that supply brain-boosting ingredients. We've also added an optional menu plan for a detoxification week, if this is something you are interested in pursuing.

### Low-Glycemic-Index Meals

The meals planned for Week 1 feature carbohydrates low on the glycemic index, making the meals unlikely to spike your blood sugar levels but adequate in energy to feed a hungry brain. Even the choices that include some gluten or more refined grains tend to be bundled with a protein and vegetable to extend the glycemic effect. These meals deliver a steady supply of energy throughout the day. Fasting times are not too long because you don't want to engage the adrenal glands, which come to your rescue when your blood sugar crashes. We also want to keep your brain happy so that your concentration and mood are on an even keel. These planned meals also ensure that your need for amino acids from protein is met, as that, too, is a source of the brain's power.

## Antioxidant Meals

In Week 2, several forms of antioxidant and protective substances are delivered to the body and to the brain every day. These come from plentiful portions of fruits and vegetables, accompanied by enhancing ingredients, such as sage and walnut. Turmeric is used to make curries because this spice directly addresses some of the inflammation that can damage the central nervous system. We begin to recognize the aggregate effect of daily and weekly diet choices. These meals are also crafted to provide ample nutrients so that the body can manufacture its own antioxidants, where possible.

## Healthy Fats Meals

The meals in Week 3 include a variety of dietary fats, which are important for the health of the vascular system. They are also rich in fiber, which helps lower cholesterol. In addition, the same components that help with detoxification and oxidative stress will help with the protection of the inner lining of the blood vessels. This diet has many components that ought to lower inflammatory activity at the site of a blood vessel plaque (including the very vital blood vessels of the brain), which is a key factor in slowing down the progression of atherosclerosis. At the same time, some of the diet components (the proanthocyanidins) help to strengthen collagen structures. This is always a good idea for improving the integrity of the brain vascular supply. Sources of omega-3 fats are provided throughout the week. This is deliberate, as a natural way to supply the fat. We also encourage the use of omega-3 eggs (hopefully organic and free-range). The use of omega-6s from deep-frying or excessive snack food is discouraged. Fresh foods made in your own kitchen, and lots of seafood, are encouraged.

## Meals for Brain-Boosting Synergy

Week 4 features deliberate menu choices that help supply brain-boosting ingredients, such as cinnamon, sage, walnuts, strawberries, blueberries, chocolate, and various vitamins. These are all brain boosters that seem to enhance cognitive activity.

Taken alone, they are not a single-agent treatment for advanced dementia, but together they have a synergistic effect in providing a powerful suite of brain-healthy foods. These are the nutritious, safe, and delicious foods we promote.

## Optional Detoxification Meals

These meals deliberately enhance our detoxification capacity by delivering many foods from the cruciferous family (such as broccoli) that have strong biochemical impact in the liver and kidneys. The diet also supplies the co-factors that are needed to power phase I and phase II detoxification — such as the B vitamins and vitamin C. A food like broccoli has the ability to switch on certain genes that increase detoxification pathways. In this way, certain foods can increase our overall capacity for detoxification. The fiber content of this diet is important as well. Fiber (along with water intake and exercise) helps maintain good bowel activity. This is important for moving toxins out of the body. Many end products of detoxification are released into the gut, via the bile, from the gallbladder and liver.

# Choose Organic

We encourage you to purchase organic foods, especially when choosing foods that tend to be sprayed with more pesticides or herbicides. Strawberries, for example, tend to be one of the more heavily sprayed crops. However, out-of-season organic crops can be very pricey, so buying organic is not always feasible. Instead of creating a hard and fast rule, we simply encourage you to make the organic choice often. This helps preserve the soil and reduces the amount of agricultural chemicals on your food.

Nutrient content can vary between organic and non-organic, and there isn't always a clear winner, but many people find the taste of organic foods superior. When using non-organic foods, wash them thoroughly (although this practice is a good idea for organic foods too, in terms of food safety).

By making the healthy choice but avoiding extremes, your decisions about organic produce, grains, dairy, eggs and meat can add up to beneficial and practical choices.

# Make Mealtimes a Special Event

Eating is a time for people to be together and to enjoy good food in good company. North Americans have pushed food to the periphery of our lives, even though we collectively consume too much of it. We eat food hastily, often in the car or as we are walking down the street or working at our desk. According to Dr. Mary Pritchard, author of *The Death of the Family Meal*, 40% of adults who regularly eat dinner with their children report that the television is on. At least they are eating dinner together.

We recommend a return to the old ways, to a ritual that has been practiced for millennia across virtually all cultures. Making mealtimes a special event doesn't mean the meals need to be fancy, formal, or expensive. It simply means that you regularly set time aside to eat meals with others whose company you enjoy, whether they are your family, your friends, or your colleagues. Shared mealtimes allow for communication, sharing, and merriment, and they take us away from a "convenience food" mentality and give us a renewed appreciation of good-quality food.

> **Q**
> **A**
>
> **What if I do not have a family to share meals with?**
>
> Instead of feeling dejected about this, make your solitary meals something to savor by preparing your favorite meals, just the way you like them, and revel in the fact that you don't have to worry about accommodating anyone else's tastes or dietary restrictions. Invite your friends to celebrate special occasions. Become the person who cooks Thanksgiving dinner every year for other single people. Volunteer to deliver meals to those in your community who are in need or who have difficulty preparing their own meals.

We hope you enjoy the following nutritious, safe, and delicious menus and recipes we have compiled for your mental and physical health and well-being. In implementing these menu plans, there are many principles to keep in mind, the first being: If at first you don't succeed … try again.

# Week 1 Menu Plan

| Meal | Monday | Tuesday | Wednesday | |
|------|--------|---------|-----------|---|
| **Breakfast** | Avocado and Egg Breakfast Wraps* <br><br> 1/3 cup (75 mL) applesauce <br><br> 6 oz (175 mL) milk** | Hot Breakfast Cereal Mix* <br><br> 1/3 cup (75 mL) blueberries <br><br> 1/2 cup (125 mL) unsweetened plain yogurt <br><br> 6 oz (175 mL) unclarified purple grape juice | Power Granola* <br><br> 1 banana <br><br> 6 oz (175 mL) milk** | |
| **Morning snack** | 1 apple <br><br> 2 oz (60 mL) low-fat cheese | Cranberry Walnut Muffin* | 1/2 cup (125 mL) sliced peaches <br><br> 1/2 cup (125 mL) cottage cheese | |
| **Lunch** | Turkey Apple Meatloaf * | Tuna Salad Melt* | Three-Bean Chili* | |
| **Afternoon snack** | 1/2 cup (125 mL) mixed walnuts and raisins <br><br> 4 oz (125 mL) green tea | Chunky Guacamole* with 8 to 10 tortilla chips <br><br> 4 oz (125 mL) oolong tea | 1/2 cup (125 mL) mixed walnuts and raisins <br><br> 4 oz (125 mL) green tea | |
| **Dinner** | Red Curry Chicken with Snap Peas and Cashews* <br><br> Green Beans and Carrots with Aromatic Spices* | Mushroom Spinach Quiche* <br><br> Everyday Salad* | Rosemary Chicken Breasts with Sweet Potatoes and Onions* <br><br> Couscous Salad with Basil and Pine Nuts* | |
| **Evening snack** | 1 apple | Dark Chocolate Mousse* | 1 orange | |

* The recipe is in the book; unless otherwise indicated, the amount is 1 serving.

** For the milk, select either low-fat organic milk, or almond or rice milk fortified with calcium and vitamin D.

| Thursday | Friday | Saturday | Sunday |
|---|---|---|---|
| Home-Style Pancakes*<br><br>$\frac{1}{3}$ cup (75 mL) strawberries<br><br>$\frac{1}{2}$ cup (125 mL) unsweetened plain yogurt<br><br>6 oz (175 mL) unclarified purple grape juice | Power Granola*<br><br>2 oz (60 mL) low-fat cheese<br><br>6 oz (175 mL) milk** | Hot Breakfast Cereal Mix*<br><br>$\frac{1}{2}$ cup (125 mL) unsweetened plain yogurt<br><br>6 oz (175 mL) unclarified purple grape juice | Home-Style Pancakes*<br><br>$\frac{1}{2}$ cup (125 mL) unsweetened plain yogurt<br><br>6 oz (175 mL) milk** |
| Cranberry Walnut Muffin* | 1 apple<br><br>2 oz (60 mL) low-fat cheese | Super Antioxidant Smoothie* | Super Antioxidant Smoothie* |
| Salmon Oasis* | Shrimp and Corn Bisque* | Cream of Broccoli Soup* | Saffron Paella Soup* |
| Chunky Guacamole* with 8 to 10 tortilla chips<br><br>4 oz (125 mL) oolong tea | Cranberry, Carrot and Apple Teff Muffin*<br><br>4 oz (125 mL) oolong tea | $\frac{1}{2}$ cup (125 mL) carrot sticks<br><br>2 oz (60 mL) low-fat cheese | $\frac{1}{3}$ cup (75 mL) roasted almonds |
| Orange Ginger Beef*<br><br>Home-Style Skillet Rice with Tomato Crust* | Red Lentil Curry with Coconut and Cilantro*<br><br>Baked Risotto with Spinach* | Tomato Onion Curry of Brown Lentils*<br><br>Fragrant Rice-Stuffed Peppers* | Yellow Tomato Gazpacho with Cilantro Oil*<br><br>Turkey Apple Meatloaf*<br><br>Saffron Mash* |
| $\frac{1}{3}$ cup (75 mL) blueberries | $\frac{1}{3}$ cup (75 mL) blueberries | Blueberry Lemon Bundt* | Chocolate Ganache Stout Cake* |

# Week 2 Menu Plan

| Meal | Monday | Tuesday | Wednesday | |
|---|---|---|---|---|
| Breakfast | Cranberry Quinoa Porridge* <br><br> ½ cup (125 mL) unsweetened plain yogurt <br><br> 6 oz (175 mL) unclarified purple grape juice | Hot Breakfast Cereal Mix* <br><br> 1 banana <br><br> 6 oz (175 mL) milk** | Cranberry Quinoa Porridge* <br><br> ½ cup (125 mL) unsweetened plain yogurt <br><br> 6 oz (175 mL) unclarified purple grape juice | |
| Morning snack | ½ cup (125 mL) mixed walnuts and raisins | Cranberry, Carrot and Apple Teff Muffin* | ½ cup (125 mL) sliced peaches <br><br> 2 oz (60 mL) low-fat cheese | |
| Lunch | 2 Creamy Mushroom Walnut Toasts* | Open-Face Salmon Salad Sandwich with Apple and Ginger* | Curried Chicken Salad Wrap* | |
| Afternoon snack | ¼ cup (60 mL) hummus <br><br> 6 gluten-free rice crackers <br><br> 4 oz (125 mL) green tea | ⅓ cup (75 mL) roasted almonds <br><br> 4 oz (125 mL) oolong tea | ¼ cup (60 mL) hummus <br><br> 6 gluten-free rice crackers <br><br> 4 oz (125 mL) green tea | |
| Dinner | Spaghetti with Sun-Dried Tomatoes and Broccoli* <br><br> Insalata Caprese* | Chicken Paprika with Noodles* <br><br> Broccoli Carrot Slaw with Cranberries and Sunflower Seeds* | Three-Spice Chicken with Potatoes* <br><br> Creamy Broccoli Curry* | |
| Evening snack | Chocolate Ganache Stout Cake* | 1 apple | Chocolate Cherry Drop* | |

\* The recipe is in the book; unless otherwise indicated, the amount is 1 serving.

\*\* For the milk, select either low-fat organic milk, or almond or rice milk fortified with calcium and vitamin D.

| | Thursday | Friday | Saturday | Sunday |
|---|---|---|---|---|
| | Hot Breakfast Cereal Mix* <br><br> 1 banana <br><br> 6 oz (175 mL) milk** | Chocolate Chip Oat Breakfast Biscuit* <br><br> ½ cup (125 mL) unsweetened plain yogurt <br><br> 6 oz (175 mL) unclarified purple grape juice | French-Herbed Strata* <br><br> ½ cup (125 mL) unsweetened plain yogurt <br><br> 6 oz (175 mL) unclarified purple grape juice | French-Herbed Strata* <br><br> ⅓ cup (75 mL) applesauce <br><br> 6 oz (175 mL) milk** |
| | ½ cup (125 mL) mixed walnuts and raisins | 1 apple <br><br> 2 oz (60 mL) low-fat cheese | Super Antioxidant Smoothie* | Super Antioxidant Smoothie* |
| | Lunch Box Peachy Sweet Potato and Couscous* | Lunch Box Peachy Sweet Potato and Couscous* | Creamy Roasted Garlic, Chicken and Mushroom Soup* | Tomato Basil Soup* |
| | Super Antioxidant Smoothie* | 4 oz (125 mL) green tea | 1 apple <br><br> 2 oz (60 mL) low-fat cheese | Cranberry, Carrot and Apple Teff Muffin* |
| | Sage and Savory Mushroom Frittata* <br><br> Sweet Cinnamon Waldorf Salad* | Salmon over White and Black Bean Salsa* <br><br> New Orleans Braised Onions* | Vegetable Moussaka* <br><br> Vegetable Salad with Feta Dressing* | Three-Pepper Tamale Pie* <br><br> Avocado Salad* |
| | 1 peach | 1 apple | 8 oz (250 g) popcorn with 1 tsp (5 mL) butter | Cinnamon Cake with Whipped Mocha Frosting* |

# Week 3 Menu Plan

| Meal | Monday | Tuesday | Wednesday | |
|------|--------|---------|-----------|---|
| **Breakfast** | Cranberry Quinoa Porridge*<br><br>⅓ cup (75 mL) applesauce<br><br>6 oz (175 mL) unclarified purple grape juice | Avocado and Egg Breakfast Wrap*<br><br>½ cup (125 mL) grapes<br><br>6 oz (175 mL) milk** | Cranberry Quinoa Porridge*<br><br>⅓ cup (75 mL) applesauce<br><br>6 oz (175 mL) unclarified purple grape juice | |
| **Morning snack** | ½ cup (125 mL) mixed walnuts and raisins | Peanut Butter and Chocolate Rice Crisp Bar* | Peanut Butter and Chocolate Rice Crisp Bar* | |
| **Lunch** | Vegetable Quinoa Salad* | Refreshing Lentil Salad* | Tomato Basil Soup*<br><br>Holy Smokes Pita Chips* | |
| **Afternoon snack** | Super Antioxidant Smoothie* | Super Antioxidant Smoothie* | Trail Mix*<br><br>4 oz (125 mL) green tea | |
| **Dinner** | Cream of Broccoli Soup*<br><br>Parmesan Herb Baked Fish Fillets*<br><br>Pasta Salad with Apricots, Dates and Orange Dressing* | Cream of Broccoli Soup*<br><br>Vegetable Cheese Loaf with Lemon Tomato Sauce*<br><br>Spaghetti Squash with Mushrooms* | Curry-Roasted Squash and Apple Soup*<br><br>Beef with Broccoli* | |
| **Evening snack** | Cinnamon Cake with Whipped Mocha Frosting* | 1 apple | Old-Fashioned Dark Chocolate Pudding* | |

\* The recipe is in the book; unless otherwise indicated, the amount is 1 serving.

\*\* For the milk, select either low-fat organic milk, or almond or rice milk fortified with calcium and vitamin D.

| Thursday | Friday | Saturday | Sunday |
|---|---|---|---|
| Walnut Flax Waffles* <br> ½ cup (125 mL) unsweetened plain yogurt <br> ½ cup (125 mL) grapes <br> 6 oz (175 mL) milk** | Cranberry Quinoa Porridge* <br> ⅓ cup (75 mL) applesauce <br> 6 oz (175 mL) unclarified purple grape juice | Crêpes with Sweet Ricotta and Strawberries* <br> 6 oz (175 mL) milk** | French-Herbed Strata* <br> 1 banana <br> 6 oz (175 mL) unclarified purple grape juice |
| Trail Mix* | Peanut Butter and Chocolate Rice Crisp Bar* | Trail Mix* | Super Antioxidant Smoothie* |
| Tabbouleh* | Pasta Salad with Apricots, Dates and Orange Dressing* | Green Macaroni and Cheese* <br> Roasted Butternut Squash Chowder with Sage Butter* | Salmon Chowder* |
| Date and Walnut Muffin* <br> 4 oz (125 mL) oolong tea | Date and Walnut Muffin* <br> 4 oz (125 mL) green tea | Cinnamon Apple Chips* | Cinnamon Apple Chips* |
| Lamb Tagine with Chickpeas and Apricots* <br> Exotic Spiced Roasties* | Peppery Meatloaf with Quinoa* <br> Spinach Salad with Oranges and Mushrooms* | Shrimp, Vegetables and Whole Wheat Pasta* <br> Everyday Salad* | Turkey Cutlets in Gingery Lemon Sauce with Cranberry Rice* <br> Vegetable Quinoa Salad* |
| ½ cup (125 mL) grapes | 1 apple | 8 oz (250 g) popcorn with 1 tsp (5 mL) butter | Chocolate Chili Cupcake* |

# Week 4 Menu Plan

| Meal | Monday | Tuesday | Wednesday | |
|------|--------|---------|-----------|---|
| **Breakfast** | Power Pita with Eggs and Vegetables*<br><br>1 banana<br><br>6 oz (175 mL) milk** | Power Granola*<br><br>½ cup (125 mL) unsweetened plain yogurt<br><br>6 oz (175 mL) unclarified purple grape juice | Toasted Oat Muesli with Dried Fruit and Pecans*<br><br>½ cup (125 mL) grapes<br><br>6 oz (175 mL) milk** | |
| **Morning snack** | Trail Mix* | Cinnamon Apple Chips* | Millet and Flax Muffin* | |
| **Lunch** | Cranberry Mandarin Coleslaw with Walnuts and Raisins* | Curried Sweet Potato and Millet Soup* | Quinoa Salad* | |
| **Afternoon snack** | Cinnamon Apple Chips*<br><br>4 oz (125 mL) green tea | Millet and Flax Muffin*<br><br>4 oz (125 mL) oolong tea | PB&J Energy Ball*<br><br>4 oz (125 mL) green tea | |
| **Dinner** | Shrimp Risotto with Artichoke Hearts and Parmesan* | Shepherd's Pie with Creamy Corn Filling*<br><br>Roasted Beet Taco with Marinated Shredded Kale* | Mandarin Rice and Walnut–Stuffed Acorn Squash*<br><br>Oriental Coleslaw* | |
| **Evening snack** | Chocolate Chili Cupcake* | 1 apple | 1 nectarine | |

\* The recipe is in the book; unless otherwise indicated, the amount is 1 serving.

\*\* For the milk, select either low-fat organic milk, or almond or rice milk fortified with calcium and vitamin D.

| Thursday | Friday | Saturday | Sunday |
|----------|--------|----------|--------|
| Power Granola*<br><br>½ cup (125 mL) unsweetened plain yogurt<br><br>6 oz (175 mL) milk** | Toasted Oat Muesli with Dried Fruit and Pecans*<br><br>½ cup (125 mL) unsweetened plain yogurt<br><br>6 oz (175 mL) unclarified purple grape juice | Home-Style Pancakes*<br><br>½ cup (125 mL) unsweetened plain yogurt<br><br>6 oz (175 mL) unclarified purple grape juice | Tomato and Asiago Cheese Strata*<br><br>⅓ cup (75 mL) strawberries<br><br>6 oz (175 mL) milk** |
| PB&J Energy Ball* | Millet and Flax Muffin* | Super Antioxidant Smoothie* | Super Antioxidant Smoothie* |
| Quinoa Chili* | Couscous Salad with Basil and Pine Nuts* | 2 Creamy Mushroom Walnut Toasts* | Couscous Salad with Basil and Pine Nuts*<br><br>Minestrone* |
| Chunky Guacamole*<br><br>Holy Smokes Pita Chips*<br><br>4 oz (125 mL) oolong tea | Trail Mix*<br><br>4 oz (125 mL) green tea | Trail Mix* | Cinnamon Apple Chips* |
| Peppery Shrimp with Quinoa*<br><br>Roasted Beet and Beet Greens Salad* | Pasta with Shrimp and Peas*<br><br>Roasted Peppers Antipasto* | Tandoori Chicken*<br><br>Red Lentil Curry with Coconut and Cilantro* | Tuna Casserole*<br><br>Broccoli Carrot Slaw with Cranberries and Sunflower Seeds* |
| Rhubarb Strawberry Cobbler* | ½ cup (125 mL) grapes | 8 oz (250 g) popcorn with 1 tsp (5 mL) butter | Perfect Chocolate Bundt* |

# Optional Detox Week Menu Plan

| Meal | Monday | Tuesday | Wednesday | |
|------|--------|---------|-----------|---|
| **Breakfast** | Tofu Quinoa Scramble* | Spiced Fruit and Grain Cereal* | Tofu Quinoa Scramble* | |
| **Morning snack** | Cran Apple Juice* | Orange Zinger Juice* | C Blitz* | |
| **Lunch** | Roasted Garlic and Lentil Soup* | Quinoa Vegetable Cakes* | Moroccan Pumpkin Soup* | |
| **Afternoon snack** | Dandelion Slam Dunk* | Chickpeas with Kiwi and Avocado Salsa* | 2 tbsp (30 mL) cashew butter<br><br>6 rice crackers | |
| **Dinner** | Winter Greens with Split Yellow Peas*<br><br>Beef and Quinoa Power Burgers* | Moroccan Pumpkin Soup*<br><br>Baked Cranberry Tofu with Creamed Asparagus and Leeks*<br><br>Everyday Salad* | Brown Chickpea Curry*<br><br>Perfect Steamed Rice* | |
| **Evening snack** | 1 apple | 1/2 cup (125 mL) grapes | 1/2 cup (125 mL) grapes | |

\*   The recipe is in the book; unless otherwise indicated, the amount is 1 serving.

| Thursday | Friday | Saturday | Sunday |
|---|---|---|---|
| Spiced Fruit and Grain Cereal* | Broccoli, Quinoa, and Feta Omelet* | Cell Support Juice* | Cell Support Juice* |
| Cherry Juice* | Spiced Carrot* | Green Energy* | Green Energy* |
| Jerusalem Artichoke Stew* | Jerusalem Artichoke Stew* | Gingered Beet and Quinoa Soup* | Browned Butter Cauliflower Quinoa Omelet* |
| Slippery Beet* | 1/2 cup (125 mL) mixed walnuts and raisins | Cruciferous Chiller* | 1/2 cup (125 mL) mixed walnuts and raisins |
| Rice Noodles with Spicy Spaghetti Sauce*  Everyday Salad* | Bengali Chicken Stew*  Green Bean, Pecan and Pomegranate Salad* | Rice Noodles with Roasted Mediterranean Vegetables*  Roasted Beet and Beet Greens Salad* | Pad Thai*  Oriental Coleslaw* |
| 1 apple | 1/2 cup (125 mL) grapes | Dark Chocolate Mouse* | Dark Chocolate Mouse* |

# About the Nutrient Analyses

The nutrient analysis done on the recipes in this book was derived from the Food Processor SQL Nutrition Analysis Software, version 10.9, ESHA Research (2011). Where necessary, data was supplemented using the USDA National Nutrient Database for Standard Reference, Release #26 (2014), retrieved January 2014, from the USDA Agricultural Research Service website: www.nal.usda.gov/fnic/foodcomp/search.

Recipes were evaluated as follows:

- The larger number of servings was used where there is a range.
- Where alternatives are given, the first ingredient and amount listed were used.
- Optional ingredients and ingredients that are not quantified were not included.
- Calculations were based on imperial measures and weights.
- Nutrient values were rounded to the nearest whole number for calories, fat, carbohydrate, protein, vitamin C, vitamin D, vitamin E, niacin, folate and selenium.
- Nutrient values were rounded to one decimal point for vitamin $B_6$, vitamin $B_{12}$ and zinc.
- The smaller quantity of an ingredient was used where a range is provided.
- Reduced-sodium broth, 1% milk, light mayonnaise and light sour cream were used where these ingredients are listed as broth, milk, mayonnaise and sour cream.
- Calculations involving meat and poultry used lean portions.
- Canola oil was used where the type of fat was not specified.
- Recipes were analyzed prior to cooking.

It is important to note that the cooking method used to prepare the recipe may alter the nutrient content per serving, as may ingredient substitutions and differences among brand-name products.

# BREAKFAST

# Power Granola

*This recipe provides a steady source of energy at the beginning of the day, or as a snack. Whole grains are an excellent way to sustain an even blood sugar level, and this is a delicious and convenient way to get some whole grains first thing in the morning.*

## Makes about 3½ cups (875 mL)

## Tip

Look for packages of ready-ground flax seeds, which may be labeled "flaxseed meal," or use a spice or coffee grinder to grind whole flax seeds to a very fine meal.

- Preheat oven to 300°F (150°C)
- Large rimmed baking sheet, lined with parchment paper

| | | |
|---|---|---|
| 2 cups | large-flake (old-fashioned) rolled oats | 500 mL |
| ½ cup | chopped pecans | 125 mL |
| ⅓ cup | ground flax seeds (flaxseed meal) | 75 mL |
| 2 tsp | ground cinnamon | 10 mL |
| ½ cup | unsweetened apple juice | 125 mL |
| ½ cup | brown rice syrup or liquid honey | 125 mL |
| 1 tbsp | vegetable oil | 15 mL |
| 2 tsp | vanilla extract | 10 mL |
| ½ cup | dried blueberries, cranberries or cherries | 125 mL |

1. In a large bowl, whisk together oats, pecans, flax seeds and cinnamon.

2. In a medium bowl, whisk together apple juice, brown rice syrup, oil and vanilla until well blended.

3. Add the apple juice mixture to the oats mixture and stir until well coated. Spread mixture in a single layer on prepared baking sheet.

4. Bake in preheated oven for 20 to 25 minutes or until oats are golden brown. Let cool completely on pan.

5. Transfer granola to an airtight container and stir in blueberries. Store at room temperature for up to 2 weeks.

### ▶ Health Tip

Berries are a great source of antioxidants — some of the best nature provides — flaxseeds and walnuts provide brain-boosting omega-3 fats, and cinnamon helps regulate blood sugar. This recipe is a winner.

## Nutrients per ¼ cup (60 mL)

| | |
|---|---|
| Calories | 204 |
| Fat | 7 g |
| Carbohydrate | 31 g |
| Protein | 5 g |
| Vitamin C | 0 mg |
| Vitamin D | 0 IU |
| Vitamin E | 0 mg |
| Niacin | 0 mg |
| Folate | 16 mcg |
| Vitamin $B_6$ | 0.1 mg |
| Vitamin $B_{12}$ | 0.0 mcg |
| Zinc | 0.2 mg |
| Selenium | 1 mcg |

# Toasted Oat Muesli with Dried Fruit and Pecans

*This convenient breakfast cereal delivers slow-burning energy so you won't feel faint or famished an hour later.*

---

**Makes about 6 cups (1.5 L)**

## Tip

Some bran cereals are high in sugar, and although some sugar content is acceptable, make sure to read the ingredients list on the bran cereal you choose for this recipe — no high-fructose corn syrup allowed!

- **Preheat oven to 350°F (180°C)**
- **Large rimmed baking sheet, lined with parchment paper**

| | | |
|---|---|---|
| 3 cups | large-flake (old-fashioned) rolled oats | 750 mL |
| ½ cup | chopped pecans | 125 mL |
| 1 cup | bran cereal (such as All-Bran) | 250 mL |
| 1½ cups | chopped mixed dried fruit | 375 mL |
| ½ cup | ground flax seeds (flaxseed meal) | 125 mL |

**Suggested Accompaniments**

Skim milk, non-dairy milk or nonfat plain yogurt (regular or Greek)

Liquid honey or agave nectar

1. Spread oats and pecans in a single layer on prepared baking sheet. Bake in preheated oven for 7 to 8 minutes or until golden and fragrant. Let cool completely on pan.

2. In an airtight container, combine oat mixture, bran cereal, dried fruit and flax seeds. Store in the refrigerator for up to 1 month.

3. Serve with any of the suggested accompaniments, as desired.

> ### ▶ Health Tip
>
> Grinding flax seeds into flaxmeal releases their many benefits: high fiber, lignans (which can reduce cholesterol), omega-3 fats and more. This recipe does toast the muesli but does not overheat it, so the value of the flaxmeal and its compounds is preserved.

## Nutrients per ¼ cup (60 mL)

| | |
|---|---|
| Calories | 107 |
| Fat | 3 g |
| Carbohydrate | 18 g |
| Protein | 3 g |
| Vitamin C | 1 mg |
| Vitamin D | 3 IU |
| Vitamin E | 0 mg |
| Niacin | 1 mg |
| Folate | 34 mcg |
| Vitamin B$_6$ | 0.3 mg |
| Vitamin B$_{12}$ | 0.5 mcg |
| Zinc | 0.4 mg |
| Selenium | 0 mcg |

# Spiced Fruit and Grain Cereal

*Centuries ago, wars were fought over spices, and when you taste this recipe, you'll be reminded of why. Spices give us great flavor, but also digestive support and health benefits.*

### Makes 2 servings

## Tip

Toast walnut halves in a dry skillet over low heat, stirring constantly, for 3 to 4 minutes or until fragrant. Transfer the toasted nuts to a plate and let cool before chopping.

| | | |
|---|---|---|
| ½ cup | quinoa, rinsed | 125 mL |
| ⅛ tsp | fine sea salt | 0.5 mL |
| 1 cup | water | 250 mL |
| ¾ cup | milk or plain non-dairy milk (such as soy, almond, rice or hemp) | 175 mL |
| ½ cup | large-flake (old-fashioned) rolled oats | 125 mL |
| 3 tbsp | chopped dried figs or dried apricots | 45 mL |
| 2 tbsp | ground flax seeds (flaxseed meal) | 30 mL |
| ¼ tsp | ground ginger | 1 mL |
| ¼ tsp | ground cloves | 1 mL |
| 2 tbsp | chopped toasted walnuts | 30 mL |
| 2 tbsp | liquid honey | 30 mL |

1. In a medium saucepan, combine quinoa, salt, water and milk. Bring to a boil over medium-high heat. Reduce heat to low, cover and simmer for 10 minutes.

2. Stir in oats, figs, flax seeds, ginger and cloves. Cover and simmer for 5 to 8 minutes or until most of the liquid is absorbed and quinoa and oats are cooked through. Stir in walnuts and drizzle with honey.

## ▸ Health Tip

Ginger contains compounds that are anti-inflammatory and improve digestion and stomach health, cloves are a source of antioxidants, and walnuts are a brain-supportive food.

## Nutrients per serving

| | |
|---|---|
| Calories | 536 |
| Fat | 14 g |
| Carbohydrate | 89 g |
| Protein | 19 g |
| Vitamin C | 1 mg |
| Vitamin D | 44 IU |
| Vitamin E | 0 mg |
| Niacin | 1 mg |
| Folate | 37 mcg |
| Vitamin $B_6$ | 0.2 mg |
| Vitamin $B_{12}$ | 0.4 mcg |
| Zinc | 2.6 mg |
| Selenium | 7 mcg |

# Hot Breakfast Cereal Mix

*The taste, texture and simplicity of rolled oats, the fiber of bran and protein from soy make this cereal a great way to stay on an even keel — and you can make your own additions at the breakfast table too!*

## Makes 1 serving

| | | |
|---|---|---|
| 2 tbsp | large-flake (old-fashioned) rolled oats | 30 mL |
| 2 tbsp | wheat bran | 30 mL |
| 1 tbsp | wheat germ | 15 mL |
| 1 tbsp | soy beverage powder | 15 mL |

**1.** In a small, microwave-safe cup, stir together oats, bran, wheat germ and soy beverage powder. Stir in $1/2$ cup (125 mL) water. Microwave on High for 1 to $1^1/_2$ minutes or until oats are tender.

## Variations

Add nuts and/or fresh or dried fruits of your choice.

Stir in fortified soy beverage or low-fat milk.

Sweeten with brown sugar or maple syrup.

*This recipe courtesy of David Shaikh.*

## Tips

For a wholesome breakfast, serve with nuts, fruit and milk or soy beverage on the side.

Enjoy this with a cup of ginger tea. Simply fill a microwave-safe mug with water and add 2 thin slices of peeled gingerroot. Microwave on High for 2 minutes. Remove the ginger and stir in 1 tsp (5 mL) liquid honey, if desired.

> ▸ **Health Tip**
>
> Wheat germ is an excellent natural source of Vitamin E — a great antioxidant with uses across the body and of particular interest in patients at risk for dementia.

## Nutrients per serving

| | |
|---|---|
| Calories | 137 |
| Fat | 2 g |
| Carbohydrate | 21 g |
| Protein | 11 g |
| Vitamin C | 0 mg |
| Vitamin D | 0 IU |
| Vitamin E | 1 mg |
| Niacin | 2 mg |
| Folate | 37 mcg |
| Vitamin $B_6$ | 0.2 mg |
| Vitamin $B_{12}$ | 0 mcg |
| Zinc | 2.2 mg |
| Selenium | 11 mcg |

# Cranberry Quinoa Porridge

*Forget about boring, lumpy porridges — this dish will give you a great start to the day with the energy and protein boost of quinoa and some nutritious natural sweetness from cranberries and honey or maple syrup.*

## Makes 6 servings

## Tip

Unless you have a stove with a true simmer, after reducing the heat to low place a heat diffuser under the pot to prevent the mixture from boiling. This device also helps ensure that the grains will cook evenly and prevents hot spots, which might cause scorching, from forming. Heat diffusers are available at kitchen supply and hardware stores and are made to work on gas or electric stoves.

| | | |
|---|---|---|
| 3 cups | water | 750 mL |
| 1 cup | quinoa, rinsed | 250 mL |
| 1/2 cup | dried cranberries | 125 mL |
| | Maple syrup or honey | |
| | Milk or non-dairy alternative (optional) | |

**1.** In a saucepan over medium heat, bring water to a boil. Stir in quinoa and cranberries and return to a boil. Reduce heat to low. Cover and simmer until quinoa is cooked (look for a white line around the seeds), about 15 minutes. Remove from heat and let stand, covered, about 5 minutes. Serve with maple syrup and milk or non-dairy alternative (if using).

## Variations

Substitute dried cherries or blueberries or raisins for the cranberries.

Use red quinoa for a change.

### ▸ Health Tip

Quinoa contains all of the essential amino acids and is a good protein source.

| Nutrients per serving | |
|---|---|
| Calories | 135 |
| Fat | 2 g |
| Carbohydrate | 27 g |
| Protein | 4 g |
| Vitamin C | 0 mg |
| Vitamin D | 0 IU |
| Vitamin E | 2 mg |
| Niacin | 1 mg |
| Folate | 52 mcg |
| Vitamin B$_6$ | 0.1 mg |
| Vitamin B$_{12}$ | 0 mcg |
| Zinc | 0.9 mg |
| Selenium | 3 mcg |

# Power Pitas with Eggs and Vegetables

*This dish is an easy-to-prepare breakfast that goes beyond the cereal and toast regimen. It will satisfy but leaves the grease and fat behind.*

## Tip

If using salsa, select a brand that has a short list of easily identifiable ingredients, for the best flavor and nutrition.

| | | |
|---|---|---|
| 3 | large egg whites | 3 |
| 1 | large egg | 1 |
| ½ cup | drained silken tofu, crumbled | 125 mL |
| 1 tsp | extra virgin olive oil | 5 mL |
| ½ cup | chopped fresh or thawed frozen broccoli florets | 125 mL |
| ½ cup | chopped red bell pepper | 125 mL |
| 2 | 6-inch (15 cm) whole wheat pitas, warmed | 2 |
| ¼ cup | reduced-sodium salsa (optional) | 60 mL |

1. In a small bowl, beat egg whites and egg until blended. Stir in tofu.

2. In a small skillet, heat oil over medium-high heat. Add broccoli and red pepper; cook, stirring, for 4 to 5 minutes or until softened. Reduce heat to medium. Pour egg mixture over vegetables and cook, stirring gently with a spatula, for 2 to 4 minutes or until eggs are set.

3. Spoon egg mixture onto warm pitas and top with salsa, if desired. Fold in half and serve right away or wrap in foil to eat on the go.

## ▶ Health Tip

Eggs are a fantastic high-value protein and the addition of tofu offers beneficial soy isoflavones. Broccoli and red peppers ensure that this counts as a serving of vegetables — ones that have excellent detoxification and antioxidant properties.

### Nutrients per serving

| | |
|---|---|
| Calories | 306 |
| Fat | 8 g |
| Carbohydrate | 41 g |
| Protein | 20 g |
| Vitamin C | 67 mg |
| Vitamin D | 21 IU |
| Vitamin E | 2 mg |
| Niacin | 3 mg |
| Folate | 67 mcg |
| Vitamin $B_6$ | 0.4 mg |
| Vitamin $B_{12}$ | 0.3 mcg |
| Zinc | 1.8 mg |
| Selenium | 46 mcg |

# Avocado and Egg Breakfast Wraps

*Avocado is a versatile food that has grown in popularity. This dish combines it with the savory taste of goat cheese in what could be described as a spinach omelet in a pita.*

## Tip

Hass avocados (sometimes called Haas avocados) are dark-skinned avocados with a nutty, buttery flesh and a longer shelf life than other varieties, making them the most popular avocado in North America. To determine whether a Hass avocado is ripe, look for purple-black skin and gently press the top — a ripe one will give slightly.

| | | |
|---|---|---|
| 2 | large eggs | 2 |
| 2 | large egg whites | 2 |
| Pinch | fine sea salt | Pinch |
| $\frac{1}{4}$ tsp | freshly ground black pepper | 1 mL |
| 1 tsp | extra virgin olive oil | 5 mL |
| 3 cups | loosely packed spinach, chopped | 750 mL |
| 2 tsp | water | 10 mL |
| 2 | 6-inch (15 cm) whole wheat tortillas, warmed | 2 |
| 2 tbsp | crumbled soft goat cheese | 30 mL |
| $\frac{1}{2}$ | small ripe Hass avocado, sliced | $\frac{1}{2}$ |

1. In a small bowl, beat eggs, egg whites, salt and pepper until blended.

2. In a small skillet, heat oil over medium-high heat. Add spinach and water; cook, stirring, until leaves are wilted. Reduce heat to medium. Pour egg mixture over spinach. Cook, stirring gently with a spatula, for 2 to 4 minutes or until eggs are set.

3. Place half the egg mixture in the center of each warm tortilla and sprinkle each with 1 tbsp (15 mL) goat cheese. Top with avocado and fold or roll up.

> ### ▶ Health Tip
>
> Avocado is rich in healthy fats and increases absorption of carotenoids, the great antioxidant molecules in spinach that give it its green color.

| Nutrients per serving | |
|---|---|
| Calories | 315 |
| Fat | 20 g |
| Carbohydrate | 22 g |
| Protein | 14 g |
| Vitamin C | 18 mg |
| Vitamin D | 43 IU |
| Vitamin E | 3 mg |
| Niacin | 2 mg |
| Folate | 157 mcg |
| Vitamin $B_6$ | 0.4 mg |
| Vitamin $B_{12}$ | 0.5 mcg |
| Zinc | 1.5 mg |
| Selenium | 23 mcg |

# Tofu Quinoa Scramble

*This is a heart-friendly high-energy breakfast that combines the protein of tofu with the protein and energy of quinoa, with a serving of tasty vegetables to boot.*

## Makes 4 servings

### Tip

To wash or not wash mushrooms? You can either wipe them with a damp cloth or quickly rinse them under cold water and immediately wrap in a clean, dry kitchen towel or paper towels to absorb excess moisture.

| | | |
|---|---|---|
| 1 tbsp | extra virgin olive oil | 15 mL |
| 1 | large red bell pepper, chopped | 1 |
| 1 cup | chopped mushrooms | 250 mL |
| 16 oz | extra-firm or firm tofu, drained and coarsely mashed with a fork | 500 g |
| 1 cup | cooked quinoa, cooled | 250 mL |
| 1/4 cup | chopped green onions | 60 mL |
| 1 tbsp | reduced-sodium tamari or soy sauce | 15 mL |
| Pinch | freshly ground black pepper | Pinch |

1. In a small skillet, heat oil over medium-high heat. Add red pepper and mushrooms; cook, stirring, for 4 to 5 minutes or until softened. Add tofu, quinoa, green onions and tamari; cook, stirring, for 5 to 6 minutes or until tofu is golden brown. Season with pepper.

> ### ▶ Health Tip
>
> Soy products like tofu offer cardiovascular benefits and are more natural than the textured vegetable proteins in some processed foods or the heat-altered soy proteins in many snack bars.

## Nutrients per serving

| | |
|---|---|
| Calories | 207 |
| Fat | 11 g |
| Carbohydrate | 16 g |
| Protein | 15 g |
| Vitamin C | 40 mg |
| Vitamin D | 2 IU |
| Vitamin E | 1 mg |
| Niacin | 2 mg |
| Folate | 63 mcg |
| Vitamin $B_6$ | 0.3 mg |
| Vitamin $B_{12}$ | 0.0 mcg |
| Zinc | 2.0 mg |
| Selenium | 20 mcg |

# Broccoli, Quinoa and Feta Omelet

*Who said omelets had to be the same old ham and cheese? This omelet is a superfood package — with several key foods of this menu plan incorporated into it.*

## Makes 4 servings

### Tip

To keep quinoa as fresh as possible, store it in an airtight container in the refrigerator for up to 6 months or in the freezer for up to 1 year.

| | | |
|---|---|---|
| 5 | large eggs | 5 |
| 1/4 tsp | fine sea salt | 1 mL |
| 1/4 tsp | freshly cracked black pepper | 1 mL |
| 2 tsp | extra virgin olive oil | 10 mL |
| 2 cups | coarsely chopped broccoli florets | 500 mL |
| 2 | cloves garlic, minced | 2 |
| 1 1/4 cups | cooked quinoa, cooled | 300 mL |
| 1/2 cup | crumbled feta cheese | 125 mL |
| 1/4 cup | packed fresh flat-leaf (Italian) parsley leaves | 60 mL |

1. In a large bowl, beat eggs, salt and pepper until blended. Set aside.

2. In a large skillet, heat oil over medium-high heat. Add broccoli and cook, stirring, for 4 to 5 minutes or until tender. Reduce heat to medium and add garlic and quinoa; cook, stirring, for 30 seconds.

3. Pour egg mixture over broccoli mixture. Cook, lifting edges to allow uncooked eggs to run underneath and shaking skillet occasionally to loosen omelet, for 4 to 5 minutes or until almost set. Slide out onto a large plate.

4. Invert skillet over omelet and, using pot holders, firmly hold plate and skillet together. Invert omelet back into skillet and cook for 1 to 2 minutes to set eggs. Slide out onto plate and sprinkle with cheese and parsley.

## Nutrients per serving

| | |
|---|---|
| Calories | 247 |
| Fat | 14 g |
| Carbohydrate | 17 g |
| Protein | 15 g |
| Vitamin C | 45 mg |
| Vitamin D | 54 IU |
| Vitamin E | 2 mg |
| Niacin | 1 mg |
| Folate | 93 mcg |
| Vitamin B$_6$ | 0.4 mg |
| Vitamin B$_{12}$ | 0.9 mcg |
| Zinc | 2.2 mg |
| Selenium | 25 mcg |

### ▶ Health Tip

Broccoli has the ability to encourage our cells to create more defensive antioxidant proteins — enzymes we need to fight aging and prevent cellular damage.

# Browned Butter Cauliflower Quinoa Omelet

*This is another way to start the day already ahead of the nutrient curve and with lots of fuel in your body — and after this dish, with its cauliflower browned in butter, you'll never want to settle for soggy overcooked cauliflower again.*

**Makes 4 servings**

## Tip

To keep parsley fresh, wrap it in several layers of paper towels and place in a plastic bag. Store in the warmest part of your refrigerator — in the butter keeper, for example, or the side door.

| | | |
|---|---|---|
| 6 | large eggs | 6 |
| ½ tsp | fine sea salt | 2 mL |
| ¼ tsp | freshly cracked black pepper | 1 mL |
| 1 tbsp | unsalted butter | 15 mL |
| 2 cups | coarsely chopped cauliflower florets | 500 mL |
| 1½ cups | cooked quinoa, cooled | 375 mL |
| 2 | cloves garlic, minced | 2 |
| ½ cup | grated manchego, Romano or Parmesan cheese | 125 mL |
| ¼ cup | packed fresh flat-leaf (Italian) parsley leaves, chopped | 60 mL |

1. In a large bowl, whisk together eggs, salt and pepper. Set aside.

2. In a large skillet, melt butter over medium-high heat. Add cauliflower and cook, stirring, for 7 to 10 minutes or until browned and tender. Reduce heat to medium and add quinoa and garlic; cook, stirring, for 1 minute.

3. Pour egg mixture over quinoa mixture. Cook, lifting edges to allow uncooked eggs to run underneath and shaking skillet occasionally to loosen omelet, for 4 to 5 minutes or until almost set. Slide out onto a large plate.

4. Invert skillet over omelet and, using pot holders, firmly hold plate and skillet together. Invert omelet back into skillet and cook for 1 to 2 minutes to set eggs. Slide out onto plate and sprinkle with cheese and parsley.

> ▶ **Health Tip**
>
> Cauliflower contains glucosinolates, which boost detoxification.

### Nutrients per serving

| | |
|---|---|
| Calories | 276 |
| Fat | 14 g |
| Carbohydrate | 19 g |
| Protein | 18 g |
| Vitamin C | 31 mg |
| Vitamin D | 66 IU |
| Vitamin E | 1 mg |
| Niacin | 1 mg |
| Folate | 102 mcg |
| Vitamin B$_6$ | 0.3 mg |
| Vitamin B$_{12}$ | 0.9 mcg |
| Zinc | 2.3 mg |
| Selenium | 27 mcg |

# Sage and Savory Mushroom Frittata

*There is no lack of flavor in this dish, with shallots, mushrooms and sage livening up a protein-packed tofu-based frittata.*

**Makes 6 to 8 servings**

## Tip

You can substitute 1 tsp (5 mL) dried sage for 1 tbsp (15 mL) fresh sage.

- Preheat oven to 350°F (180°C)
- Cast-iron or other ovenproof skillet
- Food processor

| | | |
|---|---|---|
| 2 tbsp | olive oil | 30 mL |
| 1 lb | mushrooms, sliced | 500 g |
| ¼ cup | sliced shallots (about 2 large) | 60 mL |
| 1 tbsp | vegan hard margarine | 15 mL |
| 1 tbsp | chopped fresh sage leaves (see tip, at left) | 15 mL |
| 1 lb | firm tofu, drained and crumbled | 500 g |
| 1 | package (12.3 oz/350 g) firm silken tofu | 1 |
| ¼ cup | plain soy milk | 60 mL |
| 2 tbsp | nutritional yeast | 30 mL |
| 1 tbsp | cornstarch | 15 mL |
| ¾ tsp | ground turmeric | 3 mL |
| ¾ tsp | salt | 3 mL |
| ½ tsp | freshly ground black pepper | 2 mL |

1. Place skillet over medium-high heat and let pan get hot. Add oil and tip pan to coat. Add mushrooms and shallots. Reduce heat to medium and cook, stirring, until softened and lightly browned, 6 to 8 minutes. Add margarine, sage and firm tofu and cook, stirring, for 2 to 3 minutes to let flavors combine. Remove from heat and gently distribute mixture evenly in pan.

2. In food processor, combine silken tofu, soy milk, nutritional yeast, cornstarch, turmeric, salt and pepper and process until smooth. Pour mixture evenly over vegetable mixture in pan, gently lifting and stirring to combine ingredients.

3. Bake in preheated oven until top is firm and golden, 25 to 30 minutes. Let frittata cool slightly, cut into wedges and serve.

## Nutrients per 1 of 8 servings

| | |
|---|---|
| Calories | 192 |
| Fat | 11 g |
| Carbohydrate | 11 g |
| Protein | 15 g |
| Vitamin C | 1 mg |
| Vitamin D | 14 IU |
| Vitamin E | 1 mg |
| Niacin | 9 mg |
| Folate | 92 mcg |
| Vitamin B$_6$ | 0.2 mg |
| Vitamin B$_{12}$ | 0.1 mcg |
| Zinc | 1.7 mg |
| Selenium | 12 mcg |

> ▶ **Health Tip**
>
> Sage is a brain-boosting food that has been shown to improve cognition.

# Tomato and Asiago Cheese Strata

*This is a more traditional strata with eggs and cheese. This dish is rich but not greasy and has a Mediterranean aspect due to garlic, onions, olive oil and plum tomatoes.*

---

**Makes 4 to 6 servings**

## Tip

If bread is fresh, place on a baking sheet and toast in 350°F (180°C) oven for 8 to 10 minutes or until crisp around edges.

## Variation

Instead of fresh basil, substitute 2 tbsp (30 mL) parsley and add 1 tsp (5 mL) dried basil to onions when cooking.

### Nutrients per 1 of 6 servings

| | |
|---|---|
| Calories | 403 |
| Fat | 18 g |
| Carbohydrate | 42 g |
| Protein | 20 g |
| Vitamin C | 11 mg |
| Vitamin D | 34 IU |
| Vitamin E | 2 mg |
| Niacin | 4 mg |
| Folate | 49 mcg |
| Vitamin B$_6$ | 0.2 mg |
| Vitamin B$_{12}$ | 0.8 mcg |
| Zinc | 2.2 mg |
| Selenium | 32 mcg |

- Preheat oven to 350°F (180°C)
- 8-inch (20 cm) square baking dish, well greased

| | | |
|---|---|---|
| 2 tbsp | olive oil | 30 mL |
| 1 cup | chopped Spanish onion | 250 mL |
| 2 | cloves garlic, finely chopped | 2 |
| 2 cups | chopped seeded plum (Roma) tomatoes (about 5 to 6) | 500 mL |
| 1/2 tsp | salt | 2 mL |
| 1/4 tsp | freshly ground black pepper | 1 mL |
| 2 tbsp | chopped fresh basil | 30 mL |
| 6 cups | cubed stale Italian or French bread (see tip, at left) | 1.5 L |
| 1 1/2 cups | shredded Asiago or fontina cheese | 375 mL |
| 4 | large eggs | 4 |
| 1 cup | ready-to-use vegetable or chicken broth | 250 mL |

1. In a large nonstick skillet, heat oil over medium-high heat. Cook onion and garlic, stirring, for 2 minutes. Stir in tomatoes, salt and pepper; cook, stirring often, for 5 minutes or until tomatoes are sauce-like. Stir in basil.

2. Layer half of the bread cubes in prepared baking dish. Top with half of the tomato mixture and sprinkle with half of the cheese. Layer with remaining bread and tomato mixture.

3. In a bowl, beat eggs with broth; pour over bread mixture. Sprinkle with remaining cheese. Let stand for 10 minutes for bread to absorb egg mixture. (Can be made a day ahead; cover and refrigerate.)

4. Bake in preheated oven for 35 to 40 minutes (5 to 10 minutes longer if refrigerated), until top is golden and center is set when tested with a knife. Serve warm or at room temperature.

> ▶ **Health Tip**
>
> Tomatoes are a great source of lycopene, a potent antioxidant and cell protector (cancer prevention antioxidant) molecule.

# French-Herbed Strata

*A strata is a layered dish using bread as the backbone, and* vive les herbes — *this flavorful dish will nourish and satisfy.*

## Tip

Leeks are grown in sand and are sometimes difficult to clean. A good method of cleaning is to vertically slice through the white and light green leaves, leaving most of the dark green leaves intact. Grasp the leek by the dark green leaves, fan out the bottom white and light green portions, exposing much of the inside of the leek, and run under cold water.

### Nutrients per 1 of 10 servings

| | |
|---|---|
| Calories | 215 |
| Fat | 4 g |
| Carbohydrate | 34 g |
| Protein | 10 g |
| Vitamin C | 5 mg |
| Vitamin D | 11 IU |
| Vitamin E | 1 mg |
| Niacin | 3 mg |
| Folate | 42 mcg |
| Vitamin B$_6$ | 0.1 mg |
| Vitamin B$_{12}$ | 0.2 mcg |
| Zinc | 1.0 mg |
| Selenium | 15 mcg |

- **10-cup (2.5 L) baking dish, lightly oiled**
- **Food processor**

| | | |
|---|---|---|
| 1 tbsp | olive oil | 15 mL |
| 2 | large leeks, thoroughly washed (see tip, at left) and sliced | 2 |
| 8 oz | thin asparagus, ends trimmed, cut into 3-inch (7.5 cm) pieces | 250 g |
| 3 | cloves garlic, chopped | 3 |
| 1 tbsp | freshly squeezed lemon juice | 15 mL |
| 1 tsp | salt, divided | 5 mL |
| $\frac{1}{2}$ tsp | freshly ground black pepper | 2 mL |
| $\frac{1}{2}$ | loaf (1 lb/500 g) day-old vegan French bread, cut into 2-inch (5 cm) pieces | $\frac{1}{2}$ |
| 1 | package (12.3 oz/350 g) firm silken tofu | 1 |
| 4 oz | medium regular tofu | 125 g |
| 1 cup | plain non-dairy milk | 250 mL |
| $\frac{1}{4}$ cup | dry white wine | 60 mL |
| 2 tbsp | cornstarch | 30 mL |
| 2 tsp | Dijon mustard | 10 mL |
| 1 tsp | onion powder | 5 mL |
| $\frac{1}{4}$ tsp | ground turmeric | 1 mL |
| 1 tbsp | fresh tarragon leaves | 15 mL |
| 1 tsp | herbes de Provence | 5 mL |

1. Place a large skillet over medium heat and let pan get hot. Add oil and tip pan to coat. Add leeks and cook, stirring occasionally, for 3 to 4 minutes. Add asparagus, garlic, lemon juice, $\frac{1}{2}$ tsp (2 mL) of the salt and pepper and cook until asparagus turns bright green, 2 to 3 minutes. Remove from heat, stir in bread and transfer to prepared baking dish.

## Tip

Choose your favorite non-dairy milk, such as soy, almond, rice or hemp.

**2.** In food processor, combine silken and medium tofu, milk, wine, cornstarch, mustard, onion powder, $\frac{1}{2}$ tsp (2 mL) of salt and turmeric and process until very smooth. Add tarragon and herbes de Provence and process until blended. Pour mixture over vegetables and bread. Cover strata and refrigerate for at least 2 hours or up to overnight for bread to absorb custard.

**3.** Preheat oven to 350°F (180°C).

**4.** Remove strata from refrigerator and allow it to warm to room temperature. Uncover and bake in preheated oven until slightly puffed and firm, 45 minutes to 1 hour. Let stand for 6 to 8 minutes before cutting to serve.

---

▸ **Health Tip**

Tarragon has a very high antioxidant value.

---

# Mushroom Spinach Quiche

*Quiche is a hearty breakfast, or a meal in itself at other times of the day. Use your favorite mushrooms in this dish to impart the flavors you love.*

**Makes 6 servings**

## Tip

To wash or not wash mushrooms? You can either wipe them with a damp cloth or quickly rinse them under cold water and immediately wrap in a clean, dry kitchen towel or paper towels to absorb excess moisture.

- 9-inch (23 cm) pie plate or quiche dish
- Pie weights or dried beans

| | Pastry for a single-crust 9-inch (23 cm) pie | |
|---|---|---|
| 8 cups | lightly packed fresh baby spinach (6 oz/175 g) | 2 L |
| 1 tbsp | butter | 15 mL |
| 1 | small onion, finely chopped | 1 |
| 1½ cups | chopped assorted mushrooms (such as cremini, shiitake and white button) | 375 mL |
| ¼ tsp | dried thyme | 1 mL |
| ¾ cup | shredded Jarlsberg or Cheddar cheese | 175 mL |
| 3 | large eggs | 3 |
| 1 cup | milk or light (5%) cream | 250 mL |
| ¼ tsp | salt | 1 mL |
| ¼ tsp | freshly ground black pepper | 1 mL |
| | Freshly grated nutmeg | |

1. On a lightly floured surface, roll out pastry to a 12-inch (30 cm) round. Fit into pie plate and trim edge, leaving a generous ½-inch (1 cm) overhang. Turn pastry edge under and crimp edge. Prick pastry bottom in several places with a fork. Refrigerate for 30 minutes.

2. Preheat oven to 425°F (220°C) and arrange oven rack in bottom third of oven.

3. Line pastry with a sheet of parchment paper or foil and fill with pie weights. Bake in lower third of oven for 10 minutes. Remove pie weights and bake for 5 minutes more or until edges are golden. Place on rack to cool. Reduce oven temperature to 375°F (190°C).

4. Rinse spinach and shake off excess water. Heat a large nonstick skillet over medium-high heat. Cook spinach, stirring often, until just wilted. (Or place in covered casserole dish and microwave on High for 1½ to 2 minutes.) Squeeze out excess moisture and chop. (There should be ½ cup/125 mL.) Set aside.

| Nutrients per serving | |
|---|---|
| Calories | 245 |
| Fat | 14 g |
| Carbohydrate | 20 g |
| Protein | 12 g |
| Vitamin C | 12 mg |
| Vitamin D | 44 IU |
| Vitamin E | 1 mg |
| Niacin | 2 mg |
| Folate | 109 mcg |
| Vitamin B$_6$ | 0 mg |
| Vitamin B$_{12}$ | 0.5 mcg |
| Zinc | 1.2 mg |
| Selenium | 17 mcg |

The taste of freshly grated nutmeg is so much better than the preground variety. Whole nutmeg can be found in the spice section of your supermarket or bulk food store. Use a rasp grater (such as a Microplane) to grate nutmeg.

**5.** In same nonstick skillet, melt butter over medium-high heat. Add onion, mushrooms and thyme and cook, stirring, for 3 to 4 minutes or until mushrooms are softened. Let cool slightly.

**6.** Sprinkle pastry with cheese, then with mushroom mixture and spinach. In a bowl, whisk together eggs, milk, salt, pepper and nutmeg to taste. Pour evenly into pie crust.

**7.** Bake for about 35 minutes or until a knife inserted in the center comes out clean. Transfer to a rack and let stand for 10 minutes before serving.

## Variation

*Broccoli Mushroom Quiche:* Instead of spinach, substitute $1\frac{1}{2}$ cups (375 mL) small broccoli florets. Blanch broccoli in boiling water for 1 minute or until crisp and bright green. (Or place in a covered glass dish with 2 tbsp/30 mL water and microwave on High for 1 to $1\frac{1}{2}$ minutes, until crisp and bright green.) Plunge into cold water to chill, then drain. Add to pie shell along with mushrooms.

> ### ▸ Health Tip
>
> In traditional medical systems, nutmeg has been used for centuries to support the digestive system — it is rich in essential oils and antioxidant compounds.

# Home-Style Pancakes

*This dish is a whole-grain dream, and about as far away from white flour, high-glycemic-index pancakes as you can get. The flavors here come from vanilla and the natural nutty flavor of the grains.*

## Tip

Choose your favorite gluten-free non-dairy milk, such as soy, rice, almond or potato-based milk, or if you can tolerate lactose, use regular 1% milk.

| | | |
|---|---|---:|
| ½ cup | sorghum flour | 125 mL |
| ½ cup | brown rice flour | 125 mL |
| 2 tbsp | psyllium husks | 30 mL |
| 1 tsp | gluten-free baking powder | 5 mL |
| ¼ tsp | baking soda | 1 mL |
| ¼ tsp | salt | 1 mL |
| 1 | large egg | 1 |
| 1 cup | fortified gluten-free non-dairy milk or lactose-free 1% milk | 250 mL |
| 1 tbsp | liquid honey, pure maple syrup or agave nectar | 15 mL |
| 2 tsp | grapeseed oil | 10 mL |
| 1 tsp | vanilla extract | 5 mL |
| | Butter or grapeseed oil | |

1. In a large bowl, combine sorghum flour, brown rice flour, psyllium, baking powder, baking soda and salt.

2. In another bowl, beat egg, milk, honey, oil and vanilla. Pour into flour mixture and whisk for about 1 minute or until smooth.

3. On a griddle or in a nonstick skillet, melt 1 tsp (5 mL) butter over medium heat. For each pancake, pour in ¼ cup (60 mL) batter. Cook for 1 to 2 minutes or until bubbles start to form and edges are firm. Flip over and cook other side for 1 to 2 minutes or until bottom is golden. Transfer to a plate and keep warm. Repeat with the remaining batter, greasing griddle and adjusting heat between batches as needed.

## ▸ Health Tip

This dish is an excellent source of dietary fiber. Not only does that help regulate the GI tract, but sources of fiber like whole grains and psyllium help bind some toxins in the gut and whisk them out of the body before they can be reabsorbed.

### Nutrients per pancake

| | |
|---|---:|
| Calories | 139 |
| Fat | 3 g |
| Carbohydrate | 24 g |
| Protein | 4 g |
| Vitamin C | 0 mg |
| Vitamin D | 21 IU |
| Vitamin E | 1 mg |
| Niacin | 1 mg |
| Folate | 8 mcg |
| Vitamin B6 | 0.1 mg |
| Vitamin B12 | 0.4 mcg |
| Zinc | 0.5 mg |
| Selenium | 3 mcg |

# Walnut Flax Waffles

*This is a hearty waffle that has the flavors of maple syrup and vanilla (very comforting) and the crunch of walnuts.*

## Makes 8 waffles

### Tip

Look for packages of ready-ground flax seeds, which may be labeled "flaxseed meal," or use a spice or coffee grinder to grind whole flax seeds to a very fine meal.

- Preheat waffle maker to medium-high
- Blender

| | | |
|---|---|---|
| 1$\frac{1}{2}$ cups | plain almond milk | 375 mL |
| 2 tbsp | vegetable oil | 30 mL |
| 1 tbsp | pure maple syrup | 15 mL |
| 2 tsp | vanilla extract | 10 mL |
| 1$\frac{1}{2}$ tsp | cider vinegar | 7 mL |
| 3 tbsp | ground flax seeds (flaxseed meal) | 45 mL |
| 1 cup | whole wheat flour | 250 mL |
| 1$\frac{1}{2}$ tsp | baking powder | 7 mL |
| $\frac{1}{2}$ tsp | baking soda | 2 mL |
| $\frac{1}{8}$ tsp | fine sea salt | 0.5 mL |
| $\frac{1}{2}$ cup | chopped toasted walnuts | 125 mL |
| | Nonstick cooking spray | |

1. In blender, combine almond milk, oil, maple syrup, vanilla and vinegar. Let stand for 10 minutes. Add flax seeds and blend for 1 minute or until slightly frothy.

2. In a large bowl, whisk together flour, baking powder, baking soda and salt. Add almond milk mixture and stir until just blended. Gently stir in walnuts.

3. Spray preheated waffle maker with cooking spray. For each waffle, pour about $\frac{1}{3}$ cup (75 mL) batter into waffle maker. Cook according to manufacturer's instructions until golden brown.

## Nutrients per waffle

| | |
|---|---|
| Calories | 165 |
| Fat | 10 g |
| Carbohydrate | 16 g |
| Protein | 5 g |
| Vitamin C | 0 mg |
| Vitamin D | 19 IU |
| Vitamin E | 1 mg |
| Niacin | 1 mg |
| Folate | 11 mcg |
| Vitamin B$_6$ | 0.1 mg |
| Vitamin B$_{12}$ | 0.0 mcg |
| Zinc | 0.8 mg |
| Selenium | 11 mcg |

### ▶ Health Tip

Walnuts are a good source of omega-3 fats and one of our top brain-boosting foods. Flax meal, which can be purchased vacuum-packed and kept in the fridge, is yet another good omega-3 source.

# Crêpes with Sweet Ricotta and Strawberries

*This is an intense and sweet dish, but one that makes breakfast a special event.*

## Tips

It is important to quickly pour measured batter into hot pan all at once. Use a ¼-cup (60 mL) measure and fill halfway with batter to measure 2 tbsp (30 mL).

Crêpes should not stick in a nonstick pan, but if they do, add 1 tsp (5 mL) canola oil to pan.

- Blender
- Baking sheet, lined with parchment paper

### Crêpes

| | | |
|---|---|---|
| 1 cup | all-purpose flour | 250 mL |
| 3 tbsp | packed brown sugar | 45 mL |
| ¼ tsp | salt | 1 mL |
| 1¼ cups | plain non-dairy milk | 300 mL |
| ¼ cup | canola oil | 60 mL |
| 1½ tsp | vanilla extract | 7 mL |
| 1 tsp | almond extract | 5 mL |

### Filling

| | | |
|---|---|---|
| 1½ cups | Basic Ricotta (see recipe, opposite) | 375 mL |
| 3 cups | strawberries, chopped, divided | 750 mL |
| ¼ cup | confectioners' (icing) sugar (or to taste) | 60 mL |
| 1 tsp | ground cinnamon | 5 mL |
| 1½ cups | vegan crème fraîche | 375 mL |

1. *Crêpes:* In blender, combine flour, brown sugar, salt, milk, oil and vanilla and almond extracts and pulse until just combined, about 10 seconds. Transfer batter to an airtight container and refrigerate for at least 1 hour or up to 24 hours.

2. *Filling:* In a bowl, combine ricotta, ¾ cup (175 mL) of the strawberries, sugar and cinnamon and set aside.

3. Place nonstick skillet over medium heat and let pan get hot. Pour 2 tbsp (30 mL) batter into center of pan, tipping pan to spread batter out to a 5-inch (12.5 cm) crêpe. (If batter is a little thick, adjust before pouring next crêpe by thinning with milk or water.) Cook until golden, about 30 seconds. Flip and cook for another 15 seconds. Transfer crêpes to prepared baking sheet and let cool. Repeat process with remaining batter, adjusting heat as necessary between crêpes.

| Nutrients per serving | |
|---|---|
| Calories | 601 |
| Fat | 30 g |
| Carbohydrate | 69 g |
| Protein | 16 g |
| Vitamin C | 74 mg |
| Vitamin D | 33 IU |
| Vitamin E | 4 mg |
| Niacin | 3 mg |
| Folate | 108 mcg |
| Vitamin B$_6$ | 0.2 mg |
| Vitamin B$_{12}$ | 0.7 mcg |
| Zinc | 1.5 mg |
| Selenium | 11 mcg |

## Tip

Cooked and unfilled crêpes may be stacked, divided by sheets of waxed paper, wrapped and refrigerated for up to 2 days or frozen for up to 2 months.

**4.** To serve, spoon 2 to 3 tbsp (30 to 45 mL) of ricotta filling down one side of crêpe and roll, starting at filled side. Spoon 2 tbsp (30 mL) of the crème fraîche over each crêpe, top with chopped strawberries and serve immediately.

> ▶ **Health Tip**
>
> Strawberries are a brain-friendly food. Make sure to wash them well, or just use organic strawberries, as this is a crop that is sprayed with many pesticides. Cinnamon is a good blood sugar regulator and balances the high carb and high sugar content of this dish.

# Basic Ricotta

*Whip up this basic ricotta in a snap. It is neither sweet nor savory, thus perfectly suited as a base for recipes.*

### Makes about 3¾ cups (925 mL)

• **Immersion blender**

| 16 oz | extra-firm tofu, in water, drained | 500 g |
|---|---|---|
| 8 oz | firm or extra-firm silken tofu, drained | 250 g |
| 1 tsp | granulated sugar | 5 mL |
| 1 tsp | freshly squeezed lemon juice | 5 mL |
| 2 tsp | grapeseed oil | 10 mL |
| ¾ tsp | salt | 3 mL |

**1.** In a large bowl, combine extra-firm and silken tofus and, using a potato masher, mash into small crumbs.

**2.** In a small bowl, combine sugar, lemon juice, oil and salt. Add to tofu mixture. Using immersion blender, pulse on and off until mixture is semi-smooth but still very grainy. (If immersion blender is not available, continue with potato masher.)

**3.** Refrigerate in an airtight container for up to 10 days.

### Nutrients per ½ cup (125 mL)

| | |
|---|---|
| Calories | 119 |
| Fat | 7 g |
| Carbohydrate | 4 g |
| Protein | 12 g |
| Vitamin C | 0 mg |
| Vitamin D | 0 IU |
| Vitamin E | 0 mg |
| Niacin | 0 mg |
| Folate | 18 mcg |
| Vitamin B$_6$ | 0.0 mg |
| Vitamin B$_{12}$ | 0.0 mcg |
| Zinc | 1.1 mg |
| Selenium | 11 mcg |

# Chocolate Chip Oat Breakfast Biscuits

*Here is a quick breakfast energy source that is easy to get interested in.*

**Makes 8 biscuits**

## Tips

Ragged dough looks moistened but doesn't form a ball.

This recipe can be doubled. The biscuits can also be patted out into a circle and cut into pie-shaped wedges or cut into hearts or circles with biscuit or cookie cutters.

- **Preheat oven to 400°F (200°C)**
- **Baking sheet, lined with parchment paper**

| | | |
|---|---|---:|
| 1½ cups | all-purpose flour | 375 mL |
| ¾ cup | large-flake (old-fashioned) rolled oats | 175 mL |
| ½ cup | semisweet chocolate chips | 125 mL |
| ¼ cup | granulated sugar | 60 mL |
| 1 tbsp | baking powder | 15 mL |
| ¼ tsp | salt | 1 mL |
| 1¼ cups | heavy or whipping (35%) cream | 300 mL |

### Topping (Optional)

| | | |
|---|---|---:|
| 2 tbsp | heavy or whipping (35%) cream | 30 mL |

### Glaze

| | | |
|---|---|---:|
| ¾ cup | confectioners' (icing) sugar, sifted | 175 mL |
| 4 tsp | orange juice | 20 mL |

1. In a large bowl, mix together flour, oats, chocolate chips, sugar, baking powder and salt.

2. Stir in cream, mixing just until dough is soft and ragged (see tip, at left).

3. Turn out dough onto a lightly floured work surface and gently shape into an 8- by 6-inch (20 by 15 cm) rectangle. Using a sharp knife, cut into 8 pieces. Transfer biscuits to prepared baking sheet, making sure they do not touch or overlap.

4. *Topping:* If desired, lightly brush the tops with cream.

5. Bake in preheated oven for about 20 minutes or until crisp and golden brown. Transfer biscuits to a rack to cool.

6. *Glaze:* In a medium bowl, whisk together confectioners' sugar and orange juice until smooth. Dip tops of cooled biscuits in glaze or drizzle glaze over top. Let biscuits stand on a rack until glaze hardens.

### Nutrients per biscuit

| | |
|---|---:|
| Calories | 393 |
| Fat | 18 g |
| Carbohydrate | 54 g |
| Protein | 6 g |
| Vitamin C | 2 mg |
| Vitamin D | 10 IU |
| Vitamin E | 0 mg |
| Niacin | 2 mg |
| Folate | 55 mcg |
| Vitamin B$_6$ | 0.0 mg |
| Vitamin B$_{12}$ | 0.1 mcg |
| Zinc | 1.0 mg |
| Selenium | 1 mcg |

> ▸ **Health Tip**
>
> Oats provide a balancing whole grain — but clearly this dish is more about fun.

# SNACKS AND APPETIZERS

# Cranberry Walnut Muffins

*The cranberry is praised as a sauce at the Thanksgiving table, but the ruby fruit is just as delicious when baked into muffins.*

**Makes 12 muffins**

## Tips

Look for packages of ready-ground flax seeds, which may be labeled "flaxseed meal," or use a spice or coffee grinder to grind whole flax seeds to a very fine meal.

Toast walnut halves in a dry skillet over low heat, stirring constantly, for 3 to 4 minutes or until fragrant. Transfer the toasted nuts to a plate and let cool before chopping.

- **Preheat oven to 350°F (180°C)**
- **12-cup muffin pan, greased**

| | | |
|---|---|---|
| 1¼ cups | whole wheat pastry flour | 300 mL |
| ¼ cup | wheat germ | 60 mL |
| 1½ tsp | baking powder | 7 mL |
| 1 tsp | ground cinnamon | 5 mL |
| ½ tsp | salt | 2 mL |
| ¼ tsp | baking soda | 1 mL |
| 2 | large eggs | 2 |
| ¼ cup | ground flax seeds (flaxseed meal) | 60 mL |
| ½ cup | agave nectar | 125 mL |
| ⅓ cup | low-fat (1%) plain yogurt | 75 mL |
| ¼ cup | vegetable oil | 60 mL |
| 1 tsp | vanilla extract | 5 mL |
| 1 cup | fresh cranberries, coarsely chopped | 250 mL |
| 1 cup | chopped toasted walnuts | 250 mL |

1. In a large bowl, whisk together flour, wheat germ, baking powder, cinnamon, salt and baking soda.

2. In a medium bowl, whisk together eggs, flax seeds, agave nectar, yogurt, oil and vanilla until well blended.

3. Add the egg mixture to the flour mixture and stir until just blended. Gently fold in cranberries and walnuts.

4. Divide batter equally among prepared muffin cups.

5. Bake in preheated oven for 20 to 25 minutes or until tops are golden and a toothpick inserted in the center comes out clean. Let cool in pan on a wire rack for 5 minutes, then transfer to the rack to cool.

> ▸ **Health Tip**
>
> Cranberries are loaded with disease-fighting antioxidants and are a good source of vitamin C, fiber, manganese and potassium.

## Nutrients per muffin

| | |
|---|---|
| Calories | 235 |
| Fat | 13 g |
| Carbohydrate | 25 g |
| Protein | 6 g |
| Vitamin C | 2 mg |
| Vitamin D | 7 IU |
| Vitamin E | 1 mg |
| Niacin | 0 mg |
| Folate | 21 mcg |
| Vitamin B$_6$ | 0.1 mg |
| Vitamin B$_{12}$ | 0.1 mcg |
| Zinc | 0.9 mg |
| Selenium | 7 mcg |

# Cranberry, Carrot and Apple Teff Muffins

*Here is a gluten-free muffin recipe that has a host of brain-supportive nutrients and is easy to prepare.*

**Makes 12 muffins**

## Tip

Toast pecan halves in a dry skillet over low heat, stirring constantly, for 3 to 4 minutes or until fragrant. Transfer the toasted nuts to a plate and let cool before chopping.

- Preheat oven to 350°F (180°C)
- 12-cup muffin pan, greased

| | | |
|---|---|---|
| 2 cups | teff flour | 500 mL |
| ½ cup | tapioca flour | 125 mL |
| 2 tsp | gluten-free baking powder | 10 mL |
| 1 tsp | pumpkin pie spice | 5 mL |
| 1 tsp | xanthan gum | 5 mL |
| ½ tsp | baking soda | 2 mL |
| ½ tsp | salt | 2 mL |
| 1 | large egg | 1 |
| ½ cup | unsweetened apple juice | 125 mL |
| ½ cup | unsweetened applesauce | 125 mL |
| ½ cup | pure maple syrup | 125 mL |
| ⅓ cup | vegetable oil | 75 mL |
| 1 cup | finely shredded carrots | 250 mL |
| 1 cup | chopped peeled apple | 250 mL |
| ½ cup | chopped toasted pecans | 125 mL |
| ½ cup | dried cranberries | 125 mL |

1. In a large bowl, whisk together teff flour, tapioca flour, baking powder, pumpkin pie spice, xanthan gum, baking soda and salt.

2. In a medium bowl, whisk together egg, apple juice, applesauce, maple syrup and oil until well blended.

3. Add the egg mixture to the flour mixture and stir until just blended. Gently fold in carrots, apple, pecans and cranberries.

4. Divide batter equally among prepared muffin cups.

5. Bake in preheated oven for 25 to 30 minutes or until a toothpick inserted in the center comes out clean. Let cool in pan on a wire rack for 5 minutes, then transfer to the rack to cool.

### Nutrients per muffin

| | |
|---|---|
| Calories | 254 |
| Fat | 11 g |
| Carbohydrate | 38 g |
| Protein | 4 g |
| Vitamin C | 1 mg |
| Vitamin D | 3 IU |
| Vitamin E | 1 mg |
| Niacin | 1 mg |
| Folate | 5 mcg |
| Vitamin $B_6$ | 0.2 mg |
| Vitamin $B_{12}$ | 0.0 mcg |
| Zinc | 1.7 mg |
| Selenium | 3 mcg |

# Date and Walnut Muffins

*This gluten-free muffin provides a great energy boost and healthy snacks for a few days, or for one hungry family.*

**Makes 12 muffins**

> ▶ **Health Tip**
>
> Walnuts have lots of vitamin E in a rather unusual form, gamma-tocopherol, which has cardiovascular benefits.

- Preheat oven to 350°F (180°C)
- 12-cup muffin pan, lined with paper liners

| | | |
|---|---|---|
| ¾ cup | chopped dates | 175 mL |
| ⅔ cup | boiling water | 150 mL |
| 1½ cups | Brown Rice Flour Blend (see recipe, opposite) | 375 mL |
| 1 tsp | xanthan gum | 5 mL |
| ¾ tsp | gluten-free baking powder | 3 mL |
| ¾ tsp | baking soda | 3 mL |
| ¾ tsp | ground cinnamon | 3 mL |
| ½ tsp | salt | 2 mL |
| ¾ cup | packed dark brown sugar | 175 mL |
| 6 tbsp | unsalted butter, softened | 90 mL |
| 2 | large eggs | 2 |
| 1 tsp | vanilla extract | 5 mL |
| ¾ cup | chopped toasted walnuts | 175 mL |

1. In a small bowl, combine dates and boiling water. Let stand for 10 minutes (do not drain).

2. In a medium bowl, whisk together flour blend, xanthan gum, baking powder, baking soda, cinnamon and salt.

3. In a large bowl, using an electric mixer on medium speed, beat brown sugar and butter until light and fluffy. Beat in eggs, one at a time, until well blended. Beat in vanilla until blended. Beat in date mixture.

4. Add the flour mixture to the egg mixture and, using a wooden spoon, stir until just blended. Gently fold in walnuts.

5. Divide batter equally among prepared muffin cups.

6. Bake in preheated oven for 16 to 20 minutes or until a toothpick inserted in the center comes out clean. Let cool in pan on a wire rack for 5 minutes, then transfer to the rack to cool.

**Nutrients** per muffin

| | |
|---|---|
| Calories | 263 |
| Fat | 12 g |
| Carbohydrate | 38 g |
| Protein | 4 g |
| Vitamin C | 0 mg |
| Vitamin D | 11 IU |
| Vitamin E | 1 mg |
| Niacin | 1 mg |
| Folate | 11 mcg |
| Vitamin $B_6$ | 0.2 mg |
| Vitamin $B_{12}$ | 0.1 mcg |
| Zinc | 0.7 mg |
| Selenium | 4 mcg |

# Brown Rice Flour Blend

*If you are going to do some gluten-free baking, this is a key component for some of the recipes in this book. You can also purchase blends at many supermarkets and certainly at gluten-free shops or health food stores.*

**Makes 3 cups (750 mL)**

## Tips

You can also make the blend in smaller amounts by using the basic proportions: 2 parts finely ground brown rice flour, $\frac{2}{3}$ part potato starch and $\frac{1}{3}$ part tapioca starch.

You can double, triple or quadruple the recipe to have it on hand.

| | | |
|---|---|---|
| 2 cups | finely ground brown rice flour | 500 mL |
| $\frac{2}{3}$ cup | potato starch | 150 mL |
| $\frac{1}{3}$ cup | tapioca starch | 75 mL |

**1.** In a bowl, whisk together brown rice flour, potato starch and tapioca starch.

**2.** Store in an airtight container in the refrigerator for up to 4 months, or in the freezer for up to 1 year. Let warm to room temperature before using.

> ▶ **Health Tip**
>
> Flour made from a whole grain, like brown rice flour, still contains most of its original vitamins and minerals.

## Nutrients per 2 tbsp (30 mL)

| | |
|---|---|
| Calories | 68 |
| Fat | 0 g |
| Carbohydrate | 15 g |
| Protein | 1 g |
| Vitamin C | 0 mg |
| Vitamin D | 0 IU |
| Vitamin E | 0 mg |
| Niacin | 1 mg |
| Folate | 3 mcg |
| Vitamin $B_6$ | 0.1 mg |
| Vitamin $B_{12}$ | 0.0 mcg |
| Zinc | 0.3 mg |
| Selenium | 0 mcg |

# Millet and Flax Muffins

*When muffins have great flavor, as these do, it's easy to forget they're a healthier alternative. Serve them to accompany any chicken dish when you want to wow your friends.*

## Tip

Choose your favorite gluten-free non-dairy milk, such as soy, rice, almond or potato-based milk, or if you tolerate lactose, use regular 1% milk.

- **Preheat oven to 350°F (180°C)**
- **12-cup muffin pan, 9 cups lined with paper liners**

| | | |
|---|---|---|
| ½ cup | millet grits | 125 mL |
| ¼ cup | brown rice flour | 60 mL |
| ¼ cup | ground flax seeds (flaxseed meal) | 60 mL |
| 2 tsp | gluten-free baking powder | 10 mL |
| 1 | large egg | 1 |
| 2 tbsp | granulated raw cane sugar | 30 mL |
| ½ cup | lactose-free 1% milk or fortified gluten-free non-dairy milk | 125 mL |
| 2 tbsp | unsweetened applesauce | 30 mL |

1. In a large bowl, whisk together millet grits, brown rice flour, flax seeds and baking powder.

2. In a medium bowl, whisk together egg, sugar, milk and applesauce until well combined. Pour over dry ingredients and stir until combined.

3. Spoon batter into prepared muffin cups, dividing equally. Bake in preheated oven for 15 to 20 minutes or until a tester inserted in the center comes out clean. Let cool in pan on a wire rack for 5 minutes. Transfer muffins to rack to cool.

> ▸ **Health Tip**
>
> Millet is a tasty gluten-free seed that is high in B-complex vitamins.

### Nutrients per muffin

| | |
|---|---|
| Calories | 102 |
| Fat | 3 g |
| Carbohydrate | 17 g |
| Protein | 3 g |
| Vitamin C | 0 mg |
| Vitamin D | 10 IU |
| Vitamin E | 0 mg |
| Niacin | 1 mg |
| Folate | 17 mcg |
| Vitamin B$_6$ | 0.1 mg |
| Vitamin B$_{12}$ | 0.2 mcg |
| Zinc | 0.6 mg |
| Selenium | 3 mcg |

# Trail Mix

*You don't need to be hiking to enjoy this trail mix — it's an excellent high-energy snack where every bite counts nutritionally.*

**Makes 3½ cups (875 mL)**

## Tip

Start with this basic recipe and sub in other ingredients depending on what strikes your fancy and what you have on hand. Good additions include raisins, shredded coconut, hazelnuts and even chunks of dark chocolate. Be creative — trail mix can be a little different every time you make it!

| | | |
|---|---|---|
| ½ cup | dried apricots, cut into quarters | 125 mL |
| ½ cup | dried cranberries | 125 mL |
| ½ cup | dried goji berries (optional) | 125 mL |
| ½ cup | whole almonds | 125 mL |
| ½ cup | chopped walnuts | 125 mL |
| ½ cup | unsalted sunflower seeds | 125 mL |
| ½ cup | raw green pumpkin seeds (pepitas) | 125 mL |

1. In a large bowl, combine apricots, cranberries, goji berries (if using), almonds, walnuts, sunflower seeds and pumpkin seeds.

2. Store in an airtight container at room temperature for up 1 month.

> ▸ **Health Tip**
>
> Every ingredient in this trail mix is a concentrated source of antioxidants or healthy fats. This high-energy pick-me-up will leave your body better nourished and get you through your afternoon.

**Nutrients** per ¼ cup (60 mL)

| | |
|---|---|
| Calories | 144 |
| Fat | 11 g |
| Carbohydrate | 10 g |
| Protein | 5 g |
| Vitamin C | 0 mg |
| Vitamin D | 0 IU |
| Vitamin E | 3 mg |
| Niacin | 1 mg |
| Folate | 15 mcg |
| Vitamin $B_6$ | 0.1 mg |
| Vitamin $B_{12}$ | 0 mcg |
| Zinc | 0.6 mg |
| Selenium | 5 mcg |

# Cinnamon Apple Chips

*Combining the tart and sweet flavor of apples with the natural sweetness of stevia and cinnamon, this is an enjoyable but low-glycemic-index treat.*

## Makes 8 servings

## Tip

Be sure to transfer the chips from the parchment paper to a wire rack while still warm, or they will stick.

- **Preheat oven to 325°F (160°C)**
- **2 rimmed baking sheets, lined with parchment paper**

| | | |
|---|---|---|
| 4 | large tart-sweet apples (such as Braeburn, Gala or Pippin), halved and cored | 4 |
| 4 tsp | stevia powder | 20 mL |
| ½ tsp | ground cinnamon | 2 mL |
| | Nonstick cooking spray (preferably olive oil) | |

1. Using a very sharp knife or a mandoline, cut apples into ⅛-inch (3 mm) thick slices.

2. In a small bowl, combine stevia and cinnamon.

3. Arrange apple slices in a single layer on prepared baking sheets. Spray with cooking spray and sprinkle with stevia mixture.

4. Bake in preheated oven for 35 to 40 minutes or until edges are browned and slices are dry and crispy. Transfer chips to a wire rack and let cool completely (they will crisp more as they cool). Store in an airtight container at room temperature for up to 1 week.

## Variation

*Pear Chips:* Use 4 medium Bosc pears, halved and cored, in place of the apples.

---

> ▶ **Health Tip**
>
> Recent studies indicate that eating as little as ½ tsp (2 mL) of ground cinnamon per day can boost cognitive function and memory.

### Nutrients per serving

| | |
|---|---|
| Calories | 59 |
| Fat | 0 g |
| Carbohydrate | 16 g |
| Protein | 0 g |
| Vitamin C | 5 mg |
| Vitamin D | 0 IU |
| Vitamin E | 0 mg |
| Niacin | 0 mg |
| Folate | 3 mcg |
| Vitamin $B_6$ | 0.1 mg |
| Vitamin $B_{12}$ | 0.0 mcg |
| Zinc | 0.1 mg |
| Selenium | 0 mcg |

# Holy Smokes Pita Chips

*These are the perfect accompaniment to guacamole, instead of fried nacho chips. Or serve with Warm Green Goddess Dip (page 213).*

(page 213)

**Makes 48 wedges**

## Tips

For ease in cutting, stack 2 to 3 pitas together before cutting them into wedges.

These chips will stay crisp in a sealable plastic bag or airtight container for up to 7 days.

- Preheat oven to 375°F (190°C)

| | | |
|---|---|---:|
| 2 | cloves garlic, finely minced | 2 |
| 2 tsp | ground cumin | 10 mL |
| 1/2 tsp | chili powder | 2 mL |
| 1/2 tsp | paprika | 2 mL |
| 1/2 tsp | curry powder | 2 mL |
| 1/2 tsp | freshly ground black pepper | 2 mL |
| 1/4 tsp | salt | 1 mL |
| 1 to 2 tbsp | canola oil | 15 to 30 mL |
| 2 to 3 | drops hot pepper sauce | 2 to 3 |
| 6 | 6-inch (15 cm) whole wheat pitas | 6 |

1. In a small bowl, combine garlic, cumin, chili powder, paprika, curry powder, black pepper, salt, oil and hot pepper sauce to taste.

2. Using a pastry brush, coat both sides of each pita with spice mixture and cut each into 8 wedges. Spread wedges in a single layer on two baking sheets.

3. Bake in preheated oven, turning once, for 8 to 10 minutes or until pitas are brown and crisp. Let cool completely on pans on a wire rack.

*This recipe courtesy of dietitian Mary Sue Waisman.*

### Nutrients per 4 wedges

| | |
|---|---:|
| Calories | 98 |
| Fat | 2 g |
| Carbohydrate | 18 g |
| Protein | 3 g |
| Vitamin C | 0 mg |
| Vitamin D | 0 IU |
| Vitamin E | 1 mg |
| Niacin | 1 mg |
| Folate | 12 mcg |
| Vitamin $B_6$ | 0.1 mg |
| Vitamin $B_{12}$ | 0.0 mcg |
| Zinc | 0.5 mg |
| Selenium | 14 mcg |

# PB&J Energy Balls

*Peanuts and dried blueberries share more than an affinity for each other in this delicious snack: they both contain a naturally occurring compound called resveratrol. According to recent studies, resveratrol appears to reduce fat stores in the human body.*

**Makes 24 balls**

## Tips

Look for roasted peanuts lightly seasoned with sea salt.

Store energy balls in an airtight container in the refrigerator for up to 1 week. Or wrap them in plastic wrap, then foil, completely enclosing them, and freeze for up to 6 months. Let thaw at room temperature for 1 hour before serving.

- **Food processor**

| | | |
|---|---|---|
| 2½ cups | large-flake (old-fashioned) rolled oats, divided | 625 mL |
| ⅔ cup | dried blueberries, cranberries or cherries | 150 mL |
| Pinch | fine sea salt | Pinch |
| ½ cup | unsweetened natural peanut butter | 125 mL |
| 3 tbsp | brown rice syrup or liquid honey | 45 mL |
| 1 tsp | vanilla extract | 5 mL |
| ½ cup | lightly salted roasted peanuts, chopped | 125 mL |

1. In food processor, pulse ½ cup (125 mL) of the oats until powdery. Transfer to a small dish.
2. In food processor (no need to clean it), pulse the remaining oats until finely chopped. Add blueberries, salt, peanut butter, brown rice syrup and vanilla; pulse until mixture forms a dough.
3. Transfer dough to a medium bowl and knead in peanuts.
4. Roll dough into 24 balls of equal size. Roll balls in ground oats to coat. Transfer to an airtight container and refrigerate for 1 hour.

> ▸ **Health Tip**
>
> Peanuts contain high levels of niacin, which may help protect against Alzheimer's disease and age-related cognitive problems.

## Nutrients per ball

| | |
|---|---|
| Calories | 142 |
| Fat | 6 g |
| Carbohydrate | 18 g |
| Protein | 5 g |
| Vitamin C | 0 mg |
| Vitamin D | 0 IU |
| Vitamin E | 1 mg |
| Niacin | 2 mg |
| Folate | 18 mcg |
| Vitamin $B_6$ | 0.1 mg |
| Vitamin $B_{12}$ | 0.0 mcg |
| Zinc | 1.0 mg |
| Selenium | 3 mcg |

# Cashew Butter

*Easy and delicious, this nut butter is great for breakfast on toasted whole wheat bread. It is also a very good substitute for tahini, a sesame paste, because it is milder than peanut butter, which is often used to replace tahini.*

## Makes 2½ cups (625 mL)

## Tip

Brown rice syrup has a light, mild flavor and a similar appearance to honey, though it is less sweet.

### Blender or food processor

| | | |
|---|---|---|
| ½ cup | unsweetened apple juice | 125 mL |
| 2 cups | lightly salted roasted cashews | 500 mL |
| 2 tbsp | brown rice syrup | 30 mL |
| 2 tbsp | freshly squeezed lemon juice | 30 mL |

1. In blender, combine apple juice, cashews, rice syrup and lemon juice. Blend until smooth.
2. Transfer to a clean container with lid. Store spread, tightly covered, in the refrigerator for up to 1 week.

## Nutrients per 1 tbsp (15 mL)

| | |
|---|---|
| Calories | 42 |
| Fat | 3 g |
| Carbohydrate | 3 g |
| Protein | 1 g |
| Vitamin C | 0 mg |
| Vitamin D | 0 IU |
| Vitamin E | 0 mg |
| Niacin | 0 mg |
| Folate | 5 mcg |
| Vitamin $B_6$ | 0.0 mg |
| Vitamin $B_{12}$ | 0.0 mcg |
| Zinc | 0.4 mg |
| Selenium | 1 mcg |

# Chunky Guacamole

*This rich and creamy guacamole has a full-bodied flavor that will add life to whatever it accompanies. Serve with tortilla chips, crackers or fresh vegetables.*

## Tips

Use 1 tbsp (15 mL) finely chopped pickled jalapeño peppers if fresh are not available. The added vinegar in the peppers will alter the taste slightly, so taste before adding the full tablespoon (15 mL) of pickled peppers.

If you prefer a smoother consistency, make the guacamole in a food processor.

| | | |
|---|---|---|
| 2 | avocados, peeled, pitted and quartered | 2 |
| 2 | cloves garlic, minced (about 2 tsp/10 mL) | 2 |
| 1 | small tomato, seeded and finely diced | 1 |
| 1½ tsp | freshly squeezed lime juice | 7 mL |
| 1 | jalapeño pepper, seeded and finely chopped (optional) | 1 |
| ½ tsp | hot pepper sauce (or to taste) | 2 mL |
| | Salt and freshly ground black pepper | |

**1.** In a bowl, using a fork or potato masher, mash avocados until the desired consistency is reached. Add garlic, tomato, lime juice, jalapeño pepper (if using) and hot pepper sauce. Mix well and season with salt and freshly ground black pepper to taste. Serve immediately or cover and chill. Guacamole is best eaten within a day.

### Nutrients per 2 tbsp (30 mL)

| | |
|---|---|
| Calories | 84 |
| Fat | 7 g |
| Carbohydrate | 5 g |
| Protein | 1 g |
| Vitamin C | 7 mg |
| Vitamin D | 0 IU |
| Vitamin E | 1 mg |
| Niacin | 1 mg |
| Folate | 43 mcg |
| Vitamin $B_6$ | 0.2 mg |
| Vitamin $B_{12}$ | 0.0 mcg |
| Zinc | 0.4 mg |
| Selenium | 0 mcg |

# Warm Green Goddess Dip

*Warm from the oven, this dip is sure to impress guests with its flavor and texture.*

## Makes about 2 cups (500 mL)

## Tips

To thaw frozen spinach, remove it from the package, place it in a microwave-safe bowl and defrost in the microwave until thawed, stirring occasionally. When thawed, drain and squeeze out excess water.

Serve with Holy Smokes Pita Chips (page 209) or a platter of cut-up fresh vegetables.

### Nutrients per 2 tbsp (30 mL)

| | |
|---|---|
| Calories | 77 |
| Fat | 4 g |
| Carbohydrate | 6 g |
| Protein | 4 g |
| Vitamin C | 8 mg |
| Vitamin D | 1 IU |
| Vitamin E | 1 mg |
| Niacin | 0 mg |
| Folate | 42 mcg |
| Vitamin B$_6$ | 0.1 mg |
| Vitamin B$_{12}$ | 0.1 mcg |
| Zinc | 0.4 mg |
| Selenium | 2 mcg |

- Preheat oven to 375°F (190°C)
- 8-inch (20 cm) square glass baking dish, greased

| | | |
|---|---|---|
| 1 tbsp | canola oil | 15 mL |
| 1 cup | finely chopped onion | 250 mL |
| 1/2 cup | finely chopped green onion | 125 mL |
| 1/4 cup | finely chopped red bell pepper | 60 mL |
| 3 | cloves garlic, finely minced | 3 |
| 1 | can (14 oz/398 mL) artichoke hearts, drained, patted dry and coarsely chopped | 1 |
| 1 | package (10 oz/300 g) frozen chopped spinach, thawed, squeezed dry and coarsely chopped | 1 |
| 1/4 cup | finely chopped fresh parsley, divided | 60 mL |
| 1/2 cup | light sour cream | 125 mL |
| 1/2 cup | light herb-and-garlic-flavored cream cheese | 125 mL |
| 2 tbsp | light mayonnaise | 30 mL |
| 1/4 tsp | salt | 1 mL |
| 1/4 tsp | freshly ground black pepper | 1 mL |
| 1/2 cup | shredded part-skim mozzarella cheese | 125 mL |
| 1/4 cup | freshly grated Parmesan cheese | 60 mL |

1. In a medium skillet, heat oil over medium-high heat. Sauté onion, green onion and red pepper for 3 to 5 minutes or until softened. Add garlic and sauté for 30 seconds. Remove from heat and let cool.

2. In a large bowl, combine artichoke hearts, spinach, 2 tbsp (30 mL) of the parsley, sour cream, cream cheese, mayonnaise, salt and pepper. Stir in the cooled onion mixture. Transfer to prepared baking dish.

3. Bake in preheated oven for about 20 minutes or until heated through. Remove from oven and sprinkle with the remaining parsley and the mozzarella and Parmesan. Bake for about 5 minutes or until cheese is slightly melted.

*This recipe courtesy of dietitian Mary Sue Waisman.*

# Creamy Mushroom Walnut Toasts

*This dish will satisfy and impress guests as an appetizer — or just liven up a Sunday afternoon.*

## Tip

*To make crostini:* Cut 1 thin baguette into $\frac{1}{3}$-inch (8 mm) thick slices. Arrange on baking sheet; brush lightly with 2 tbsp (30 mL) olive oil or melted butter. Bake in 375°F (190°C) oven for 5 minutes or until edges are lightly toasted.

- **Preheat oven to 375°F (190°C)**
- **Food processor**

| | | |
|---|---|---|
| 1 lb | mushrooms (an assortment of white, oyster and portobello), coarsely chopped | 500 g |
| 2 tbsp | butter | 30 mL |
| $\frac{1}{3}$ cup | finely chopped green onions | 75 mL |
| 2 | cloves garlic, minced | 2 |
| $\frac{1}{2}$ tsp | dried thyme | 2 mL |
| 4 oz | cream cheese or goat cheese, cut into pieces | 125 g |
| $\frac{1}{3}$ cup | freshly grated Parmesan cheese (plus extra for topping) | 75 mL |
| $\frac{1}{3}$ cup | finely chopped walnuts | 75 mL |
| 2 tbsp | finely chopped fresh parsley | 30 mL |
| | Salt and freshly ground black pepper | |
| 40 | crostini (see tip, at left) | 40 |

1. In food processor, finely chop mushrooms in batches using on-off turns.

2. In a large skillet, heat butter over medium-high heat. Add mushrooms, green onions, garlic and thyme; cook for 5 to 7 minutes or until mushrooms are softened. Cook 1 to 2 minutes more, if necessary, until all moisture has evaporated. (Mixture should be dry and almost crumbly.) Remove from heat.

3. Add cream cheese, stirring until smooth. Add Parmesan cheese, walnuts and parsley. Season with salt and pepper to taste. Transfer to a bowl; cover and let cool.

## Nutrients per appetizer

| | |
|---|---|
| Calories | 39 |
| Fat | 2 g |
| Carbohydrate | 3 g |
| Protein | 1 g |
| Vitamin C | 1 mg |
| Vitamin D | 2 IU |
| Vitamin E | 0 mg |
| Niacin | 1 mg |
| Folate | 7 mcg |
| Vitamin B$_6$ | 0.0 mg |
| Vitamin B$_{12}$ | 0.0 mcg |
| Zinc | 0.2 mg |
| Selenium | 1 mcg |

## Tips

Spread toasts with mushroom mixture just before baking to prevent them from turning soggy.

Mushroom-walnut filling can be frozen for up to 1 month.

**4.** Spread crostini with a generous teaspoonful (5 to 7 mL) of mushroom mixture. Arrange on baking sheet. Sprinkle tops with additional Parmesan cheese. Bake in preheated oven for 8 to 10 minutes or until edges are toasted.

> ### ▸ Health Tip
>
> Walnuts are a good source of the mineral manganese (not magnesium — manganese), which is important for joint health and is part of a very important antioxidant system that protects the cells in our body.

# Roasted Peppers Antipasto

*Go Mediterranean with this appetizer that brings out the wonderful sweetness of bell peppers.*

## Tips

To save time and trouble, core and cut peppers in half before roasting or grilling. This tends to dehydrate and shrink the flesh a little, making it fragile, but it's a heck of a lot easier.

For parties, try serving these peppers with black olives, sun-dried tomatoes, capers, sliced ripe tomatoes, mozzarella or bocconcini cheese, artichoke hearts and marinated mushrooms to create a real Italian appetizer extravaganza.

### Nutrients per serving

| | |
|---|---|
| Calories | 231 |
| Fat | 20 g |
| Carbohydrate | 7 g |
| Protein | 6 g |
| Vitamin C | 115 mg |
| Vitamin D | 3 IU |
| Vitamin E | 3 mg |
| Niacin | 1 mg |
| Folate | 44 mcg |
| Vitamin B$_6$ | 0.3 mg |
| Vitamin B$_{12}$ | 0.3 mcg |
| Zinc | 0.8 mg |
| Selenium | 3 mcg |

• **Preheat oven to 400°F (200°C)**

| | | |
|---|---|---|
| 3 | bell peppers, preferably different colors (e.g., green, red and yellow) | 3 |
| 1 tsp | vegetable oil | 5 mL |
| 1 tbsp | balsamic vinegar | 15 mL |
| 1/4 cup | extra virgin olive oil | 60 mL |
| | Salt and freshly ground black pepper | |
| 2 oz | Parmesan cheese, shaved | 60 g |
| 1/4 cup | thinly sliced red onion | 60 mL |
| | Few sprigs of fresh basil and/or parsley, chopped | |

1. Cut peppers in half lengthwise, then core and deseed them. Brush their skins with the vegetable oil, and arrange the peppers (without crowding) in an oven pan, skin side up. Roast in preheated oven for 20 to 25 minutes, just until the skin has crinkled but before it has blackened. (If you wait until the skin turns black, the flesh of these halved peppers will totally disintegrate.) Remove peppers from oven and let cool for 5 to 10 minutes.

2. Using a spatula, pry the cooled peppers from the pan and transfer them to a work surface. Remove the skins (they should come off easily and more or less in one piece). Cut each into 5 or 6 strips and transfer to a plate.

3. Moisten the pepper strips with vinegar, then douse them with olive oil. Season to taste with salt and pepper. Decorate with Parmesan shavings, onions and basil and/or parsley just prior to serving. The oiled peppers will wait (and improve) for up to 1 hour.

> ## ▸ Health Tip
>
> Balasmic vinegar concentrates some of the powerful antioxidant molecules from grapes, known collectively as polyphenols.

# SOUPS

# Gingered Beet and Quinoa Soup

*This extremely nutritious soup provides a very satisfying meatless meal but complements a main dish too.*

## Tips

If you prefer a silken texture, you can purée the finished soup. Working in batches, transfer soup to food processor or blender (or use immersion blender in pot) and purée until smooth. Return soup to pot (if necessary) and heat over low heat, uncovered, for 4 to 5 minutes or until warm.

Store the cooled soup in an airtight container in the refrigerator for up to 2 days or in the freezer for up to 6 months.

| | | |
|---|---|---|
| 4 cups | diced peeled beets | 1 L |
| 6 cups | ready-to-use reduced-sodium vegetable or chicken broth, divided | 1.5 L |
| 1 tbsp | extra virgin olive oil | 15 mL |
| 2 cups | chopped onions | 500 mL |
| 1½ tbsp | ground ginger | 22 mL |
| ⅔ cup | quinoa, rinsed | 150 mL |
| | Fine sea salt and freshly ground black pepper | |
| ½ cup | plain Greek yogurt | 125 mL |
| ⅓ cup | packed fresh mint leaves, chopped | 75 mL |

**1.** In a microwave-safe bowl, combine beets and 2 cups (500 mL) of the broth. Cover loosely and microwave on High for 15 minutes or until beets are tender. Set aside.

**2.** Meanwhile, in a large pot, heat oil over medium-high heat. Add onions and cook, stirring, for 6 to 8 minutes or until softened. Add ginger and cook, stirring, for 30 seconds.

**3.** Stir in beet mixture, quinoa and the remaining broth; bring to a boil. Reduce heat to low, cover and simmer for 15 to 20 minutes or until quinoa is tender. Season to taste with salt and pepper. Serve dolloped with yogurt and sprinkled with mint.

> ▸ **Health Tip**
>
> Beets give us a great taste but also a health-promoting substance — pigments collectively called betalains that support detoxification in the body and may also reduce the chemical changes to the LDL particle (cholesterol) that can make it more reactive to the body.

### Nutrients per serving

| | |
|---|---|
| Calories | 188 |
| Fat | 4 g |
| Carbohydrate | 33 g |
| Protein | 7 g |
| Vitamin C | 9 mg |
| Vitamin D | 0 IU |
| Vitamin E | 1 mg |
| Niacin | 1 mg |
| Folate | 137 mcg |
| Vitamin $B_6$ | 0.2 mg |
| Vitamin $B_{12}$ | 0.0 mcg |
| Zinc | 1.1 mg |
| Selenium | 3 mcg |

# Cream of Broccoli Soup

*This flavorful soup derives protein and fats from cashews and offers a non-meat and non-dairy savory soup option.*

**Makes 6 servings**

## Variations

Add ⅛ tsp (0.5 mL) ground nutmeg or allspice or more to taste.

Refrigerate and serve soup chilled.

- Food processor

| | | |
|---|---|---|
| 1 cup | raw cashews | 250 mL |
| 1 lb | broccoli | 500 g |
| 2 tsp | olive oil | 10 mL |
| ½ | onion, chopped | ½ |
| 5 cups | ready-to-use vegetable broth | 1.25 L |
| 1 | russet (Idaho) potato, peeled and cut into 1-inch (2.5 cm) cubes | 1 |
| ¼ tsp | freshly ground black pepper | 1 mL |
| ½ tsp | salt | 2 mL |

1. Place cashews in a bowl and add water to cover by 3 inches (7.5 cm). Cover bowl and let soak for at least 2 hours.

2. Cut broccoli into 2-inch (5 cm) florets. Peel stalk and cut in half lengthwise and then crosswise into 1-inch (2.5 cm) pieces. You should have about 8 cups (2 L) total. Set aside.

3. Place cashews and 2 tbsp (30 mL) of the soaking water into food processor and process to a semi-smooth paste. Leave in processor and set aside.

4. Place a large saucepan over medium heat and let pan get hot. Add oil and tip pan to coat. Add onion and cook, stirring occasionally, until softened, 3 to 4 minutes. Add vegetable broth and potato, increase heat to high and bring to a boil. Reduce heat and simmer until slightly softened, 5 to 6 minutes. Add broccoli and black pepper, increase heat to high and bring to a boil. Reduce heat and simmer until potatoes and broccoli are tender, 6 to 8 minutes.

5. Let cool slightly. Working in batches, ladle soup into food processor with cashews and blend until smooth. Return to pan. Stir in salt. Taste and adjust seasonings and heat over low heat, stirring often, until soup is heated through. Serve hot.

### ▶ Health Tip

A class of plant compounds called glycosinolates help give broccoli its powerful role in supporting detoxification and helping the body eliminate some toxins that can promote the aging processes in the brain.

### Nutrients per serving

| | |
|---|---|
| Calories | 206 |
| Fat | 12 g |
| Carbohydrate | 21 g |
| Protein | 7 g |
| Vitamin C | 73 mg |
| Vitamin D | 0 IU |
| Vitamin E | 1 mg |
| Niacin | 1 mg |
| Folate | 78 mcg |
| Vitamin B$_6$ | 0.3 mg |
| Vitamin B$_{12}$ | 0.0 mcg |
| Zinc | 1.7 mg |
| Selenium | 5 mcg |

SOUPS **219**

# Yellow Tomato Gazpacho with Cilantro Oil

*This chilled soup shines when tomatoes are in season and is an easy and light alternative to traditional Spanish gazpacho. With no bread or olive oil, it's low in fat — but it's big in flavor.*

**Makes 6 servings**

## Tip

If yellow tomatoes are not available, red ones work just as well.

- **Food processor or blender**

| | | |
|---|---|---|
| 1 | yellow bell pepper, chopped | 1 |
| ½ | English cucumber, peeled, seeded and chopped | ½ |
| 1½ lbs | yellow tomatoes (about 5 medium), chopped | 750 g |
| ½ cup | chopped sweet onion (such as Vidalia) | 125 mL |
| 1 tsp | minced garlic | 5 mL |
| 2 tbsp | sherry vinegar | 30 mL |
| | Salt and freshly ground black pepper | |
| | Cilantro Oil (see recipe, opposite) | |

1. In food processor, in batches if necessary, process yellow pepper, cucumber, tomatoes, onion and garlic until almost smooth. Transfer to a bowl and stir in vinegar. Season to taste with salt and pepper. Cover and refrigerate until cold, about 3 hours. Taste and adjust seasoning with vinegar, salt and pepper, if necessary.

2. Ladle into chilled bowls and drizzle with Cilantro Oil.

> ### ▸ Health Tip
>
> Yellow tomatoes are a good source of iron, potassium, folate and other nutrients.

| Nutrients per serving | |
|---|---|
| Calories | 36 |
| Fat | 0 g |
| Carbohydrate | 7 g |
| Protein | 2 g |
| Vitamin C | 69 mg |
| Vitamin D | 0 IU |
| Vitamin E | 0 mg |
| Niacin | 1.6 mg |
| Folate | 47 mcg |
| Vitamin B$_6$ | 0.1 mg |
| Vitamin B$_{12}$ | 0.0 mcg |
| Zinc | 0.4 mg |
| Selenium | 1 mcg |

# Cilantro Oil

*Cilantro provides a good source of many health-promoting antioxidants.*

**Makes about 1 cup (250 mL)**

## Tip

Store in an airtight container in the refrigerator for up to 3 days.

- **Blender**

| | | |
|---|---|---|
| 2 cups | packed fresh cilantro leaves | 500 mL |
| ½ cup | olive oil | 125 mL |
| ½ cup | vegetable oil | 125 mL |

**1.** Bring a large saucepan of water to a boil. Add cilantro and blanch for 5 seconds. Drain and immediately plunge into a bowl of ice water. Drain well and squeeze out all liquid.

**2.** In blender, purée cilantro, olive oil and vegetable oil until smooth. Strain through several layers of cheesecloth or a paper coffee filter into a squeeze bottle, discarding solids.

## Nutrients per 1 tbsp (15 mL)

| | |
|---|---|
| Calories | 114 |
| Fat | 13 g |
| Carbohydrate | 0 g |
| Protein | 0 g |
| Vitamin C | 0 mg |
| Vitamin D | 0 IU |
| Vitamin E | 2 mg |
| Niacin | 0 mg |
| Folate | 0 mcg |
| Vitamin $B_6$ | 0.0 mg |
| Vitamin $B_{12}$ | 0.0 mcg |
| Zinc | 0.0 mg |
| Selenium | 0 mcg |

# Tomato Basil Soup

*This is an easy-to-prepare version of a classic, ideal for busy cooks.*

**Makes 4 servings**

## Tip

To keep basil fresh, like other fresh herbs (including parsley), wrap it in several layers of paper towel and place in a plastic bag; store in the warmest part of your fridge — in the butter keeper, for example, or the side door.

- **Food processor**

| | | |
|---|---|---|
| 2 tsp | olive oil | 10 mL |
| ½ | onion, chopped | ½ |
| 1 | can (28 oz/796 mL) whole tomatoes, with juice | 1 |
| 2 cups | ready-to-use vegetable broth | 500 mL |
| 2 cups | tomato marinara sauce | 500 mL |
| ½ tsp | salt | 2 mL |
| ½ tsp | freshly ground black pepper | 2 mL |
| ½ cup | packed fresh basil leaves, divided | 125 mL |
| ¼ cup | toasted pine nuts | 60 mL |

1. Place a medium saucepan over medium heat and let pan get hot. Add oil and tip pan to coat. Add onion and cook, stirring occasionally, until softened but not browned, 3 to 4 minutes. Add tomatoes, vegetable broth, marinara sauce, salt and pepper. Reduce heat to low and simmer, stirring occasionally and breaking up tomatoes with the back of a spoon, about 10 minutes. Stir in ¼ cup (60 mL) of the basil. Let cool.

2. Transfer soup to a food processor and blend until smooth, 20 to 30 seconds. Return soup to saucepan, taste and adjust seasonings. Turn heat to low and simmer until soup is hot throughout. Chiffonade remaining basil leaves. Serve soup hot, topped with a scattering of basil and a sprinkle of pine nuts.

> ▶ **Health Tip**
>
> Basil contains the brain-protective flavonoids orientin and vicenin, which are just some of the amazing compounds in this commonly used herb.

## Nutrients per serving

| | |
|---|---|
| Calories | 151 |
| Fat | 9 g |
| Carbohydrate | 18 g |
| Protein | 5 g |
| Vitamin C | 29 mg |
| Vitamin D | 0 IU |
| Vitamin E | 4 mg |
| Niacin | 3 mg |
| Folate | 38 mcg |
| Vitamin B$_6$ | 0.4 mg |
| Vitamin B$_{12}$ | 0.0 mcg |
| Zinc | 1.1 mg |
| Selenium | 1 mcg |

# Curried Sweet Potato and Millet Soup

*Leave humdrum vegetable soups behind with this garden of veggies and sweet potatoes.*

**Makes 6 servings**

## Tips

To get this quantity of puréed sweet potato, bake, peel and mash 2 medium sweet potatoes, each about 6 oz (175 g). You can also use a can (14 oz/398 mL) of sweet potato purée.

Toasting brings out millet's pleasantly nutty flavor. To toast, heat in a dry skillet over medium heat, stirring constantly, until it crackles and releases its aroma, for 5 minutes.

| | | |
|---|---|---|
| 1 tbsp | vegetable oil | 15 mL |
| 2 | onions, finely chopped | 2 |
| 2 | carrots, peeled and diced | 2 |
| 2 | stalks celery, diced | 2 |
| 2 | cloves garlic, minced | 2 |
| 2 tsp | minced gingerroot | 10 mL |
| 2 tsp | curry powder | 10 mL |
| 1 tsp | freshly grated orange zest | 5 mL |
| 2 cups | sweet potato purée (see tip, at left) | 500 mL |
| 6 cups | ready-to-use reduced-sodium vegetable or chicken broth | 1.5 L |
| ¾ cup | millet, toasted (see tip, at left) | 175 mL |
| 1 cup | freshly squeezed orange juice | 250 mL |
| ¼ cup | pure maple syrup | 60 mL |
| | Salt and freshly ground black pepper | |
| | Toasted chopped walnuts or sliced almonds | |
| | Plain yogurt (optional) | |

1. In a large saucepan or stockpot, heat oil over medium heat for 30 seconds. Add onions, carrots and celery and cook, stirring, until carrots have softened, about 7 minutes.

2. Add garlic, ginger, curry powder and orange zest and cook, stirring, for 1 minute. Add sweet potato and broth and stir well. Bring to a boil. Stir in millet. Reduce heat to low. Cover and simmer until millet is tender and flavors have blended, about 30 minutes.

3. Add orange juice and maple syrup and heat through. Season to taste with salt and pepper. Ladle into bowls and garnish with toasted walnuts and, if desired, a drizzle of yogurt.

> ▶ **Health Tip**
>
> Sweet potatoes are an unbeatable source of beta-carotene — a safe form of pre-vitamin A and great antioxidant in its own right.

### Nutrients per serving

| | |
|---|---|
| Calories | 291 |
| Fat | 4 g |
| Carbohydrate | 60 g |
| Protein | 6 g |
| Vitamin C | 30 mg |
| Vitamin D | 0 IU |
| Vitamin E | 2 mg |
| Niacin | 3 mg |
| Folate | 60 mcg |
| Vitamin $B_6$ | 0.4 mg |
| Vitamin $B_{12}$ | 0.0 mcg |
| Zinc | 1.0 mg |
| Selenium | 2 mcg |

# Moroccan Pumpkin Soup

*Pumpkin is a wildly popular flavor these days, but almost always in conjunction with aromatic spices. This dish delivers on that count and more!*

## Tips

Any small, thick-skinned cooking pumpkin or a butternut squash will work in this recipe.

Pressed curry powder is available in cubes and can usually be found in gourmet or natural food stores.

- **Blender**

| | | |
|---|---|---|
| 1 tsp | whole cumin seeds | 5 mL |
| 1 tsp | whole coriander seeds | 5 mL |
| ½ tsp | whole fennel seeds | 2 mL |
| 3 tbsp | olive oil, divided | 45 mL |
| 2 | red onions, chopped | 2 |
| 1 tbsp | blackstrap molasses | 15 mL |
| 1 | onion, sliced | 1 |
| 1 | leek, white and green parts, sliced | 1 |
| 1 tbsp | organic cane sugar | 15 mL |
| 1 | sweet or pie pumpkin (2 lbs/1 kg), peeled and cut into 1-inch (2.5 cm) cubes | 1 |
| 2 | apples, chopped | 2 |
| 1 tbsp | curry powder or cube (see tip, at left) | 15 mL |
| 1 tsp | ground turmeric | 5 mL |
| ½ tsp | ground cinnamon | 2 mL |
| 4 cups | ready-to-use vegetable broth or water | 1 L |
| 1 cup | rice milk | 250 mL |
| ½ cup | cashews | 125 mL |

1. In a large saucepan, toast cumin, coriander and fennel seeds over high heat until the seeds begin to pop and their fragrance is released, about 2 minutes. Do not allow to smoke or burn. Add 2 tbsp (30 mL) of the oil to pan and heat. Stir in red onions. Reduce heat to medium and cook, stirring frequently, for 10 minutes or until onions are soft and caramelized. Transfer ¾ cup (175 mL) to a bowl and add molasses. Stir and set aside.

## Nutrients per serving

| | |
|---|---|
| Calories | 277 |
| Fat | 13 g |
| Carbohydrate | 40 g |
| Protein | 5 g |
| Vitamin C | 22 mg |
| Vitamin D | 17 IU |
| Vitamin E | 3 mg |
| Niacin | 2 mg |
| Folate | 55 mcg |
| Vitamin B$_6$ | 0.3 mg |
| Vitamin B$_{12}$ | 0.3 mcg |
| Zinc | 1.4 mg |
| Selenium | 4 mcg |

## Tip

Leeks are grown in sand and are sometimes difficult to clean. A good method of cleaning is to vertically slice through the white and light green leaves, leaving most of the dark green leaves intact. Grasp the leek by the dark green leaves, fan out the bottom white and light green portions, exposing much of the inside of the leek, and run under cold water.

**2.** Add remaining oil to onions in pan and heat over high heat. Stir in leek. Reduce heat to medium and cook, stirring frequently, for 6 minutes or until soft. One at a time, add sugar, pumpkin, apples, curry powder, turmeric and cinnamon, stirring after each addition. Cook, stirring, for 1 minute. Add vegetable broth and bring to a gentle boil over high heat. Cover, reduce heat to medium-low and gently boil for 40 minutes or until vegetables are tender when pierced with the tip of a knife.

**3.** In blender, combine rice milk and cashews. Blend until smooth. Ladle 2 cups (500 mL) of the soup mixture into blender. Blend with nut mixture until smooth. Stir into soup and heat through. Ladle soup into bowls and float 2 tbsp (30 mL) of the reserved red onion on top of each.

> ### ▶ Health Tip
>
> Cumin, coriander and fennel are potent digestive tonics. Blackstrap molasses is a great source of iron, calcium, manganese and other nutrients.

# Curry-Roasted Squash and Apple Soup

*This spicy and warming soup tastes great and will stimulate your digestion with its array of active spices and flavors.*

---

## Makes 8 servings

### Tip

To peel butternut squash, cut it in half crosswise to create two flat surfaces. Place each half on its flat surface and use a sharp knife to remove the tough peel.

- Preheat oven to 450°F (230°C)
- Rimmed baking sheet, ungreased
- Immersion blender or upright blender

| | | |
|---|---|---|
| 2 tsp | salt | 10 mL |
| 1 tsp | ground coriander | 5 mL |
| 1 tsp | ground cumin | 5 mL |
| 1/2 tsp | ground turmeric | 2 mL |
| 1/4 tsp | ground cinnamon | 1 mL |
| 1/4 tsp | freshly ground black pepper | 1 mL |
| 1/4 cup | vegetable oil | 60 mL |
| 2 tbsp | cider vinegar or white wine vinegar | 30 mL |
| 4 | cloves garlic | 4 |
| 2 | tart apples, peeled and chopped | 2 |
| 1 | butternut squash, peeled and cut into 1/2-inch (1 cm) pieces (about 8 cups/2 L) | 1 |
| 1 | large onion, chopped | 1 |
| 6 cups | water (approx.) | 1.5 L |
| 1/2 tsp | garam masala, divided | 2 mL |
| | Salt and freshly ground black pepper | |

1. In a small bowl, combine salt, coriander, cumin, turmeric, cinnamon, pepper, oil and vinegar.

2. On baking sheet, combine garlic, apples, squash and onion. Drizzle with spice mixture and toss to coat evenly. Roast in preheated oven, stirring twice, for about 45 minutes or until softened and golden brown.

3. Transfer roasted vegetables to a large pot. Add water and bring to a boil over medium-high heat. Reduce heat and simmer, stirring occasionally, until vegetables are very soft and liquid is reduced by about one-third, about 30 minutes. Remove from heat.

### Nutrients per serving

| | |
|---|---|
| Calories | 161 |
| Fat | 7 g |
| Carbohydrate | 25 g |
| Protein | 2 g |
| Vitamin C | 33 mg |
| Vitamin D | 0 IU |
| Vitamin E | 3 mg |
| Niacin | 2 mg |
| Folate | 43 mcg |
| Vitamin B$_6$ | 0.3 mg |
| Vitamin B$_{12}$ | 0.0 mcg |
| Zinc | 0.3 mg |
| Selenium | 1 mcg |

## Tip

The soup can be made ahead, cooled, covered and refrigerated for up to 2 days or frozen for up to 2 months (thaw overnight in the refrigerator). Reheat over medium heat until steaming and season to taste before serving.

**4.** Using an immersion blender in pot or transferring soup in batches to an upright blender, purée until very smooth. Return to pot, if necessary.

**5.** Reheat over medium heat until steaming, stirring often. Thin with a little water, if necessary, to desired consistency. Stir in half the garam masala and season to taste with salt and pepper. Ladle into warmed bowls and serve sprinkled with remaining garam masala.

## Variation

Replace squash with 2 large sweet potatoes, peeled and cut into $\frac{1}{2}$-inch (1 cm) pieces.

> ▶ **Health Tip**
>
> Coriander and cinnamon are promising agents for regulating blood sugar.

# Roasted Butternut Squash Chowder with Sage Butter

*This is a deeply flavored dish that contains white wine as well as garlic and onions, with a flavorful topping.*

---

**Makes 6 servings**

## Tip

You can use $1\frac{1}{2}$ cups (375 mL) table (18%) cream instead of the half-and-half and whipping creams.

- Preheat oven to 400°F (200°C)
- Rimmed baking sheet, lined with parchment paper

| | | |
|---|---|---|
| 1 | butternut squash ($3\frac{1}{2}$ to 4 lbs/1.75 to 2 kg), halved lengthwise and seeded | 1 |
| $\frac{1}{4}$ cup | olive oil, divided | 60 mL |
| 10 | fresh sage leaves, thinly sliced | 10 |
| 1 | large onion, finely chopped | 1 |
| 1 | clove garlic, minced | 1 |
| 1 cup | dry white wine | 250 mL |
| 2 | large potatoes, peeled and cut into $\frac{1}{2}$-inch (1 cm) dice | 2 |
| 6 cups | ready-to-use vegetable or chicken broth (or a blend of the two) | 1.5 L |
| 1 tsp | salt | 5 mL |
| 1 tsp | freshly squeezed lemon juice | 5 mL |
| Pinch | cayenne pepper | Pinch |
| Pinch | ground nutmeg | Pinch |
| | Freshly ground black pepper | |
| 1 cup | half-and-half (10%) cream | 250 mL |
| $\frac{1}{2}$ cup | heavy or whipping (35%) cream | 125 mL |
| $\frac{1}{4}$ cup | unsalted butter | 60 mL |
| 12 | whole fresh sage leaves | 12 |

1. Rub the cut side of one of the squash halves with 1 tbsp (15 mL) of the oil and place cut side down on prepared baking sheet. Roast in preheated oven until a knife pierces easily into the thick part of the neck, about 40 minutes. Let cool on pan.

2. Meanwhile, peel and cut the remaining squash half into $\frac{1}{2}$-inch (1 cm) dice; set aside.

## Nutrients per serving

Calories 542 (higher calories because of the cream!)

| | |
|---|---|
| Fat | 29 g |
| Carbohydrate | 62 g |
| Protein | 7 g |
| Vitamin C | 83 mg |
| Vitamin D | 14 IU |
| Vitamin E | 6 mg |
| Niacin | 5 mg |
| Folate | 98 mcg |
| Vitamin B$_6$ | 0.8 mg |
| Vitamin B$_{12}$ | 0.2 mcg |
| Zinc | 1.1 mg |
| Selenium | 3 mcg |

## Tip

The taste of freshly grated nutmeg is so much better than the preground variety. Whole nutmeg can be found in the spice section of your supermarket or bulk food store. Use a rasp grater (such as a Microplane) to grate nutmeg.

**3.** In a large pot, heat the remaining oil over medium-high heat. Add sliced sage leaves and sauté until fragrant, about 1 minute. Add onion and sauté until softened, about 4 minutes. Add garlic and sauté until fragrant, about 1 minute. Add wine and cook until reduced by half, about 5 minutes. Add diced squash, potatoes, broth and salt; bring to a boil. Reduce heat and simmer until vegetables are tender, about 20 minutes.

**4.** Scoop roasted squash from its shell, mash it and add it to the soup. Season with lemon juice, cayenne, nutmeg and black pepper to taste. Stir in half-and-half cream and whipping cream; reheat over medium heat until steaming, stirring often. Taste and adjust seasoning with cayenne, nutmeg, salt and black pepper, if necessary.

**5.** In a skillet, melt butter over medium heat until sizzling. Add whole sage leaves and sauté until crispy and browned, about 2 minutes. Transfer sage to a plate lined with paper towels. Remove pan from heat.

**6.** Ladle chowder into heated bowls and top each with a drizzle of sage butter and 2 fried sage leaves.

> ▶ **Health Tip**
>
> Sage has been found by researchers to be both a potent antioxidant and a memory booster.

# Minestrone

*This rich minestrone provides a high level of protein and a wide variety of veggies and spices — a meal in itself.*

**Makes 6 to 8 servings**

## Tip

A 19-oz (540 mL) can of beans will yield about 2 cups (500 mL) once the beans are drained and rinsed. If you have smaller or larger cans, you can use the volume called for or just add the amount from your can.

| | | |
|---|---|---|
| 1 tbsp | grapeseed oil | 15 mL |
| 1 | clove garlic, minced | 1 |
| 1/2 cup | chopped onion | 125 mL |
| 1 tbsp | chopped fresh parsley | 15 mL |
| 1 | potato (unpeeled), chopped | 1 |
| 1 | tomato, chopped | 1 |
| 2 cups | rinsed drained canned romano beans | 500 mL |
| 1 cup | cubed cooked chicken | 250 mL |
| 1/2 cup | peas | 125 mL |
| 1/2 cup | broccoli florets | 125 mL |
| 1/2 cup | chopped celery | 125 mL |
| 1/4 cup | chopped dry-packed sun-dried tomatoes | 60 mL |
| | Salt and freshly ground black pepper | |

1. In a large saucepan, heat oil over medium heat. Sauté garlic, onion and parsley for 3 to 4 minutes or until onion is softened.

2. Stir in potato, chopped tomato, beans, chicken, peas, broccoli, celery, sun-dried tomatoes and 8 cups (2 L) water; bring to a boil over medium-high heat. Cover, leaving lid ajar, reduce heat to low and simmer, stirring occasionally, for 30 minutes or until vegetables are tender (or for up to 1 1/2 hours if you prefer a very soft texture). Season to taste with salt and pepper.

## Variations

Substitute cooked beef for the chicken.

Add 1 cup (250 mL) cooked gluten-free pasta to the finished minestrone.

> ▸ **Health Tip**
>
> Broccoli is a good source of vitamin C and vitamin K.

| Nutrients per 1 of 8 servings | |
|---|---|
| Calories | 137 |
| Fat | 3 g |
| Carbohydrate | 18 g |
| Protein | 11 g |
| Vitamin C | 16 mg |
| Vitamin D | 1 IU |
| Vitamin E | 1 mg |
| Niacin | 3 mg |
| Folate | 71 mcg |
| Vitamin $B_6$ | 0.3 mg |
| Vitamin $B_{12}$ | 0.1 mcg |
| Zinc | 1.0 mg |
| Selenium | 7 mcg |

# Roasted Garlic and Lentil Soup

*Lentils are an amazing food, full of nutrients and amino acids and adding substance to this garlic-infused soup.*

---

## Makes 6 servings

### Tips

Use fresh tomatoes in season and substitute 1 cup (250 mL) of crushed canned tomatoes in winter.

Look for red rice in gourmet or natural food stores.

You can use 2 cups (500 mL) cooked lentils plus ½ cup (125 mL) vegetable broth, instead of canned.

This soup is best if served immediately. When stored, even in the refrigerator, it thickens, absorbing the liquid.

### Nutrients per serving

| | |
|---|---|
| Calories | 354 |
| Fat | 11 g |
| Carbohydrate | 54 g |
| Protein | 13 g |
| Vitamin C | 26 mg |
| Vitamin D | 0 IU |
| Vitamin E | 2 mg |
| Niacin | 3 mg |
| Folate | 197 mcg |
| Vitamin B$_6$ | 0.6 mg |
| Vitamin B$_{12}$ | 0.0 mcg |
| Zinc | 2.2 mg |
| Selenium | 4 mcg |

- Preheat oven to 375°F (190°C)
- 10-inch (25 cm) pie plate or baking dish
- Blender

| | | |
|---|---|---|
| 10 | small (2-inch/5 cm diameter) tomatoes | 10 |
| 12 | cloves garlic | 12 |
| 4 tbsp | olive oil, divided | 60 mL |
| 1 tbsp | chopped fresh rosemary | 15 mL |
| 1 cup | chopped onion | 250 mL |
| 1 tsp | ground cumin | 5 mL |
| ½ tsp | crushed fennel seeds | 2 mL |
| ½ tsp | sea salt | 2 mL |
| Pinch | each ground ginger and ground nutmeg | Pinch |
| 1 cup | red or brown rice | 250 mL |
| 3 cups | ready-to-use vegetable broth or water (approx.), divided | 750 mL |
| 1 | can (19 oz/540 mL) lentils, with liquid | 1 |

1. In pie plate, combine tomatoes and garlic and toss with 2 tbsp (30 mL) of the oil and rosemary. Bake in preheated oven for 40 minutes or until garlic is soft. Let cool.

2. Meanwhile, in a large saucepan, heat remaining oil over medium heat. Add onion and cook, stirring occasionally, for 6 to 8 minutes or until soft. Add cumin, fennel, salt, ginger, nutmeg and rice. Cook, stirring constantly, for 1 minute. Add 2 cups (500 mL) of the vegetable broth. Increase heat to high and bring to a boil. Cover, reduce heat to low and simmer for 40 minutes or until rice is tender.

3. When tomatoes and garlic are cool enough to handle, transfer to blender and add remaining vegetable broth. Blend until smooth. Add tomato purée and lentils with liquid to rice in saucepan. Bring to a simmer and cook for 1 to 2 minutes or until heated through. Add more vegetable broth or water if a thinner soup is desired.

> ### ▶ Health Tip
>
> Garlic has many health benefits and is a food that concentrates selenium — a necessary mineral for production of glutathione, a master antioxidant and detoxification enzyme — in the body.

# Creamy Roasted Garlic, Chicken and Mushroom Soup

*This dish will warm you up on a cold winter's day and provide a creamy, savory rich soup in any season.*

## Tip

To clean mushrooms, you can either rinse them quickly in water or wipe them with a damp paper towel. Mushrooms will be much happier in your refrigerator if you store them in a paper bag.

### ▶ Health Tip

Parsley contains luteolin, one of the most potent antioxidants and under investigation for cancer prevention properties.

### Nutrients per serving

| | |
|---|---|
| Calories | 437 |
| Fat | 29 g |
| Carbohydrate | 18 g |
| Protein | 29 g |
| Vitamin C | 8 mg |
| Vitamin D | 22 IU |
| Vitamin E | 1 mg |
| Niacin | 17 mg |
| Folate | 57 mcg |
| Vitamin B$_6$ | 0.7 mg |
| Vitamin B$_{12}$ | 0.5 mcg |
| Zinc | 1.7 mg |
| Selenium | 23 mcg |

- **Preheat oven to 350°F (180°C)**
- **Small baking dish**

| | | |
|---|---|---|
| 3 | heads garlic | 3 |
| 2 tbsp | olive oil | 30 mL |
| | Salt and freshly ground black pepper | |
| 3 tbsp | unsalted butter | 45 mL |
| 2 | onions, finely chopped | 2 |
| 2 | cloves garlic, minced | 2 |
| 1 lb | mushrooms, sliced | 500 g |
| 3 tbsp | all-purpose flour | 45 mL |
| 4 cups | ready-to-use chicken broth | 1 L |
| 3 cups | shredded cooked chicken | 750 mL |
| 1 cup | heavy or whipping (35%) cream | 250 mL |
| ¼ cup | chopped fresh parsley | 60 mL |
| | Crispy Shallots (see recipe, opposite) | |

**1.** Slice the top ½ inch (1 cm) off each head of garlic. Place in baking dish, drizzle with oil and sprinkle with salt and pepper to taste. Cover dish tightly with foil and bake in preheated oven until garlic is golden brown and tender, about 45 minutes. Let cool completely. Squeeze garlic between fingertips to release cloves. Transfer cloves to small bowl and mash into a paste with a fork. Set aside.

**2.** In a large pot, melt butter over medium heat. Add onion and sauté until softened, about 6 minutes. Add minced garlic and mushrooms; sauté until mushrooms release their liquid and start to brown, about 10 minutes. Sprinkle with flour and sauté for 2 minutes.

**3.** Gradually whisk in broth and reserved roasted garlic paste; simmer for 20 minutes to blend the flavors. Stir in chicken and cream; heat until steaming, about 5 minutes, stirring often. Do not let boil. Stir in parsley. Taste and adjust seasoning with salt and pepper, if necessary.

**4.** Ladle into heated bowls and garnish with crispy shallots.

# Crispy Shallots

*Shallots are a type of onion, but smaller and very rich in flavor.*

**Makes enough to garnish 6 servings of soup**

- Candy/deep-fry thermometer

| | | |
|---|---|---|
| 1½ cups | vegetable oil | 375 mL |
| 6 | shallots, thinly sliced | 6 |
| | Salt | |

1. In a saucepan, heat oil over medium heat until it registers 350°F (180°C) on thermometer. Add shallots, in two batches, and fry, stirring frequently, until golden brown, 3 to 4 minutes. Using a slotted spoon, remove shallots to a plate lined with paper towels. Season to taste with salt. Serve hot or let cool and use within 3 hours.

> ▶ **Health Tip**
>
> All members of the allium family, including shallots, garlic and onions, confer many health benefits, and working them into daily dishes is the best way to receive these benefits.

## Nutrients per serving

| | |
|---|---|
| Calories | 84 |
| Fat | 9 g |
| Carbohydrate | 0 g |
| Protein | 0 g |
| Vitamin C | 1 mg |
| Vitamin D | 0 IU |
| Vitamin E | 2 mg |
| Niacin | 0 mg |
| Folate | 3 mcg |
| Vitamin $B_6$ | 0.0 mg |
| Vitamin $B_{12}$ | 0.0 mcg |
| Zinc | 0.0 mg |
| Selenium | 0 mcg |

# Shrimp and Corn Bisque

*You don't have to live by the sea or a fisherman's wharf to enjoy this soup, but just have fresh or frozen shrimp on hand — you'll still feel like you do when you taste this rich, nutritious dish.*

## Makes 6 servings

## Tip

Small amounts of cayenne and nutmeg add immeasurably to the flavor of soups without announcing their presence.

| | | |
|---|---|---|
| 5 tbsp | unsalted butter, divided | 75 mL |
| 2 | onions, finely chopped, divided | 2 |
| 2 | stalks celery, diced, divided | 2 |
| 1 | carrot, diced | 1 |
| 2 lbs | medium shrimp, peeled, deveined and halved lengthwise, shells reserved | 1 kg |
| 1 | clove garlic, minced | 1 |
| 6 | whole black peppercorns | 6 |
| 1 | bay leaf | 1 |
| ½ tsp | dried thyme | 2 mL |
| 4 | ears corn, kernels removed and reserved and cobs cut into quarters | 4 |
| 8 cups | ready-to-use shellfish, chicken or vegetable broth | 2 L |
| 3 tbsp | all-purpose flour | 45 mL |
| ½ tsp | salt | 2 mL |
| 1 cup | heavy or whipping (35%) cream | 250 mL |
| Pinch | ground nutmeg | Pinch |
| Pinch | cayenne pepper | Pinch |
| | Freshly ground black pepper | |
| 3 tbsp | minced fresh chives | 45 mL |

1. In a large pot, melt 2 tbsp (30 mL) of the butter over medium heat. Add half the onions, half the celery and the carrot; sauté until softened, about 6 minutes. Add shrimp shells, garlic, peppercorns, bay leaf and thyme; sauté until shells turn pink and garlic is fragrant, about 4 minutes. Add corn cobs and broth; bring to a boil. Reduce heat and simmer for 30 minutes.

2. Meanwhile, in a saucepan, melt remaining butter over medium heat. Add remaining onion and celery; sauté until softened, about 6 minutes. Add flour and salt; sauté for 2 minutes. Gradually whisk in cream and cook, stirring, until slightly thickened, about 3 minutes. Remove from heat and set aside.

| Nutrients per serving | |
|---|---|
| Calories | 472 |
| Fat | 29 g |
| Carbohydrate | 26 g |
| Protein | 31 g |
| Vitamin C | 8 mg |
| Vitamin D | 21 IU |
| Vitamin E | 3 mg |
| Niacin | 9 mg |
| Folate | 66 mcg |
| Vitamin B$_6$ | 0.4 mg |
| Vitamin B$_{12}$ | 2.1 mcg |
| Zinc | 2.4 mg |
| Selenium | 46 mcg |

## Tip

Is cutting onions bringing you to tears? Try placing them in the freezer for 10 minutes before chopping.

**3.** Strain the broth and discard all solids; return broth to the pot and bring to a simmer over medium heat. Add corn kernels and simmer until almost tender, about 5 minutes. Add shrimp and simmer until pink and opaque, about 2 minutes. Add cream mixture and bring to a simmer, stirring often. Stir in nutmeg and cayenne. Season with salt and black pepper to taste.

**4.** Ladle into heated bowls and garnish with chives.

> ### ▶ Health Tip
>
> Use shrimp that are ocean-caught (wild) or organically (certified) farm-raised, as some farm-raised shrimp are from contaminated sources — often extremely toxic ponds that are laced with antibiotics.

# Saffron Paella Soup

*We often think of soup as a starter dish, but this is a meal of a soup. The paella is a traditional dish in Mediterranean cuisine, and this recipe brings out the best of that tradition.*

## Tip

Have the fishmonger tap each mussel individually to make sure it is alive and check again just before cooking. Live mussels will close when tapped. Any mussels that do not open while cooking were dead before they were cooked and should be discarded.

### Nutrients per serving

| | |
|---|---|
| Calories | 642 |
| Fat | 36 g |
| Carbohydrate | 30 g |
| Protein | 50 g |
| Vitamin C | 44 mg |
| Vitamin D | 5 IU |
| Vitamin E | 4 mg |
| Niacin | 15 mg |
| Folate | 109 mcg |
| Vitamin B$_6$ | 0.7 mg |
| Vitamin B$_{12}$ | 6.7 mcg |
| Zinc | 5.7 mg |
| Selenium | 61 mcg |

| | | |
|---|---|---|
| 1/4 cup | olive oil, divided | 60 mL |
| 1 | large onion, chopped, divided | 1 |
| 1 lb | chicken thighs | 500 g |
| 3 | cloves garlic, minced | 3 |
| 8 cups | ready-to-use chicken broth, divided | 2 L |
| 1 | can (14 oz/398 mL) diced tomatoes, with juice | 1 |
| 1/2 cup | long-grain white rice | 125 mL |
| 1/4 tsp | salt | 1 mL |
| 1/4 tsp | saffron threads | 1 mL |
| 1 | red bell pepper, diced | 1 |
| 1 lb | smoked Spanish chorizo or andouille sausage, diced | 500 g |
| 12 | mussels, scrubbed and debearded (see tips) | 12 |
| 1 cup | frozen peas, thawed | 250 mL |
| 1 lb | large shrimp, peeled and deveined | 500 g |
| 1/4 cup | minced fresh flat-leaf (Italian) parsley | 60 mL |
| | Garlic-seasoned croutons | |

1. In a large pot, heat 3 tbsp (45 mL) of the oil over medium-high heat. Add half the onion and sauté until starting to soften, about 2 minutes. Add chicken, skin side down, and cook until browned, about 4 minutes. (Be careful not to let the onion burn.) Turn chicken over and brown the other side. Add garlic and sauté for 2 minutes. Add 5 cups (1.25 L) of the broth and tomatoes; bring to a boil. Reduce heat and simmer until juices run clear when chicken is pierced, about 30 minutes. Remove from heat.

2. Using tongs, transfer chicken to a large plate and let cool slightly. Remove skin and bones and discard. Shred the meat into bite-size pieces and set aside. Set cooking liquid aside.

## Tip

To scrub and debeard mussels, hold each mussel under cool running water and scrub the shell with a stiff-bristled brush. Next, grab the fibers of the "beard" with your fingers and pull them out, tugging toward the hinged point of the shell.

**3.** In a saucepan, bring the remaining broth to a simmer over medium heat. Add rice, salt and saffron; cover, reduce heat and simmer until rice is almost tender, about 15 minutes. Remove from heat and let stand, covered, until ready to use.

**4.** In another large pot, heat the remaining oil over medium heat. Add the remaining onion, red pepper and sausage; sauté until vegetables are softened, about 6 minutes. Add reserved cooking liquid and bring to a simmer. Add reserved chicken and rice, mussels and peas; return to a simmer. Cover, reduce heat to low and simmer gently for 5 minutes. Add shrimp, cover and simmer gently until mussels have opened and shrimp are pink and opaque, 2 to 3 minutes. Discard any mussels that do not open.

**5.** Ladle into heated bowls, making sure each bowl contains a few shrimp and 2 mussels. Garnish with parsley and croutons.

---

### ▶ Health Tip

This dish is a source of omega-3 fatty acids, which are essential for brain health. Due to toxin, parasite and antibiotic concerns, avoid farm-raised seafood unless it is truly organic and sustainable.

# Salmon Chowder

*This hearty soup creates a fantastic stock from the salmon, broth, milk and herbs.*

**Makes 5 servings**

## Tips

Hot-smoked salmon is smoked at a much higher temperature than cold-smoked salmon. This gives it a fuller, smokier flavor and a firmer texture.

If you can't find hot-smoked salmon, add hot pepper flakes to taste along with regular smoked salmon. You can also use smoked whitefish or trout.

> ▶ **Health Tip**
>
> Salmon is a source of omega-3 fats in a form that the body can very readily use.

### Nutrients per serving

| | |
|---|---|
| Calories | 172 |
| Fat | 3 g |
| Carbohydrate | 26 g |
| Protein | 12 g |
| Vitamin C | 30 mg |
| Vitamin D | 202 IU |
| Vitamin E | 1 mg |
| Niacin | 4 mg |
| Folate | 44 mcg |
| Vitamin B$_6$ | 0.3 mg |
| Vitamin B$_{12}$ | 1.3 mcg |
| Zinc | 0.9 mg |
| Selenium | 11 mcg |

- **Preheat barbecue grill or broiler**

| | | |
|---|---|---|
| 1 | small onion, cut into 1/4-inch (0.5 cm) thick slices | 1 |
| 1 | potato, cut into 1/4-inch (0.5 cm) thick slices | 1 |
| 1 | large carrot, cut lengthwise into 1/4-inch (0.5 cm) thick slices | 1 |
| ¼ | stalk celery | ¼ |
| 1 | green bell pepper, quartered and seeded | 1 |
| 2 cups | ready-to-use fish or chicken broth | 500 mL |
| ½ tsp | crumbled dried thyme | 2 mL |
| ¼ tsp | crumbled dried basil | 1 mL |
| 2 cups | 1% milk | 500 mL |
| ¼ cup | all-purpose flour | 60 mL |
| 4 oz | unsalted hot-smoked salmon or smoked whitefish | 125 g |
| ¾ cup | frozen corn kernels | 175 mL |
| Pinch | salt | Pinch |
| | Freshly ground black pepper | |

1. Place onion, potato, carrot, celery and green pepper on barbecue or under broiler; cook, turning occasionally, until distinct grill marks are visible and pepper skin is blackened. Place vegetables in plastic bag; seal and let stand for 20 minutes.

2. Peel skins off peppers; dice peppers. Dice remaining roasted vegetables and place in large saucepan. Add 1 cup (250 mL) broth, thyme and basil; bring to a boil. Add remaining broth and 1½ cups (375 mL) milk; bring just to simmer. Stir flour with remaining milk until smooth; gradually stir into soup. Simmer over low heat for 5 minutes.

3. Remove skin and any bones from fish; cut into ¼-inch (0.5 cm) cubes. Add to soup along with corn; cook for 10 minutes. Season with salt, and pepper to taste. Serve hot.

*This recipe courtesy of chef Dean Mitchell and dietitian Suzanne Journault-Hemstock.*

# SALADS

# Everyday Salad

*This salad is a quickly prepared standby that delivers more than a full serving of fresh vegetables.*

**Makes 4 servings**

## Tip

For the dried herbs, try dried Italian seasoning. You can also use basil or thyme, or a combination.

| | | |
|---|---|---:|
| 4 cups | packed baby spinach (about 6 oz/175 g) | 1 L |
| 1/2 cup | shredded red cabbage | 125 mL |
| 1/2 cup | sliced peeled cucumber | 125 mL |
| 1/2 cup | chopped yellow bell pepper | 125 mL |
| 1/4 cup | chopped red bell pepper | 60 mL |
| 20 | cherry tomatoes | 20 |
| 2 tbsp | balsamic vinegar | 30 mL |
| 1 1/2 tbsp | extra virgin olive oil | 22 mL |
| 1 tsp | dried herbs (see tip, at left) | 5 mL |
| | Salt and freshly ground black pepper | |

1. In a large bowl, combine spinach, cabbage, cucumber, yellow pepper, red pepper and tomatoes.

2. In a small bowl, whisk together vinegar, oil and herbs. Drizzle over salad and toss to coat. Season to taste with salt and pepper.

> ▸ **Health Tip**
>
> The spinach and bell peppers deliver a host of carotenoids, which have major antioxidant roles to play in the body and are best consumed as a mixed carotenoid package as they naturally occur in foods.

## Nutrients per serving

| | |
|---|---:|
| Calories | 89 |
| Fat | 6 g |
| Carbohydrate | 9 g |
| Protein | 2 g |
| Vitamin C | 63 mg |
| Vitamin D | 0 IU |
| Vitamin E | 2 mg |
| Niacin | 1 mg |
| Folate | 89 mcg |
| Vitamin B$_6$ | 0.2 mg |
| Vitamin B$_{12}$ | 0.0 mcg |
| Zinc | 0.4 mg |
| Selenium | 0 mcg |

# Spinach Salad with Oranges and Mushrooms

*Toasted almonds and water chestnuts give this salad a crunch factor.*

**Makes 6 servings**

## Tips

Use 1½ cups (375 mL) canned drained mandarins to replace the orange.

Oyster mushrooms or other wild mushrooms are exceptionally tasty.

Prepare salad early in the day, keeping refrigerated. Prepare dressing up to 2 days ahead. Pour over salad just before serving.

### Salad

| | | |
|---|---|---|
| 8 cups | packed fresh spinach, washed, dried and torn into bite-sized pieces | 2 L |
| 1½ cups | sliced mushrooms | 375 mL |
| ¾ cup | sliced water chestnuts | 175 mL |
| ½ cup | sliced red onions | 125 mL |
| ¼ cup | raisins | 60 mL |
| 2 tbsp | sliced or chopped almonds, toasted | 30 mL |
| 1 | orange, peeled and sections cut into pieces | 1 |

### Dressing

| | | |
|---|---|---|
| 3 tbsp | olive oil | 45 mL |
| 3 tbsp | balsamic vinegar | 45 mL |
| 2 tbsp | orange juice concentrate, thawed | 30 mL |
| 1 tbsp | liquid honey | 15 mL |
| 1 tsp | grated orange zest | 5 mL |
| 1 tsp | minced garlic | 5 mL |

1. *Salad:* In large serving bowl, combine spinach, mushrooms, water chestnuts, red onions, raisins, almonds and orange pieces; toss well.

2. *Dressing:* In small bowl, whisk together olive oil, balsamic vinegar, orange juice concentrate, honey, orange zest and garlic; pour over salad and toss.

### ▶ Health Tip

Although drying somewhat decreases the antioxidant powers of raisins versus the grapes they started out as, the beneficial molecules, including flavanols, are still present in valuable amounts.

## Nutrients per serving

| | |
|---|---|
| Calories | 163 |
| Fat | 8 g |
| Carbohydrate | 22 g |
| Protein | 3 g |
| Vitamin C | 33 mg |
| Vitamin D | 1 IU |
| Vitamin E | 3 mg |
| Niacin | 2 mg |
| Folate | 107 mcg |
| Vitamin $B_6$ | 0.2 mg |
| Vitamin $B_{12}$ | 0.0 mcg |
| Zinc | 0.5 mg |
| Selenium | 1 mcg |

# Sweet Cinnamon Waldorf Salad

*Nothing complements a special meal like a good Waldorf salad and this recipe is a winner.*

---

**Makes 6 to 8 servings**

## Tips

For a nice change, use a combination of peas and apples to total $2\frac{1}{2}$ cups (625 mL).

Prepare salad early in the day. Refrigerate and toss well just before serving. Keeps well for 2 days in refrigerator.

### Salad

| | | |
|---|---|---|
| $2\frac{1}{2}$ cups | diced apples | 625 mL |
| $\frac{3}{4}$ cup | diced celery | 175 mL |
| 1 cup | red or green seedless grapes, quartered | 250 mL |
| 1 cup | chopped red or green peppers | 250 mL |
| $\frac{1}{3}$ cup | raisins | 75 mL |
| $\frac{1}{2}$ cup | canned mandarin oranges, drained | 125 mL |
| 2 tbsp | finely chopped pecans | 30 mL |

### Dressing

| | | |
|---|---|---|
| $\frac{1}{4}$ cup | light mayonnaise | 60 mL |
| $\frac{1}{4}$ cup | light (1%) sour cream | 60 mL |
| 2 tbsp | liquid honey | 30 mL |
| 1 tbsp | freshly squeezed lemon juice | 15 mL |
| $\frac{1}{2}$ tsp | ground cinnamon | 2 mL |

1. *Salad:* In serving bowl, combine apples, celery, grapes, sweet peppers, raisins, mandarin oranges and pecans.

2. *Dressing:* In small bowl, combine mayonnaise, sour cream, honey, lemon juice and cinnamon; mix thoroughly. Pour over salad and toss.

> ▶ **Health Tip**
>
> Pecans may have cholesterol-lowering effects and cinnamon has a blood-sugar-stabilizing effect.

## Nutrients per 1 of 8 servings

| | |
|---|---|
| Calories | 128 |
| Fat | 5 g |
| Carbohydrate | 22 g |
| Protein | 1 g |
| Vitamin C | 33 mg |
| Vitamin D | 1 IU |
| Vitamin E | 1 mg |
| Niacin | 0 mg |
| Folate | 16 mcg |
| Vitamin B$_6$ | 0.1 mg |
| Vitamin B$_{12}$ | 0.0 mcg |
| Zinc | 0.3 mg |
| Selenium | 1 mcg |

# Green Bean, Pecan and Pomegranate Salad

*This is a good departure from lettuce-based salad, which we love but can become repetitive. Pomegranate and green beans give this salad flavor and crunch — add the olives for a more Mediterranean take.*

## Tip

Do not be tempted to cook the beans for more than 3 minutes or they will soften too much.

**Salad**

| | | |
|---|---|---|
| 1 lb | green beans, cut into 2-inch (5 cm) pieces | 500 g |
| 1/2 cup | diced red onion | 125 mL |
| 1 cup | whole pecans | 250 mL |
| 1 cup | pomegranate seeds | 250 mL |
| 1/4 cup | chopped green olives (optional) | 60 mL |

**Pomegranate Dressing**

| | | |
|---|---|---|
| 1/3 cup | olive oil | 75 mL |
| 3 tbsp | Pomegranate Molasses (see recipe, page 283, or store-bought) | 45 mL |
| 1 tbsp | chopped fresh parsley | 15 mL |

1. *Salad:* In a pot of boiling salted water, cook green beans for 3 minutes. Drain and rinse with cold water. Let cool to room temperature. In a bowl, combine green beans, red onion, pecans, pomegranate seeds and olives (if using).

2. *Dressing:* Meanwhile, in a jar with a tight-fitting lid, combine oil, molasses and parsley. Shake well to combine and drizzle over salad.

▶ **Health Tip**

The concentrate of pomegranate juice in the "molasses" of the dressing packs a powerful dose of vascular-protective molecules.

## Nutrients per serving

| | |
|---|---|
| Calories | 451 |
| Fat | 37 g |
| Carbohydrate | 32 g |
| Protein | 5 g |
| Vitamin C | 21 mg |
| Vitamin D | 0 IU |
| Vitamin E | 4 mg |
| Niacin | 1 mg |
| Folate | 64 mcg |
| Vitamin $B_6$ | 0.4 mg |
| Vitamin $B_{12}$ | 0.0 mcg |
| Zinc | 1.6 mg |
| Selenium | 5 mcg |

# Vegetable Salad with Feta Dressing

*The variety of vegetables in this salad, combined with the feta cheese and herbed dressing, makes it a satisfying starter that can complement a pasta or meat dish.*

**Makes 4 to 6 servings**

## Tips

Try goat cheese instead of feta for a change.

Prepare salad and dressing early in the day. Toss just before serving.

- **Food processor or blender**

### Salad

| | | |
|---|---|---|
| 2 cups | chopped celery | 500 mL |
| 2 cups | chopped English cucumbers | 500 mL |
| 2 cups | chopped red bell peppers | 500 mL |
| 2 cups | chopped plum (Roma) tomatoes | 500 mL |
| 1 cup | chopped red onions | 250 mL |
| 1/3 cup | sliced black olives | 75 mL |

### Dressing

| | | |
|---|---|---|
| 2 oz | feta cheese, crumbled | 60 g |
| 1/3 cup | light sour cream | 75 mL |
| 2 tbsp | 2% plain yogurt | 30 mL |
| 1 tbsp | freshly squeezed lemon juice | 15 mL |
| $1\frac{1}{2}$ tsp | minced garlic | 7 mL |
| $1\frac{1}{4}$ tsp | dried oregano | 6 mL |

1. *Salad:* In a serving bowl, combine celery, cucumbers, red peppers, tomatoes, red onions and olives.

2. *Dressing:* In food processor, combine feta, sour cream, yogurt, lemon juice, garlic and oregano; process until smooth.

3. Pour dressing over salad; toss to coat.

> ▶ **Health Tip**
>
> Oregano has an anti-inflammatory compound known as beta-caryophyllin, along with other beneficial effects.

### Nutrients per 1 of 6 servings

| | |
|---|---|
| Calories | 108 |
| Fat | 5 g |
| Carbohydrate | 12 g |
| Protein | 4 g |
| Vitamin C | 77 mg |
| Vitamin D | 3 IU |
| Vitamin E | 1 mg |
| Niacin | 1 mg |
| Folate | 61 mcg |
| Vitamin $B_6$ | 0.3 mg |
| Vitamin $B_{12}$ | 0.3 mcg |
| Zinc | 0.8 mg |
| Selenium | 2 mcg |

# Avocado Salad

*This easy-to-prepare salad will satisfy the growing number of avocado fans and create some new ones.*

## Tip

Hass avocados (sometimes called Haas avocados) are dark-skinned avocados with a nutty, buttery flesh and a longer shelf life than other varieties, making them the most popular avocado in North America. To determine whether a Hass avocado is ripe, look for purple-black skin and gently press the top — a ripe one will give slightly.

| | | |
|---|---|---|
| 1 tbsp | freshly squeezed lime juice | 15 mL |
| 1 | ripe avocado | 1 |
| 1/4 cup | slivered red bell peppers | 60 mL |
| 1/4 cup | slivered red onion | 60 mL |
| 2 tbsp | vegetable oil | 30 mL |
| | Salt and freshly ground black pepper | |
| | Few sprigs fresh coriander, chopped | |
| | Pico de gallo | |
| | Corn chips | |

1. Put lime juice in a small bowl. Peel avocado and cut into slices (or scoop out with a small spoon) and add to the lime juice. Toss gently until well coated. Add red peppers and onions; drizzle with oil. Toss gently until all ingredients are thoroughly combined. Season to taste with salt and pepper.

2. Transfer salad to a serving plate and spread out attractively. Garnish with chopped coriander and serve within 1 hour, accompanied by pico de gallo and corn chips.

> ## ▶ Health Tip
>
> Not only are the oils and fats in avocado nutritious in their own right, but they enhance absorption of other nutrients, such as the carotenoids from bell peppers.

| Nutrients per serving | |
|---|---|
| Calories | 298 |
| Fat | 29 g |
| Carbohydrate | 12 g |
| Protein | 2 g |
| Vitamin C | 37 mg |
| Vitamin D | 0 IU |
| Vitamin E | 5 mg |
| Niacin | 2 mg |
| Folate | 93 mcg |
| Vitamin $B_6$ | 0.3 mg |
| Vitamin $B_{12}$ | 0.0 mcg |
| Zinc | 0.7 mg |
| Selenium | 1 mcg |

# Roasted Beet and Beet Greens Salad

*For beet lovers, this dish has the sour factor from vinegar but adds the sweetness and tanginess of orange along with ample garlic.*

**Makes 4 servings**

## Tip

Any type of beet (red, golden or red-and-white-striped Chioggia) would be great in this salad. To avoid stained hands, wear plastic gloves when peeling dark-colored beets.

- Preheat oven to 400°F (200°C)
- Large rimmed baking sheet

| | | |
|---|---|---|
| 4 | beets, with greens attached (about 1½ lbs/750 g) | 4 |
| 2 | oranges | 2 |
| 2 | cloves garlic, minced | 2 |
| ½ cup | thinly sliced red onion | 125 mL |
| ½ tsp | fine sea salt | 2 mL |
| 2 tbsp | extra virgin olive oil | 30 mL |
| 1 tbsp | red wine vinegar | 15 mL |

1. Trim greens from beets. Cut off and discard stems, then coarsely chop leaves. Set beet greens aside.

2. Tightly wrap each beet in foil and place on baking sheet. Roast in preheated oven for about 90 minutes or until tender when pierced with a fork. Let cool completely in foil on baking sheet.

3. Meanwhile, in a large saucepan of boiling water, cook beet greens for 2 to 3 minutes or until tender. Drain, then let cool completely.

4. Peel beets and cut each into 8 wedges. Place beets in a medium bowl.

5. Squeeze beet greens to remove any excess water, then add to beets.

6. Grate 1 tsp (5 mL) zest from oranges. Add to beet mixture, along with garlic, red onion, salt, oil and vinegar.

7. Using a sharp knife, cut peel and pith from oranges. Working over the beet mixture, cut between membranes to release segments. Squeeze the membranes to release any remaining juice. Gently toss to coat. Let stand for at least 30 minutes or overnight to blend the flavors.

> ▸ **Health Tip**
>
> Beet greens contain lutein, a great protector of blood vessels and the retina, and beet roots are a liver-friendly food.

## Nutrients per serving

| | |
|---|---|
| Calories | 115 |
| Fat | 7 g |
| Carbohydrate | 13 g |
| Protein | 2 g |
| Vitamin C | 50 mg |
| Vitamin D | 0 IU |
| Vitamin E | 1 mg |
| Niacin | 0 mg |
| Folate | 8 mcg |
| Vitamin $B_6$ | 0.1 mg |
| Vitamin $B_{12}$ | 0.0 mcg |
| Zinc | 0.2 mg |
| Selenium | 1 mcg |

# Insalata Caprese

*This is a salad favorite, and this version definitely qualifies as "Mediterranean diet" with the addition of kalamata olives.*

## Tip

Bocconcini are fresh, golf-ball-sized mozzarella curds that must be kept in water until they are needed. They are widely available. In supermarkets, they usually sit in plastic tubs right by the ricotta and other Italian dairy products.

| | | |
|---|---|---|
| 1 lb | ripe tomatoes, sliced $1/2$ inch (1 cm) thick (about 4 tomatoes) | 500 g |
| $1/4$ cup | thinly sliced red onion | 60 mL |
| $1/4$ cup | thinly sliced green bell peppers | 60 mL |
| $1/4$ cup | extra virgin olive oil | 60 mL |
| 2 tbsp | balsamic vinegar | 30 mL |
| | Salt and freshly ground black pepper | |
| 6 oz | bocconcini (see tip, at left) | 175 g |
| $1/4$ cup | kalamata olives (about 8) | 60 mL |
| 12 | large fresh basil leaves | 12 |

1. On a large presentation plate, arrange tomato slices in one layer. Scatter sliced onions and green peppers evenly over the tomatoes.

2. In a small bowl, whisk together oil, vinegar, salt and pepper until emulsified. Pour dressing evenly over the tomatoes.

3. Drain and pat dry the bocconcini. Slice into rounds $1/4$ inch (0.5 cm) thick. Put at least one slice of cheese on top of each tomato slice.

4. Place olives decoratively among the tomatoes. Garnish with the basil leaves, and serve within 30 minutes.

> ▶ **Health Tip**
>
> Olives pack a remarkable array of beneficial phytonutrients and may be part of the reason why the Mediterranean diet is consistently proving itself beneficial.

### Nutrients per serving

| | |
|---|---|
| Calories | 282 |
| Fat | 22 g |
| Carbohydrate | 9 g |
| Protein | 13 g |
| Vitamin C | 24 mg |
| Vitamin D | 6 IU |
| Vitamin E | 3 mg |
| Niacin | 1 mg |
| Folate | 26 mcg |
| Vitamin $B_6$ | 0.2 mg |
| Vitamin $B_{12}$ | 0.4 mcg |
| Zinc | 1.6 mg |
| Selenium | 7 mcg |

# Broccoli Carrot Slaw with Cranberries and Sunflower Seeds

*This dish is a great way to get the health benefits of broccoli, sweetened and brightened with the other ingredients in this upbeat salad.*

**Makes 6 servings**

## Tip

Agave nectar (a.k.a. agave syrup) is a plant-based sweetener derived from the agave cactus, native to Mexico. Agave juice produces a light golden syrup.

| | | |
|---|---|---|
| ¼ cup | nonfat plain Greek yogurt | 60 mL |
| 2 tbsp | freshly squeezed lemon juice | 30 mL |
| 1 tbsp | agave nectar or liquid honey | 15 mL |
| 2 tsp | Dijon mustard | 10 mL |
| ⅛ tsp | fine sea salt | 0.5 mL |
| 3 cups | shredded peeled broccoli stems (from 1 large bunch) | 750 mL |
| 2 cups | shredded peeled carrots | 500 mL |
| ½ cup | chopped green onions | 125 mL |
| ⅓ cup | dried cranberries, chopped | 75 mL |
| ¼ cup | lightly salted roasted sunflower seeds | 60 mL |

1. In a small bowl, whisk together yogurt, lemon juice, agave nectar, mustard and salt.

2. In a large bowl, combine broccoli, carrots, green onions and cranberries. Add dressing and gently toss to coat. Cover and refrigerate for at least 30 minutes, until chilled, or for up to 2 hours. Just before serving, sprinkle with sunflower seeds.

---

▶ **Health Tip**

Broccoli contains compounds that switch on the body's anti-cancer and detoxification molecules.

---

| **Nutrients** per serving | |
|---|---|
| Calories | 105 |
| Fat | 3 g |
| Carbohydrate | 18 g |
| Protein | 3 g |
| Vitamin C | 36 mg |
| Vitamin D | 0 IU |
| Vitamin E | 2 mg |
| Niacin | 1 mg |
| Folate | 71 mcg |
| Vitamin B$_6$ | 0.2 mg |
| Vitamin B$_{12}$ | 0.0 mcg |
| Zinc | 0.6 mg |
| Selenium | 5 mcg |

# Cranberry Mandarin Coleslaw with Walnuts and Raisins

*This is no ordinary coleslaw — it has plenty of sweetness and lots of crunch; and a checklist of healthy ingredients.*

**Makes 8 to 10 servings**

## Tip

Pepitas are pumpkin seeds with the white hull removed, leaving the flat, dark green inner seed. They are subtly sweet and nutty, with a slightly chewy texture.

| | | |
|---|---|---|
| 3 cups | shredded red and/or green cabbage | 750 mL |
| 2 cups | shredded carrots | 500 mL |
| 1 cup | chopped celery | 250 mL |
| ½ cup | chopped green onions | 125 mL |
| 1 tbsp | freshly squeezed lemon juice | 15 mL |
| ½ cup | raisins | 125 mL |
| ½ cup | raw green pumpkin seeds (pepitas) | 125 mL |
| ½ cup | fresh cranberries | 125 mL |
| ½ cup | walnut halves | 125 mL |
| 6 tbsp | extra virgin olive oil | 90 mL |
| ¼ cup | brown or natural rice vinegar | 60 mL |
| 1 | can (10 oz/284 mL) mandarin oranges, drained | 1 |

1. In a large bowl, combine cabbage, carrots, celery and green onions. Drizzle with lemon juice and toss to coat. Toss in raisins, pumpkin seeds, cranberries and walnuts.

2. In a small bowl, whisk together oil and vinegar. Drizzle over salad and toss to coat. Top with mandarin oranges. Cover and refrigerate overnight to blend the flavors.

> ▸ **Health Tip**
>
> Just ¼ cup (60 mL) of walnuts has nearly all of the recommended daily amount of brain-nourishing omega-3 fats.

## Nutrients per 1 of 10 servings

| | |
|---|---|
| Calories | 199 |
| Fat | 15 g |
| Carbohydrate | 16 g |
| Protein | 4 g |
| Vitamin C | 22 mg |
| Vitamin D | 0 IU |
| Vitamin E | 1 mg |
| Niacin | 1 mg |
| Folate | 30 mcg |
| Vitamin B$_6$ | 0.1 mg |
| Vitamin B$_{12}$ | 0.0 mcg |
| Zinc | 0.9 mg |
| Selenium | 1 mcg |

# Oriental Coleslaw

*This Asian-inspired coleslaw delivers some of the fresh ingredients from important food families such as cabbage (cruciferous) and has loads of flavor.*

**Makes 8 to 10 servings**

## Tips

Other vegetables, such as green beans or broccoli, can replace the snow peas.

Prepare salad and dressing early in the day. Best if tossed just before serving.

### Salad

| | | |
|---|---|---|
| ¾ cup | chopped snow peas | 175 mL |
| 3 cups | shredded green cabbage | 750 mL |
| 3 cups | shredded red cabbage | 750 mL |
| 1 cup | sliced water chestnuts | 250 mL |
| 1 cup | sliced red peppers | 250 mL |
| ¾ cup | drained canned mandarin oranges | 175 mL |
| 2 | medium green onions, chopped | 2 |

### Dressing

| | | |
|---|---|---|
| 3 tbsp | brown sugar | 45 mL |
| 2 tbsp | rice wine vinegar | 30 mL |
| 2 tbsp | vegetable oil | 30 mL |
| 1 tbsp | soy sauce | 15 mL |
| 1 tbsp | sesame oil | 15 mL |
| 1 tsp | minced garlic | 5 mL |
| 1 tsp | minced gingerroot | 5 mL |

1. *Salad:* In saucepan of boiling water or microwave, blanch snow peas just until tender-crisp, approximately 1 to 2 minutes; refresh in cold water and drain. Place in serving bowl with shredded cabbage, water chestnuts, red peppers, mandarin oranges and green onions; toss well to combine.

2. *Dressing:* In small bowl, whisk together brown sugar, vinegar, vegetable oil, soy sauce, sesame oil, garlic and ginger; pour over salad and toss well.

> ▶ **Health Tip**
>
> Sesame oil contains sesamol, a very potent antioxidant.

## Nutrients per 1 of 10 servings

| | |
|---|---|
| Calories | 95 |
| Fat | 4 g |
| Carbohydrate | 13 g |
| Protein | 2 g |
| Vitamin C | 52 mg |
| Vitamin D | 0 IU |
| Vitamin E | 1 mg |
| Niacin | 1 mg |
| Folate | 28 mcg |
| Vitamin B$_6$ | 0.2 mg |
| Vitamin B$_{12}$ | 0.0 mcg |
| Zinc | 0.3 mg |
| Selenium | 1 mcg |

# Tabbouleh

*This is one of the healthiest salads around, and a great example of how flavor can meet nutritional value.*

## Tips

If you prefer a sweeter taste, add 2 tbsp (30 mL) more oil.

Leftover tabbouleh can be kept in the refrigerator, covered, for up to 3 days. Be sure to bring it back up to room temperature before serving.

| | | |
|---|---|---|
| 2 cups | packed chopped fresh parsley | 500 mL |
| 1 | onion, finely chopped | 1 |
| 1 | tomato, finely chopped | 1 |
| $\frac{1}{2}$ cup | bulgur (about 4 oz/125 g) | 125 mL |
| 6 tbsp | freshly squeezed lemon juice | 90 mL |
| $\frac{1}{4}$ cup | olive oil | 60 mL |
| | Salt and freshly ground black pepper | |

1. In a bowl, combine parsley, onion and tomato. Mix well. Set aside.

2. In a saucepan, boil bulgur wheat in plenty of water for 6 to 8 minutes, until tender. Drain and refresh with cold water. Drain again completely and add cooked bulgur to the vegetables in the bowl. Mix well.

3. Sprinkle lemon juice and olive oil over the salad. Add salt and pepper to taste. Toss to mix thoroughly. Transfer to a serving plate. The salad can be served immediately, although it'll be better if it waits up to 2 hours, covered and unrefrigerated.

> ▶ **Health Tip**
>
> Parsley contains compounds that have a natural diuretic effect on the body, and it is a fantastic source of vitamin K.

## Nutrients per serving

| | |
|---|---|
| Calories | 139 |
| Fat | 9 g |
| Carbohydrate | 13 g |
| Protein | 2 g |
| Vitamin C | 37 mg |
| Vitamin D | 0 IU |
| Vitamin E | 2 mg |
| Niacin | 1 mg |
| Folate | 42 mcg |
| Vitamin $B_6$ | 0.1 mg |
| Vitamin $B_{12}$ | 0.0 mcg |
| Zinc | 0.5 mg |
| Selenium | 0 mcg |

# Couscous Salad with Basil and Pine Nuts

*This couscous recipe packs in the vegetables and the flavor of orange zest, as well as garlic.*

---

**Makes 4 servings**

## Tips

Tender basil leaves bruise easily when chopped. Stack the leaves one on top of the other, roll up into a cigar shape and, using a sharp knife, cut into fine thin shreds.

If you can't find fresh basil, substitute ¼ cup (60 mL) chopped fresh parsley and 1 tsp (5 mL) dried basil.

| | | |
|---|---|---|
| 1 cup | couscous | 250 mL |
| 1 cup | ready-to-use low-sodium chicken or vegetable broth | 250 mL |
| 4 | green onions, chopped | 4 |
| 1 | red bell pepper, finely chopped | 1 |
| 1 | zucchini, diced | 1 |
| ¼ cup | raisins | 60 mL |
| ¼ cup | olive oil | 60 mL |
| 2 tbsp | red wine vinegar | 30 mL |
| 1 tsp | grated orange zest | 5 mL |
| 2 tbsp | freshly squeezed orange juice | 30 mL |
| 1 | large garlic clove, minced | 1 |
| ½ tsp | salt (optional) | 2 mL |
| | Freshly ground black pepper | |
| ¼ cup | chopped fresh basil | 60 mL |
| ¼ cup | toasted pine nuts (see tip, at left) | 60 mL |

1. Place couscous in a large bowl; pour broth over. Cover with a dinner plate and let stand for 5 minutes. Fluff with a fork to break up any lumps. Let cool to room temperature. Add green onions, red pepper, zucchini and raisins.

2. In a small bowl, whisk together oil, vinegar, orange zest, orange juice, garlic, salt (if using) and pepper to taste. Pour over salad; toss well. Just before serving, stir in basil and pine nuts. Serve salad at room temperature.

> ▶ **Health Tip**
>
> Pine nuts contain pinolenic acid, which may work to curb appetite.

| Nutrients per serving | |
|---|---|
| Calories | 394 |
| Fat | 20 g |
| Carbohydrate | 46 g |
| Protein | 9 g |
| Vitamin C | 46 mg |
| Vitamin D | 0 IU |
| Vitamin E | 3 mg |
| Niacin | 3 mg |
| Folate | 34 mcg |
| Vitamin $B_6$ | 0.2 mg |
| Vitamin $B_{12}$ | 0.1 mcg |
| Zinc | 1.2 mg |
| Selenium | 0 mcg |

# Quinoa Salad

*The versatile supergrain appears once again, this time as a side salad with a full complement of vegetables and herbs.*

**Makes 4 servings**

## Tip

To keep quinoa as fresh as possible, store it in an airtight container in the refrigerator for up to 6 months or in the freezer for up to 1 year.

| | | |
|---|---|---|
| 1¼ cups | ready-to-use reduced-sodium vegetable broth | 300 mL |
| ¾ cup | quinoa, rinsed | 175 mL |
| ½ cup | thawed frozen peas | 125 mL |
| ¼ cup | finely chopped orange bell pepper | 60 mL |
| ¼ cup | finely chopped yellow bell pepper | 60 mL |
| 1 tbsp | finely chopped red onion | 15 mL |
| 2 tbsp | extra virgin olive oil | 30 mL |
| 1 tbsp | chopped fresh parsley | 15 mL |
| 1 tsp | dried thyme | 5 mL |
| 1 tsp | freshly squeezed lemon juice | 5 mL |
| | Salt and freshly ground black pepper | |

1. In a saucepan, bring broth to a boil over high heat. Add quinoa, reduce heat to low, cover and simmer for 20 minutes or until quinoa is tender and liquid is almost absorbed. Remove from heat and let stand, covered, for 5 minutes or until liquid is absorbed.

2. In a large bowl, combine quinoa, peas, orange pepper, yellow pepper and red onion.

3. In a small bowl, whisk together oil, parsley, thyme and lemon juice. Drizzle over salad and toss to coat. Season to taste with salt and pepper. Serve warm or cover and refrigerate for 1 hour, until chilled, and serve cold.

## Variation

If you're making this salad for non-vegetarians, you can substitute reduced-sodium chicken or turkey broth for the vegetable broth.

> ▶ **Health Tip**
>
> Quinoa, unlike many other grains, can be considered a complete protein.

### Nutrients per serving

| | |
|---|---|
| Calories | 201 |
| Fat | 9 g |
| Carbohydrate | 25 g |
| Protein | 6 g |
| Vitamin C | 29 mg |
| Vitamin D | 0 IU |
| Vitamin E | 2 mg |
| Niacin | 1 mg |
| Folate | 79 mcg |
| Vitamin B$_6$ | 0.2 mg |
| Vitamin B$_{12}$ | 0.0 mcg |
| Zinc | 1.2 mg |
| Selenium | 3 mcg |

# Vegetable Quinoa Salad

*This simple-to-prepare salad can be accentuated with some hot pepper flakes and lavender flowers or left without, but still with plenty of pizzazz from Italian parsley, bell peppers and cucumber to accentuate the quinoa.*

**Makes 10 servings**

## Tips

If you are not a fan of the strong flavors of hot pepper and/or lavender, leave them out. You could also substitute your favorite homemade or store-bought dressing; ¼ cup (60 mL) is required to coat the salad. Remember, you do not want it soaked in dressing, just enough to enhance the natural flavors.

Only lavender that has been grown specifically for food use should be used in cooking.

### Nutrients per serving

| Calories | 106 |
|---|---|
| Fat | 5 g |
| Carbohydrate | 13 g |
| Protein | 3 g |
| Vitamin C | 11 mg |
| Vitamin D | 0 IU |
| Vitamin E | 1 mg |
| Niacin | 0 mg |
| Folate | 39 mcg |
| Vitamin B$_6$ | 0.1 mg |
| Vitamin B$_{12}$ | 0.0 mcg |
| Zinc | 0.6 mg |
| Selenium | 1 mcg |

### Salad

| 1 cup | quinoa, well rinsed and drained | 250 mL |
|---|---|---|
| 2 cups | cold water | 500 mL |
| 2 | tomatoes, chopped | 2 |
| 2 | large sprigs Italian (flat-leaf) parsley (leaves only), chopped | 2 |
| ¼ | English cucumber, chopped | ¼ |
| ⅓ cup | chopped red, green, yellow or mixed bell peppers | 75 mL |

### Vinaigrette

| 3 tbsp | extra virgin olive oil | 45 mL |
|---|---|---|
| 2 tbsp | freshly squeezed lemon juice | 30 mL |
| 1½ tsp | hot pepper flakes (optional) | 7 mL |
| ½ tsp | salt | 2 mL |
| ½ tsp | freshly ground black pepper | 2 mL |
| ½ tsp | dried lavender flowers (optional) | 2 mL |

1. *Salad:* In a medium saucepan over medium heat, bring quinoa and water to a boil. Reduce heat and boil gently for 10 to 15 minutes or until the white germ separates from the seed. Cover, remove from heat and let stand for 5 minutes. Remove lid, let cool and fluff with a fork.

2. Meanwhile, in a large bowl, combine tomatoes, parsley, cucumber and bell peppers. Stir in cooled quinoa.

3. *Vinaigrette:* In a small bowl, whisk together olive oil, lemon juice, hot pepper flakes (if using), salt, pepper and lavender (if using). Pour over salad and toss to coat.

*This recipe courtesy of Deloris Del Rio.*

> ▸ **Health Tip**
>
> Both cucumbers and bell peppers are rich sources of vitamin C.

# Refreshing Lentil Salad

*This salad comes to the table with some substance, from the lentils, but also the freshness and sweetness of oranges, cranberries and lemon juice.*

## Tips

Instead of using canned lentils, you can cook dried lentils. Place $\frac{1}{2}$ cup (125 mL) dried green or yellow lentils in a saucepan with $1\frac{1}{2}$ cups (375 mL) water. Bring to a boil, then reduce heat and simmer for 20 to 30 minutes or until tender. Check near the end of cooking and add more water if the lentils become dry. Drain well. Makes about $1\frac{1}{4}$ cups (300 mL) cooked lentils.

Serve this salad on top of mixed greens for a refreshing lunch.

| **Nutrients** per serving | |
| --- | --- |
| Calories | 167 |
| Fat | 7 g |
| Carbohydrate | 22 g |
| Protein | 6 g |
| Vitamin C | 34 mg |
| Vitamin D | 0 IU |
| Vitamin E | 2 mg |
| Niacin | 1 mg |
| Folate | 116 mcg |
| Vitamin B$_6$ | 0.2 mg |
| Vitamin B$_{12}$ | 0.0 mcg |
| Zinc | 0.9 mg |
| Selenium | 2 mcg |

| | | |
| --- | --- | --- |
| 2 | plum (Roma) tomatoes, seeded and diced | 2 |
| 2 | oranges, peeled and cut into segments | 2 |
| 1 | can (19 oz/540 mL) lentils, drained and rinsed | 1 |
| $\frac{1}{2}$ cup | sliced green onions | 125 mL |
| $\frac{1}{4}$ cup | coarsely chopped fresh cilantro | 60 mL |
| 3 tbsp | coarsely chopped dried cranberries | 45 mL |
| $\frac{1}{3}$ cup | freshly squeezed lemon juice | 75 mL |
| 2 tbsp | canola oil | 30 mL |
| $\frac{1}{2}$ tsp | freshly ground black pepper | 2 mL |
| $\frac{1}{4}$ tsp | salt | 1 mL |
| $\frac{1}{4}$ cup | toasted slivered almonds | 60 mL |

**1.** In a large bowl, combine tomatoes, oranges, lentils, green onions, cilantro and cranberries. Drizzle with lemon juice and oil; toss to coat. Sprinkle with pepper and salt. Top with toasted almonds.

*This recipe courtesy of dietitian Julie Aubé.*

> ▶ **Health Tip**
>
> Oranges are a good source of bioflavonoids, molecules that can alter inflammation in the body and also support the formation of connective tissue, including that of the arteries.

# Chickpeas with Kiwi and Avocado Salsa

*This marriage of chickpeas (sometimes galled garbanzo beans) and the delicious kiwi and avocado salsa is a match made in heaven.*

---

**Makes 4 to 6 servings**

### Tip

You can use 2 cups (500 mL) cooked chickpeas instead of canned.

| | | |
|---|---|---|
| 1 | can (14 to 19 oz/398 to 540 mL) chickpeas, drained and rinsed | 1 |
| 3 cups | Kiwi and Avocado Salsa with Pomegranate and Red Onion (see recipe, opposite) | 750 mL |

**1.** In a bowl, combine chickpeas and salsa. Recipe may be made ahead and stored, tightly covered, in the refrigerator for up to 2 days.

**Nutrients** per 1 of 6 servings

| | |
|---|---|
| Calories | 254 |
| Fat | 15 g |
| Carbohydrate | 28 g |
| Protein | 5 g |
| Vitamin C | 52 mg |
| Vitamin D | 0 IU |
| Vitamin E | 4 mg |
| Niacin | 1 mg |
| Folate | 86 mcg |
| Vitamin $B_6$ | 0.5 mg |
| Vitamin $B_{12}$ | 0.0 mcg |
| Zinc | 1.0 mg |
| Selenium | 3 mcg |

# Kiwi and Avocado Salsa with Pomegranate and Red Onion

| | | |
|---|---|---:|
| 4 | kiwifruit, peeled and chopped | 4 |
| 1 | avocado, peeled and diced | 1 |
| ½ | red onion, diced | ½ |
| ½ cup | fresh pomegranate seeds (optional) | 125 mL |
| 3 tbsp | freshly squeezed lemon juice | 45 mL |
| ¼ cup | grapeseed oil or hemp oil | 60 mL |
| 1 tbsp | Pomegranate Molasses (see recipe, page 283, or store-bought) | 15 mL |
| | Sea salt and freshly ground pepper | |

**Makes about 3 cups (750 mL)**

## Tip

Use this salsa as a garnish for baked and roasted dishes. If the ingredients are cut into a fairly small dice (close to ¼ inch/0.5 cm), the salsa will be easier to use as you might a sauce.

1. In a bowl, combine kiwis, avocado, red onion and pomegranate seeds (if using). Toss with lemon juice. Drizzle oil and molasses over the salsa and toss well to combine. Season to taste with salt and pepper.

2. Store salsa, tightly covered, in the refrigerator for up to 2 days.

---

▶ **Health Tip**

Kiwi is a fantastic source of vitamin C.

---

**Nutrients** per ½ cup (125 mL)

| | |
|---|---:|
| Calories | 176 |
| Fat | 14 g |
| Carbohydrate | 13 g |
| Protein | 1 g |
| Vitamin C | 49 mg |
| Vitamin D | 0 IU |
| Vitamin E | 4 mg |
| Niacin | 1 mg |
| Folate | 41 mcg |
| Vitamin $B_6$ | 0.2 mg |
| Vitamin $B_{12}$ | 0.0 mcg |
| Zinc | 0.3 mg |
| Selenium | 1 mcg |

# Pasta Salad with Apricots, Dates and Orange Dressing

*You may end up eating this salad as a light meal.*

## Makes 6 to 8 servings

## Tips

A delicious sweet pasta salad that goes well with a grilled fish or chicken entrée. Prunes can replace apricots or dates, or use in combination.

Prepare salad and dressing early in day. Toss just before serving.

### Salad

| | | |
|---|---|---:|
| 12 oz | medium shell pasta | 375 g |
| 1½ cups | diced red or green bell peppers | 375 mL |
| ¾ cup | diced dried apricots | 175 mL |
| ¾ cup | diced dried dates | 175 mL |
| ½ cup | chopped green onions | 125 mL |

### Dressing

| | | |
|---|---|---:|
| 3 tbsp | balsamic vinegar | 45 mL |
| 3 tbsp | frozen orange juice concentrate, thawed | 45 mL |
| 3 tbsp | olive oil | 45 mL |
| 2 tbsp | freshly squeezed lemon juice | 30 mL |
| 2 tbsp | water | 30 mL |
| 1½ tsp | crushed garlic | 7 mL |
| ½ cup | chopped fresh parsley | 125 mL |

1. *Salad:* Cook pasta in boiling water according to package instructions or until firm to the bite. Rinse with cold water. Drain and place in serving bowl.

2. Add sweet peppers, apricots, dates and green onions.

3. *Dressing:* In small bowl, combine vinegar, orange juice concentrate, oil, lemon juice, water, garlic and parsley. Pour over salad, and toss.

▶ **Health Tip**

Dates contain a variety of vitamins, and lots of the mineral potassium, which is important for nerve transmission and often needed in the diet of people taking diuretics for issues such as high blood pressure.

## Nutrients per 1 of 8 servings

| | |
|---|---:|
| Calories | 304 |
| Fat | 6 g |
| Carbohydrate | 56 g |
| Protein | 7 g |
| Vitamin C | 55 mg |
| Vitamin D | 0 IU |
| Vitamin E | 2 mg |
| Niacin | 4 mg |
| Folate | 136 mcg |
| Vitamin B$_6$ | 0.2 mg |
| Vitamin B$_{12}$ | 0.0 mcg |
| Zinc | 0.8 mg |
| Selenium | 27 mcg |

# MEATLESS MAINS

# Jerusalem Artichoke Stew

*This vegetarian stew draws on vegetable broth and wine to create a basic stock and adds a variety of vegetables.*

## Tips

When Jerusalem artichokes are not available, use potatoes instead.

You can use 2 cups (500 mL) cooked white beans, drained and rinsed, instead of canned.

| | | |
|---|---|---:|
| 1 tbsp | olive oil | 15 mL |
| 1 | onion, chopped | 1 |
| 2 | stalks celery, chopped | 2 |
| 2 | cloves garlic, finely chopped | 2 |
| 4 cups | ready-to-use vegetable broth or water | 1 L |
| 2 cups | diced Jerusalem artichokes or potatoes | 500 mL |
| 1 | carrot, diced | 1 |
| 1/2 cup | shredded rutabaga or green cabbage | 125 mL |
| 1/4 cup | dry white wine | 60 mL |
| 1 | can (14 to 19 oz/398 to 540 mL) cannellini beans or flageolets, drained and rinsed | 1 |
| 3 tbsp | chopped fresh parsley | 45 mL |
| 2 tbsp | freshly squeezed lemon juice | 30 mL |
| | Sea salt and freshly ground pepper | |

**1.** In a large saucepan, heat oil over medium heat. Add onion and celery and cook, stirring occasionally, for 6 to 8 minutes or until soft. Add garlic and cook, stirring frequently, for 2 minutes. Add broth. Increase heat to high and bring to a boil. Add Jerusalem artichokes, carrot, rutabaga and white wine. Cover, reduce heat to medium-low and simmer, stirring once or twice, for 15 minutes or until vegetables are tender when pierced with the tip of a knife.

**2.** Add beans, parsley and lemon juice and heat through. Season to taste with salt and pepper. Using a potato masher, mash some of the vegetables to thicken the stew.

## ▶ Health Tip

Jerusalem artichokes are a good source of minerals, supplying magnesium, potassium and iron — all important for the nervous system and the transport of oxygen to the nervous system.

### Nutrients per serving

| | |
|---|---:|
| Calories | 146 |
| Fat | 3 g |
| Carbohydrate | 25 g |
| Protein | 5 g |
| Vitamin C | 12 mg |
| Vitamin D | 0 IU |
| Vitamin E | 1 mg |
| Niacin | 1 mg |
| Folate | 46 mcg |
| Vitamin $B_6$ | 0.2 mg |
| Vitamin $B_{12}$ | 0.0 mcg |
| Zinc | 0.5 mg |
| Selenium | 1 mcg |

# Roasted Beet Tacos with Marinated Shredded Kale

*Who said tacos had to be a shell that contains ground meat? This vegetarian version delivers on flavor and nutrients.*

**Makes 4 to 6 servings**

**▶ Health Tip**

Kale contains isothiocyanates — the compounds that induce production of the body's protective enzymes — and kale's vitamin K content is off the charts.

### Nutrients per 1 of 6 servings

| | |
| --- | --- |
| Calories | 235 |
| Fat | 15 g |
| Carbohydrate | 25 g |
| Protein | 5 g |
| Vitamin C | 87 mg |
| Vitamin D | 0 IU |
| Vitamin E | 2 mg |
| Niacin | 1 mg |
| Folate | 108 mcg |
| Vitamin B$_6$ | 0.3 mg |
| Vitamin B$_{12}$ | 0.0 mcg |
| Zinc | 0.7 mg |
| Selenium | 1 mcg |

- **Preheat oven to 400°F (200°C)**
- **11- by 7-inch (28 by 18 cm) glass baking dish, lightly oiled**
- **Baking sheet, lined with parchment paper**

| | | |
| --- | --- | --- |
| 2 | large onions, thinly sliced | 2 |
| 6 tbsp | olive oil, divided | 90 mL |
| | Salt | |
| 4 | medium red or golden beets, with greens | 4 |
| ½ tsp | freshly ground black pepper, divided | 2 mL |
| | Grated zest and juice of 1 lemon | |
| 6 cups | shredded kale (½ large bunch) | 1.5 L |
| 6 to 8 | 4-inch (10 cm) corn tortillas, warmed | 6 to 8 |

1. Arrange racks in oven to accommodate both a baking sheet and shallow baking dish.

2. In prepared baking dish, combine onions, 2 tbsp (30 mL) of the oil and 1 tsp (5 mL) of salt. Cover with foil and roast in preheated oven, stirring occasionally, until golden brown and caramelized, 1 to 1½ hours.

3. Meanwhile, trim greens from beets. Discard stems and chop greens. Set greens aside. Peel beets and cut into ¼-inch (0.5 cm) dice. In a bowl, toss beets with 2 tbsp (30 mL) of olive oil, 1 tsp (5 mL) of salt and ¼ tsp (1 mL) of black pepper. Spread beets onto prepared baking sheet and roast, stirring occasionally, until beets are fork-tender, 20 to 25 minutes.

4. Meanwhile, in a large bowl, whisk together lemon zest, 2 tbsp (30 mL) of the lemon juice, remaining 2 tbsp (30 mL) of oil, pinch of salt and remaining ¼ tsp (1 mL) of black pepper. Add shredded kale and beet green tops and toss to coat. Cover and refrigerate until needed.

5. To serve, spoon a generous amount of caramelized onion down center of each warmed tortilla; top with roasted beets and marinated shredded kale and beet greens.

# Three-Pepper Tamale Pie

*This satisfying, chile-spiced dish provides a break from animal sources of protein.*

**Makes 4 to 6 servings**

## Tip

Vegan hard margarine, such as Earth Balance vegan buttery flavor sticks, has almost half as much saturated fat as regular butter and no cholesterol. Where butter is called for in a recipe, vegan hard margarine can be a heart-healthy, delicious alternative.

### Nutrients per 1 of 6 servings

| | |
|---|---|
| Calories | 309 |
| Fat | 11 g |
| Carbohydrate | 46 g |
| Protein | 9 g |
| Vitamin C | 38 mg |
| Vitamin D | 20 IU |
| Vitamin E | 3 mg |
| Niacin | 3 mg |
| Folate | 142 mcg |
| Vitamin B$_6$ | 0.3 mcg |
| Vitamin B$_{12}$ | 0.0 mcg |
| Zinc | 1.2 mg |
| Selenium | 8 mcg |

• **8-cup (2 L) glass baking dish, lightly oiled**

| | | |
|---|---|---|
| 2 tbsp | olive oil | 30 mL |
| 1 | onion, chopped | 1 |
| 1 | red bell pepper, chopped | 1 |
| 2 | cloves garlic, minced | 2 |
| 1½ cups | drained cooked pinto beans | 375 mL |
| 1 cup | drained cooked kidney beans | 250 mL |
| 1 cup | frozen roasted corn kernels | 250 mL |
| 1 | can (4 oz/127 mL) diced roasted mild green chiles | 1 |
| 1 cup | canned diced tomatoes, with juice | 250 mL |
| 1 cup | tomato sauce | 250 mL |
| 2 tsp | New Mexico red chile powder | 10 mL |
| 2 tsp | ground cumin | 10 mL |
| ¾ tsp | salt | 3 mL |

**Topping**

| | | |
|---|---|---|
| ¾ cup | cornmeal | 175 mL |
| 2 cups | water | 500 mL |
| ¾ tsp | salt | 3 mL |
| ¾ tsp | chipotle chile powder (optional) | 3 mL |
| 2 tbsp | vegan hard margarine | 30 mL |
| ½ cup | pitted black olives | 125 mL |

1. Place a large heavy-bottomed skillet over medium heat and let pan get hot. Add oil and tip pan to coat. Add onion, bell pepper and garlic and cook, stirring, until softened and slightly browned, 6 to 8 minutes.

2. Increase heat to medium-high. Stir in pinto beans, kidney beans, corn, green chiles, tomatoes, tomato sauce, chile powder, cumin and salt and bring just to a boil. Reduce heat and simmer until thickened, 20 to 25 minutes. Transfer to baking dish. Preheat oven to 375°F (190°C).

## Variation

For a spicier tamale pie, add 2 chopped chipotle chiles and 1 tbsp (15 mL) adobo sauce from canned chipotles when you add the green chiles.

**3.** *Topping:* In a small saucepan, whisk together cornmeal and water. Whisk in salt and chipotle chile powder (if using). Bring to a boil over medium-high heat. Reduce heat and simmer, stirring frequently, until thickened, 8 to 10 minutes. Whisk in margarine. Spread mixture evenly over filling and dot top with olives.

**4.** Bake in preheated oven until filling is bubbly and top is golden brown, 35 to 45 minutes. Let tamale pie cool slightly before cutting and serving.

---

▶ **Health Tip**

Chiles are in the capsicum family and have numerous health benefits, including cancer prevention and cardiovascular uses, due to the presence of capsaicin (the heat-producing compound).

# Vegetable Cheese Loaf with Lemon Tomato Sauce

*This meat(less) loaf packs plenty of flavor and is topped with a tangy sauce.*

**Makes 6 servings**

## Tip

When buying celery, look for heads that are tight. Avoid any that are discolored or cracked, as they are not fresh. In this recipe, celery is used to flavor the vegetable loaf. But celery is also one of the all-time great healthy snacks. Keep plenty on hand, as it keeps well, refrigerated.

| Nutrients per serving | |
| --- | --- |
| Calories | 327 |
| Fat | 19 g |
| Carbohydrate | 24 g |
| Protein | 15 g |
| Vitamin C | 37 mg |
| Vitamin D | 26 IU |
| Vitamin E | 1 mg |
| Niacin | 1 mg |
| Folate | 61 mcg |
| Vitamin $B_6$ | 0.2 mg |
| Vitamin $B_{12}$ | 0.7 mcg |
| Zinc | 0.8 mg |
| Selenium | 15 mcg |

- Preheat oven to 350°F (180°C)
- 9- by 5-inch (23 by 12.5 cm) loaf pan, lightly greased

| | | |
| --- | --- | --- |
| ¾ cup | finely chopped onion | 175 mL |
| 3 tbsp | butter or margarine | 45 mL |
| ¾ cup | finely chopped celery | 175 mL |
| 2 | carrots, peeled and grated | 2 |
| 2 cups | small-curd cottage cheese | 500 mL |
| 2 cups | fresh bread crumbs | 500 mL |
| 2 | large eggs, well beaten | 2 |
| | Zest and juice of ½ lemon | |
| 1 tsp | salt | 5 mL |
| ½ tsp | freshly ground black pepper | 2 mL |
| ¼ tsp | dried basil | 1 mL |

### Lemon Tomato Sauce

| | | |
| --- | --- | --- |
| 2½ cups | tomato juice, divided | 625 mL |
| 1 | onion, cut in half | 1 |
| 4 | sprigs fresh parsley | 4 |
| 1 | bay leaf | 1 |
| 1 | whole clove | 1 |
| ½ tsp | dried basil | 2 mL |
| ½ tsp | granulated sugar | 2 mL |
| ⅓ cup | butter or margarine | 75 mL |
| ¼ cup | all-purpose flour | 60 mL |
| | Juice of ½ lemon | |

1. In a medium skillet over medium heat, cook onion in melted butter for about 5 minutes or until tender. Add celery and carrots; cook for 1 minute.

2. In a large bowl, combine cottage cheese, bread crumbs, eggs, lemon zest and juice, and seasonings. Add vegetable mixture; stir.

## Tip

To keep parsley fresh, wrap it in several layers of paper towels and place in a plastic bag. Store in the warmest part of your refrigerator — in the butter keeper, for example, or the side door.

**3.** Place in prepared baking pan. Bake in preheated oven for 35 to 40 minutes or until knife inserted in center comes out clean. Remove loaf from pan.

**4.** *Sauce:* In a medium saucepan, combine $1\frac{1}{2}$ cups (375 mL) tomato juice, onion, parsley, seasonings and sugar. Bring to a boil, reduce heat and simmer for 15 to 20 minutes. Press mixture through sieve. Reserve sieved tomato mixture.

**5.** In a small saucepan, melt butter and blend in flour; cook for 1 to 2 minutes. Gradually add remaining tomato juice. Cook, stirring constantly, for 4 to 5 minutes or until smooth and thickened. Add reserved tomato mixture and lemon juice. Reheat to serving temperature. To serve, slice loaf; pour sauce over slices.

*This recipe courtesy of Margaret McIntyre.*

> ▶ **Health Tip**
>
> Lycopene, from tomatoes, has been shown to be one of the more useful cancer prevention phytochemicals.

# Vegetable Moussaka

*Moussaka is a favorite in Balkan and Mediterranean cooking. Many readers will have had moussaka at their favorite Greek restaurant, but this version is meatless — and good.*

## Tip

To vary the flavors in this tasty dish and transform it into a great party pleaser, add grilled peppers and zucchini to the eggplant layer.

- Preheat oven to 350°F (180°C)
- Baking sheets, greased
- Food processor
- 13- by 9-inch (33 by 23 cm) baking pan, greased

| | | |
|---|---|---|
| 2 | eggplants | 2 |
| 1 tsp | salt | 5 mL |
| 1 | onion, chopped | 1 |
| 1 | clove garlic, minced | 1 |
| 1 | can (19 oz/540 mL) chickpeas, drained and rinsed | 1 |
| 1 | can (28 oz/796 mL) tomatoes | 1 |
| 1 tbsp | dried oregano | 15 mL |
| 1 tbsp | dried basil | 15 mL |
| 1/2 tsp | ground cinnamon | 2 mL |
| 1/2 tsp | freshly ground black pepper | 2 mL |
| 1/4 cup | freshly grated Parmesan cheese | 60 mL |

**Topping**

| | | |
|---|---|---|
| 1 lb | tofu | 500 g |
| 1 | onion, quartered | 1 |
| 2 | large egg whites | 2 |
| Pinch | ground nutmeg | Pinch |

**1.** Slice eggplants lengthwise into 1/4-inch (5 mm) thick slices; sprinkle with salt. Drain in colander for 30 minutes. Arrange in a single layer on prepared baking sheets. Bake in preheated oven for 15 minutes. Turn and bake for 15 minutes.

**2.** In a nonstick skillet sprayed with nonstick cooking spray, cook onion and garlic, stirring, for 2 minutes. Add chickpeas, mashing slightly. Stir in tomatoes, oregano, basil, cinnamon, pepper and 1/2 tsp (2 mL) salt; bring to a boil. Reduce heat and simmer, uncovered, for 20 minutes, stirring occasionally. Process in food processor until mixture resembles coarse meal.

| Nutrients per serving | |
|---|---|
| Calories | 246 |
| Fat | 7 g |
| Carbohydrate | 34 g |
| Protein | 17 g |
| Vitamin C | 15 mg |
| Vitamin D | 1 IU |
| Vitamin E | 1 mg |
| Niacin | 2 mg |
| Folate | 102 mcg |
| Vitamin B$_6$ | 0.5 mg |
| Vitamin B$_{12}$ | 0.1 mcg |
| Zinc | 2.2 mg |
| Selenium | 15 mcg |

## Tip

Is cutting onions bringing you to tears? Try placing them in the freezer for 10 minutes before chopping.

3. In prepared baking pan, layer half of the eggplant, then all of the chickpea mixture, half of the Parmesan, then remaining eggplant.

4. *Topping:* In food processor, purée tofu, onion, egg whites and nutmeg until smooth. Spread over moussaka. Sprinkle with remaining Parmesan. Bake in preheated oven for 30 minutes.

*This recipe courtesy of chef Mark Mogensen and dietitian Marsha Rosen.*

> ▶ **Health Tip**
>
> Chickpeas are an excellent source of fiber — key to the health of the gastrointestinal system.

# Broccoli and Quinoa Enchiladas

*This high-protein dish is meatless, but not short on taste.*

## Tip

To keep quinoa as fresh as possible, store it in an airtight container in the refrigerator for up to 6 months or in the freezer for up to 1 year.

- Preheat oven to 350°F (180°C)
- 8- or 9-inch (20 or 23 cm) square glass baking dish or metal baking pan, sprayed with nonstick cooking spray

| | | |
|---|---|---|
| 2 tsp | olive oil | 10 mL |
| 1¼ cups | chopped onions | 300 mL |
| 2 cups | finely chopped broccoli florets | 500 mL |
| 1 tsp | ground cumin | 5 mL |
| 1½ cups | picante sauce, divided | 375 mL |
| 1½ cups | cooked quinoa, cooled | 375 mL |
| 1 cup | cottage or ricotta cheese | 250 mL |
| 1 cup | shredded sharp (old) white Cheddar cheese, divided | 250 mL |
| 8 | 8-inch (20 cm) multigrain tortillas, warmed | 8 |

1. In a large skillet, heat oil over medium heat. Add onions and cook, stirring, for 6 to 8 minutes or until softened. Add broccoli, cumin and ⅓ cup (75 mL) of the picante sauce; cook, stirring, for 1 minute. Remove from heat and stir in quinoa, cottage cheese and ⅓ cup (75 mL) of the Cheddar.

2. Spoon about ⅓ cup (75 mL) of the quinoa mixture down the center of each warmed tortilla. Roll up like a cigar and place, seam side down, in prepared baking dish. Spoon the remaining picante sauce over top.

3. Cover and bake in preheated oven for 20 to 25 minutes or until heated through. Sprinkle with the remaining Cheddar. Bake, uncovered, for 5 minutes or until cheese is bubbling.

### Nutrients per serving

| | |
|---|---|
| Calories | 268 |
| Fat | 7 g |
| Carbohydrate | 38 g |
| Protein | 13 g |
| Vitamin C | 18 mg |
| Vitamin D | 1 IU |
| Vitamin E | 1 mg |
| Niacin | 2 mg |
| Folate | 85 mcg |
| Vitamin B$_6$ | 0.2 mg |
| Vitamin B$_{12}$ | 0.3 mcg |
| Zinc | 1.1 mg |
| Selenium | 16 mcg |

### ▶ Health Tip

With a history dating back thousands of years, cumin has some potent antioxidant molecules and has been used for digestive ailments.

# Lunch Box Peachy Sweet Potato and Couscous

*Here is a convenient and nutritious hot lunch with minimal prep time.*

## Tip

Pack up the ingredients you need for this meal the night before and, if you have access to a microwave, cook the meal at work or at school.

- **3-cup (750 mL) microwave-safe glass or ceramic container**

| | | |
|---|---|---|
| 1 | small sweet potato (about 6 oz/175 g) | 1 |
| 1/4 cup | couscous | 60 mL |
| 2 tbsp | raisins | 30 mL |
| 1 tsp | chicken or vegetable bouillon powder | 5 mL |
| 1/4 tsp | ground ginger | 1 mL |
| 1/8 tsp | ground cinnamon (optional) | 0.5 mL |
| 1 | can (5 oz/142 g) diced peaches, with juice | 1 |
| 1/4 cup | water | 60 mL |

**1.** Microwave sweet potato on High for 2 to 2½ minutes or until just cooked. Let cool; peel and dice into 1-inch (2.5 cm) pieces. Place in microwave-safe container.

**2.** Add couscous, raisins, chicken bouillon, ginger and cinnamon (if using). Refrigerate for up to 1 day.

**3.** When you are ready to cook, stir in peaches and water. Microwave, loosely covered, on High for 3 minutes. Stir, cover and let stand for 2 to 3 minutes. Fluff with a fork.

## Variation

For a change, substitute curry powder for the ginger and cinnamon. Add some leftover cooked pork strips, if desired.

*This recipe courtesy of dietitians Bev Callaghan and Lynn Roblin.*

### ▶ Health Tip

Sweet potatoes are loaded with carotenoids, beneficial antioxidants that can also be converted to vitamin A in the body.

| Nutrients per serving | |
|---|---|
| Calories | 317 |
| Fat | 1 g |
| Carbohydrate | 75 g |
| Protein | 6 g |
| Vitamin C | 10 mg |
| Vitamin D | 0 IU |
| Vitamin E | 1 mg |
| Niacin | 3 mg |
| Folate | 31 mcg |
| Vitamin $B_6$ | 0.5 mg |
| Vitamin $B_{12}$ | 0.0 mcg |
| Zinc | 0.8 mg |
| Selenium | 13 mcg |

# Quinoa Vegetable Cakes

*In this dish, the quinoa vegetable cake is baked, eliminating any greasy aftertaste while delivering the goods in flavor and nutrition.*

## Tips

If you prefer, an equal amount of chopped fresh cilantro, basil or flat-leaf (Italian) parsley may be used in place of the dill.

Store the quinoa cakes wrapped in foil or in an airtight container in the refrigerator for up to 2 days. Reheat in the microwave on Medium (50%) for 45 to 60 seconds or until warmed through.

| Nutrients per serving | |
| --- | --- |
| Calories | 308 |
| Fat | 7 g |
| Carbohydrate | 47 g |
| Protein | 17 g |
| Vitamin C | 10 mg |
| Vitamin D | 21 IU |
| Vitamin E | 3 mg |
| Niacin | 1 mg |
| Folate | 193 mcg |
| Vitamin B$_6$ | 0.4 mg |
| Vitamin B$_{12}$ | 0.6 mcg |
| Zinc | 2.9 mg |
| Selenium | 18 mcg |

- Preheat oven to 400°F (200°C)
- Large rimmed baking sheet, sprayed with nonstick cooking spray (preferably olive oil)

| | | |
| --- | --- | --- |
| 2 | cloves garlic, minced | 2 |
| 1 | package (10 oz/300 g) frozen chopped spinach, thawed and squeezed dry | 1 |
| 3 cups | cooked quinoa, cooled | 750 mL |
| ¾ cup | finely shredded carrots | 175 mL |
| ½ cup | finely chopped green onions | 125 mL |
| ¼ cup | quinoa flour | 60 mL |
| 1 tbsp | dried Italian seasoning | 15 mL |
| 1 tsp | baking powder | 5 mL |
| | Fine sea salt and freshly cracked black pepper | |
| 2 | large eggs, lightly beaten | 2 |
| 1 tbsp | chopped fresh dill | 15 mL |
| 1 cup | plain yogurt | 250 mL |
| 1 tbsp | freshly squeezed lemon juice | 15 mL |

1. In a large bowl, combine garlic, spinach, quinoa, carrots, green onions, quinoa flour, Italian seasoning, baking powder, ½ tsp (2 mL) salt, ½ tsp (2 mL) pepper and eggs.

2. Scoop 8 equal mounds of quinoa mixture onto prepared baking sheet. Using a spatula, flatten mounds to ½-inch (1 cm) thickness.

3. Bake in preheated oven for 15 minutes. Turn cakes over and bake for 8 to 12 minutes or until golden brown and hot in the center.

4. Meanwhile, in a small bowl, whisk together dill, yogurt and lemon juice. Season to taste with salt and pepper.

5. Serve warm quinoa cakes with yogurt sauce drizzled on top or served alongside.

> ▶ **Health Tip**
>
> Quinoa is not only rich in many nutrients, but it is very high in fiber, even for a whole grain.

# Red Lentil Curry with Coconut and Cilantro

*This dish turns up the spices with the aromatic tastes of curry.*

## Tips

Choose enriched coconut milk to increase your intake of calcium and vitamin D.

Traditionally, Indian lentil dishes such as this one are served very loose and almost soupy. You can adjust the texture to your taste by adding more water or simmering longer to thicken.

Leftovers will thicken considerably upon cooling. If reheating in the microwave or a saucepan, add boiling water before heating to return to desired consistency.

### Nutrients per serving

| | |
|---|---|
| Calories | 291 |
| Fat | 20 g |
| Carbohydrate | 23 g |
| Protein | 10 g |
| Vitamin C | 3 mg |
| Vitamin D | 0 IU |
| Vitamin E | 1 mg |
| Niacin | 1 mg |
| Folate | 77 mcg |
| Vitamin B$_6$ | 0.2 mg |
| Vitamin B$_{12}$ | 0.0 mcg |
| Zinc | 1.7 mg |
| Selenium | 3 mcg |

| | | |
|---|---|---:|
| 2 tbsp | vegetable oil | 30 mL |
| 1 | small onion, finely chopped | 1 |
| 2 | cloves garlic, minced | 2 |
| 1 tbsp | minced gingerroot | 15 mL |
| | Salt | |
| 1 tsp | ground coriander | 5 mL |
| 1 tsp | ground cumin | 5 mL |
| 1/4 tsp | ground turmeric | 1 mL |
| 1 cup | dried red lentils, rinsed | 250 mL |
| 1 | can (14 oz/400 mL) coconut milk | 1 |
| 1 cup | water | 250 mL |
| 1/4 cup | torn fresh cilantro leaves | 60 mL |
| | Garam masala | |

1. In a saucepan, heat oil over medium heat. Add onion and cook, stirring, until softened and starting to brown, about 5 minutes. Add garlic, ginger, 1 tsp (5 mL) salt, coriander, cumin and turmeric; cook, stirring, until softened and fragrant, about 2 minutes.

2. Stir in lentils until coated with spices. Stir in coconut milk and water; bring to a boil, scraping up bits stuck to pan and stirring to prevent lumps. Reduce heat to low, partially cover and simmer, stirring often, until lentils are very soft and mixture is thick, about 15 minutes.

3. Remove from heat, cover and let stand for 5 minutes. Season to taste with salt. Stir in all but a few leaves of cilantro. Serve sprinkled with remaining cilantro and garam masala.

## Variation

Add 1 or 2 hot chile peppers, minced, with the garlic.

> ### ▶ Health Tip
>
> The array of spices in this dish provide a substantial dose of antioxidants and anti-inflammatory compounds, not the least of which come from the turmeric.

# Tomato Onion Curry of Brown Lentils

*Lentils provide a substantial meal, especially when combined with a side dish of rice.*

## Tip

If ripe fresh tomatoes aren't available, substitute $1\frac{1}{2}$ cups (375 mL) drained canned diced tomatoes and reduce salt to $\frac{1}{4}$ tsp (1 mL), adding more to taste at the end if necessary.

| | | |
|---|---|---|
| 1 cup | whole brown lentils, rinsed | 250 mL |
| 5 cups | water, divided | 1.25 L |
| 2 tbsp | vegetable oil | 30 mL |
| 2 | bay leaves | 2 |
| $\frac{1}{2}$ tsp | cumin seeds | 2 mL |
| 1 | large onion, finely chopped | 1 |
| 2 | cloves garlic, minced | 2 |
| 1 | hot green chile pepper, minced | 1 |
| 1 tbsp | minced gingerroot | 15 mL |
| 1 tsp | salt | 5 mL |
| $\frac{1}{2}$ tsp | ground turmeric | 2 mL |
| 2 | tomatoes, diced | 2 |

1. In a saucepan, combine lentils and 4 cups (1 L) of the water. Bring to a boil over high heat. Reduce heat and simmer until lentils are almost tender, about 25 minutes. Drain and set aside.

2. In a skillet, heat oil over medium-high heat until hot but not smoking. Add bay leaves and cumin seeds; cook, stirring, until seeds are toasted but not yet popping, about 30 seconds. Add onion and cook, stirring, until starting to soften, about 2 minutes. Reduce heat to medium-low and cook, stirring often, until onions are very soft and golden brown, about 10 minutes.

3. Add garlic, chile pepper, ginger, salt and turmeric; cook, stirring, until softened and fragrant, about 2 minutes. Increase heat to medium and add tomatoes. Cook, stirring, until tomatoes are softened, about 2 minutes.

4. Add reserved lentils and remaining water; bring to a boil, stirring often. Reduce heat and boil gently, stirring often, until lentils are tender and most of the liquid is absorbed, 10 to 15 minutes. Discard bay leaves.

### ▶ Health Tip

A food like lentils can slowly release energy — and sugars — into the bloodstream, which is important for people who need to control their blood sugar, including those with diabetes.

## Nutrients per 1 of 6 servings

| | |
|---|---|
| Calories | 178 |
| Fat | 5 g |
| Carbohydrate | 25 g |
| Protein | 9 g |
| Vitamin C | 28 mg |
| Vitamin D | 0 IU |
| Vitamin E | 1 mg |
| Niacin | 1 mg |
| Folate | 166 mcg |
| Vitamin B$_6$ | 0.3 mg |
| Vitamin B$_{12}$ | 0.0 mcg |
| Zinc | 1.7 mg |
| Selenium | 3 mcg |

# Brown Chickpea Curry

*This is as aromatic and pungent a dish of chickpeas as you'll find, and the touch of coconut makes it extra-special.*

**Makes 4 to 6 servings**

## Tips

Sambhar powder, a South Indian spice blend, includes fenugreek, peppercorns, red chiles, coriander, cumin, mustard seeds, turmeric, curry leaves and asafetida, among other spices. It will stay fresh for 1 year if stored in the refrigerator.

Indian poppy seeds are pale-colored and will not discolor the dish as dark poppy seeds tend to do. However, if you only have dark ones, they can be substituted.

- **Blender**

| | | |
|---|---|---|
| 1 cup | chickpeas | 250 mL |
| 1 tsp | salt (or to taste) | 5 mL |
| 1/3 cup | fresh or frozen grated coconut | 75 mL |
| 2 tbsp | unsalted Thai tamarind purée | 30 mL |
| 1 tbsp | sambhar powder (see tip, at left) | 15 mL |
| 1 tsp | Indian poppy seeds (see tip, at left) | 5 mL |

**1.** Pick through and rinse chickpeas 2 to 3 times. Add water to cover by 3 inches (7.5 cm) and soak at room temperature in a bowl for 6 hours or overnight.

**2.** Drain chickpeas. Place in a saucepan with 4 cups (1 L) fresh water. Bring to a boil over high heat. Reduce heat to low and boil gently until chickpeas are tender, 20 to 25 minutes. Add salt just before chickpeas are ready and remove from heat.

**3.** With a slotted spoon, transfer 1/2 cup (125 mL) of the cooked chickpeas to blender. Add coconut, tamarind, sambhar powder and poppy seeds. Add 1/2 cup (125 mL) of the chickpea liquid and blend to a purée.

**4.** Pour purée into remaining chickpeas in saucepan and cook over medium-low heat, stirring occasionally, until gravy thickens to the consistency you prefer, 6 to 8 minutes. If not serving immediately, allow a little extra liquid to remain, as it thickens considerably as it cools.

---

### ▶ Health Tip

Coconut has a high amount of medium-chain fatty acids, which are heart-friendly and are not processed in the body the same way as long-chain fatty acids.

---

### Nutrients per 1 of 6 servings

| | |
|---|---|
| Calories | 147 |
| Fat | 4 g |
| Carbohydrate | 23 g |
| Protein | 7 g |
| Vitamin C | 2 mg |
| Vitamin D | 0 IU |
| Vitamin E | 0 mg |
| Niacin | 1 mg |
| Folate | 188 mcg |
| Vitamin $B_6$ | 0.2 mg |
| Vitamin $B_{12}$ | 0.0 mcg |
| Zinc | 1.2 mg |
| Selenium | 3 mcg |

# Winter Greens with Split Yellow Peas

*For anyone who has been turned off greens by mushy, nondescript victims of the saucepan, this dish will put them back on your good list.*

**Makes 8 servings**

## Tip

Greens, when cooked, reduce drastically in volume, so a little bit more or a little bit less will not change the dish.

---

### ▶ Health Tip

Collard greens and mustard greens have the compounds that help support the body's detoxification systems, and they are phenomenal sources of vitamin K.

---

**Nutrients** per serving

| | |
|---|---|
| Calories | 158 |
| Fat | 5 g |
| Carbohydrate | 22 g |
| Protein | 9 g |
| Vitamin C | 65 mg |
| Vitamin D | 0 IU |
| Vitamin E | 3 mg |
| Niacin | 2 mg |
| Folate | 273 mcg |
| Vitamin B$_6$ | 0.3 mg |
| Vitamin B$_{12}$ | 0.0 mcg |
| Zinc | 1.2 mg |
| Selenium | 5 mcg |

| | | |
|---|---|---|
| 1 cup | split yellow peas | 250 mL |
| ½ tsp | ground turmeric | 2 mL |
| 2½ tsp | salt (or to taste), divided | 12 mL |
| 6 to 7 cups | spinach, rinsed and chopped (see tip, at left) | 1.5 to 1.75 L |
| 6 to 7 cups | turnip greens, rinsed and chopped | 1.5 to 1.75 L |
| 6 to 7 cups | mustard or collard greens, rinsed and chopped | 1.5 to 1.75 L |
| 2 tbsp | vegetable oil | 30 mL |
| 2 tbsp | slivered gingerroot | 30 mL |
| 1 tbsp | minced green chile peppers, preferably serranos | 15 mL |
| 2 tbsp | dark mustard seeds, coarsely pounded | 30 mL |
| 1 tbsp | cumin seeds | 15 mL |
| 1½ tsp | salt (or to taste) | 7 mL |
| 2 tbsp | freshly squeezed lime or lemon juice (or to taste) | 30 mL |

1. Clean and pick through peas for any small stones and grit. Rinse several times in cold water until water is fairly clear. Soak in 2½ cups (625 mL) water in a saucepan for 15 minutes.

2. Bring peas to a boil over medium heat. Reduce heat to low. Stir in turmeric and boil gently, partially covered, until peas are soft but not mushy and water is absorbed, 20 to 25 minutes. Add 1 tsp (5 mL) of the salt in the last 5 minutes of cooking. Set aside.

3. In a large pot, combine spinach, turnip and mustard greens and 2 tbsp (30 mL) water. Cover and cook over low heat until water is absorbed, about 5 minutes.

4. Meanwhile, in a large skillet, heat oil over medium heat. Add ginger and chiles and sauté for 1 minute. Add mustard and cumin and sauté, stirring continuously, for 2 minutes.

5. Add spinach mixture, peas and remaining salt. Mix well and heat through. Add lime juice to taste. Serve with Indian bread.

# Quinoa Chili

*Quinoa makes a terrific centerpiece in this chili, along with the wonderful smokiness of chipotle pepper.*

## Tip

Like most whole-grain dishes, this chili soaks up liquid if left to sit, so keep some extra vegetable broth on hand to add if you're reheating leftovers.

### ▶ Health Tip

Quinoa is a source of iron, so in fact this vegetarian dish comes complete with iron along with many other nutrients.

### Nutrients per serving

| | |
|---|---|
| Calories | 306 |
| Fat | 6 g |
| Carbohydrate | 56 g |
| Protein | 13 g |
| Vitamin C | 52 mg |
| Vitamin D | 0 IU |
| Vitamin E | 3 mg |
| Niacin | 3 mg |
| Folate | 193 mcg |
| Vitamin B$_6$ | 0.7 mg |
| Vitamin B$_{12}$ | 0.0 mcg |
| Zinc | 2.2 mg |
| Selenium | 8 mcg |

| | | |
|---|---|---|
| 1 tbsp | olive oil | 15 mL |
| 2 | onions, finely chopped | 2 |
| 2 | stalks celery, diced | 2 |
| 1 | carrot, peeled and diced | 1 |
| 1 | green bell pepper, finely chopped | 1 |
| 4 | cloves garlic, minced | 4 |
| 2 tbsp | chili powder | 30 mL |
| 1 | chipotle pepper in adobo sauce, minced | 1 |
| 1 | can (28 oz/796 mL) no-salt-added diced tomatoes, with juice | 1 |
| 2 cups | ready-to-use reduced-sodium vegetable broth | 500 mL |
| | Salt and freshly ground black pepper | |
| 1 cup | quinoa, rinsed | 250 mL |
| 2 cups | drained rinsed cooked or canned pinto beans (see tip, at left) | 500 mL |
| 1 cup | corn kernels | 250 mL |

**1.** In a large deep skillet with a tight-fitting lid, heat oil over medium heat for 30 seconds. Add onions, celery, carrot, bell pepper and garlic and stir well. Reduce heat to low. Cover and cook until vegetables are softened, about 10 minutes.

**2.** Increase heat to medium. Add chili powder and chipotle pepper and cook, stirring, for 1 minute. Add tomatoes and broth and bring to a boil. Season to taste with salt and black pepper. Add quinoa, beans and corn and cook, stirring, until mixture returns to a boil. Reduce heat to low. Cover and simmer until quinoa is tender, about 25 minutes.

## Variations

*Millet Chili:* Substitute an equal quantity of toasted millet for the quinoa. Increase the quantity of vegetable broth to 2$\frac{1}{2}$ cups (625 mL) and increase cooking time to about 25 minutes.

Substitute red kidney, cranberry or small red beans for the pinto beans.

# Three-Bean Chili

*Who doesn't like a good bowl of chili? This version will give you all the benefits from beans, garlic, onion and spices, without the saturated fats.*

**Makes 6 to 8 servings**

## Tips

Because can sizes vary, we provide a range of amounts for beans in our recipes. If you're using 19-oz (540 mL) cans, add a bit more chili powder to taste.

Use diced tomatoes with or without seasonings.

| | | |
|---|---|---|
| 1 tbsp | vegetable oil | 15 mL |
| 1 | large onion, coarsely chopped | 1 |
| 1 | red bell pepper, cut into 1-inch (2.5 cm) cubes | 1 |
| 2 | cloves garlic, minced (about 2 tsp/10 mL) | 2 |
| 1½ tbsp | chili powder | 22 mL |
| 1½ tsp | ground cumin | 7 mL |
| ½ tsp | dried oregano | 2 mL |
| ½ tsp | ground cinnamon | 2 mL |
| ½ tsp | ground allspice | 2 mL |
| ¼ tsp | hot pepper flakes | 1 mL |
| 2 cups | ready-to-use vegetable broth | 500 mL |
| ½ cup | tomato paste | 125 mL |
| 1 | can (14 to 19 oz/398 to 540 mL) black beans, drained and rinsed | 1 |
| 1 | can (14 to 19 oz/398 to 540 mL) red kidney beans, drained and rinsed | 1 |
| 1 | can (14 to 19 oz/398 to 540 mL) navy or white kidney beans, drained and rinsed | 1 |
| 1 | can (28 oz/796 mL) diced tomatoes, with juices (see tip, at left) | 1 |
| 1 tbsp | red wine vinegar | 15 mL |

**1.** In a large pot, heat oil over medium heat for 30 seconds. Add onion and red pepper and cook, stirring, for 3 minutes or until softened. Add garlic and cook, stirring, for 1 minute. Add chili powder, cumin, oregano, cinnamon, allspice and hot pepper flakes and cook, stirring, for 1 minute.

## Nutrients per 1 of 8 servings

| | |
|---|---|
| Calories | 213 |
| Fat | 3 g |
| Carbohydrate | 38 g |
| Protein | 11 g |
| Vitamin C | 36 mg |
| Vitamin D | 0 IU |
| Vitamin E | 2 mg |
| Niacin | 3 mg |
| Folate | 92 mcg |
| Vitamin B$_6$ | 0.4 mg |
| Vitamin B$_{12}$ | 0.0 mcg |
| Zinc | 1.3 mg |
| Selenium | 4 mcg |

## Tip

Store leftovers in an airtight container in the refrigerator for up to 4 days, or in the freezer for up to 2 months.

**2.** Add vegetable broth and increase heat to medium-high. Bring to a simmer and cook for 5 minutes or until pepper is very soft. Add tomato paste and stir well. Add black, red kidney and navy beans, tomatoes and vinegar. Return to a boil. Reduce heat to low, cover and simmer for 35 minutes or until thickened.

## Variation

For a more substantial version of this chili, add 6 oz (175 g) soy ground meat alternative. In a skillet, heat 1 tbsp (15 mL) of olive oil over medium-high heat. Add meat alternative and reduce heat to medium. Cook, stirring frequently, for 5 minutes or until heated through. Add to chili along with the vinegar.

> ### ▶ Health Tip
>
> Oregano has antioxidant and antibacterial volatile oils such as thymol, pinene, limonene, carvacrol, ocimene and caryophyllene.

# Fragrant Rice-Stuffed Peppers

*This dish uses the pleasing-to-the-senses jasmine rice, along with crunchy walnuts, to create a delicious stuffed pepper.*

## Makes 4 servings

## Tips

Leaves and tender top stems of beets are often trimmed and tossed away. These leaves, also referred to as beet greens, are delicious and a source of nutritious antioxidants.

Toast walnut halves in a dry skillet over low heat, stirring constantly, for 3 to 4 minutes or until fragrant. Transfer the toasted nuts to a plate and let cool before chopping.

- Preheat oven to 425°F (220°C)
- Baking sheet, lined with parchment paper
- 13- by 9-inch (33 by 23 cm) baking dish, lightly oiled

### Filling

| | | |
|---|---|---|
| 1 cup | brown jasmine rice | 250 mL |
| 1¾ cups | ready-to-use vegetable broth | 425 mL |
| 8 | beets, trimmed and peeled, beet greens reserved | 8 |
| 5 tbsp | olive oil, divided | 75 mL |
| 3½ tsp | balsamic vinegar, divided | 17 mL |
| ½ tsp | salt, divided | 2 mL |
| ½ tsp | freshly ground black pepper, divided | 2 mL |
| 2 | green onions, white and green parts, thinly sliced | 2 |
| 2 | cloves garlic, minced | 2 |
| ¾ cup | coarsely chopped toasted walnuts | 175 mL |
| 4 | yellow or red bell peppers | 4 |

1. *Filling:* In a small saucepan over medium-high heat, combine rice and vegetable broth and bring to a boil. Reduce heat, cover and simmer for 50 minutes.

2. Cut beets into ¼-inch (0.5 cm) pieces and toss with 1 tbsp (15 mL) of the olive oil, 3 tsp (15 mL) of the balsamic vinegar, ¼ tsp (1 mL) of the salt and ¼ tsp (1 mL) of the black pepper. Spread beets onto prepared baking sheet and roast in preheated oven until softened and slightly browned, 20 to 25 minutes.

## Nutrients per serving

| | |
|---|---|
| Calories | 588 |
| Fat | 31 g |
| Carbohydrate | 69 g |
| Protein | 13 g |
| Vitamin C | 351 mg |
| Vitamin D | 0 IU |
| Vitamin E | 3 mg |
| Niacin | 2 mg |
| Folate | 236 mcg |
| Vitamin B$_6$ | 0.6 mg |
| Vitamin B$_{12}$ | 0.0 mcg |
| Zinc | 1.7 mg |
| Selenium | 6 mcg |

## Variation

Add 1 cup (250 mL) cooked lentils or black beans to add protein to this meal.

**3.** Remove and discard tough stems from beet greens, coarsely chop greens and set aside. Place a large skillet over medium-high heat and let pan get hot. Add 2 tbsp (30 mL) of oil and tip pan to coat. Add green onions and garlic and cook, stirring frequently, until softened, about 1 minute. Add beet greens, $\frac{1}{2}$ tsp (2 mL) of balsamic vinegar, $\frac{1}{4}$ tsp (1 mL) of salt and $\frac{1}{4}$ tsp (1 mL) of black pepper and cook until most of liquid has evaporated, 2 to 3 minutes. Remove from heat and stir in cooked rice, roasted beets and toasted walnuts, mixing to incorporate. Taste and adjust seasonings.

**4.** Cut tops off peppers and reserve. Remove and discard seeds and membranes and slice a thin strip off pepper bottoms to level. Arrange peppers in prepared baking dish and spoon in filling. Replace tops and drizzle peppers with remaining 2 tbsp (30 mL) of oil. Bake in preheated oven until peppers are tender and slightly charred, about 30 minutes.

> ▸ **Health Tip**
>
> Consuming walnuts has been shown to improve working memory.

# Green Macaroni and Cheese

*Here is a great combination of spinach, almonds and mac and cheese. If you have children, the color may meet with sniffs of disapproval, but the taste may win them over.*

**Makes 5 servings**

## Variations

Substitute ½ cup (125 mL) freshly grated Parmesan cheese for the Cheddar. Because of its stronger flavor, you don't need as much.

Substitute a 1-lb (500 g) container of fat-free cottage cheese for the Cheddar.

Add chopped fresh dill and extra black pepper, and use penne, rotini or fusilli in place of the macaroni.

- Food processor

| | | |
|---|---|---|
| 1 | bag (10 oz/300 g) baby spinach | 1 |
| 2 tbsp | freshly squeezed lemon juice | 30 mL |
| 1 tbsp | extra virgin olive oil | 15 mL |
| 12 oz | whole wheat macaroni | 375 g |
| 1 cup | shredded white Cheddar cheese | 250 mL |
| ½ cup | slivered almonds, toasted | 125 mL |
| | Freshly ground black pepper | |

1. In food processor, pulse spinach, lemon juice and olive oil for 15 seconds, until roughly puréed (don't overdo it).

2. Cook macaroni according to package directions until al dente (tender to the bite). Drain and return to the pot. Add spinach mixture, tossing to coat evenly. Stir in cheese and almonds. Season to taste with pepper.

*This recipe courtesy of Jody MacLean.*

> ▸ **Health Tip**
>
> Almonds seem to help control blood sugar spikes after eating.

## Nutrients per serving

| | |
|---|---|
| Calories | 428 |
| Fat | 17 g |
| Carbohydrate | 56 g |
| Protein | 20 g |
| Vitamin C | 18 mg |
| Vitamin D | 5 IU |
| Vitamin E | 4 mg |
| Niacin | 4 mg |
| Folate | 160 mcg |
| Vitamin B$_6$ | 0.3 mg |
| Vitamin B$_{12}$ | 0.2 mcg |
| Zinc | 3.0 mg |
| Selenium | 4 mcg |

# Rice Noodles with Roasted Mediterranean Vegetables

*Rice noodles have a wonderful ability to absorb flavors and sauces, and this dish provides them with plenty of inspiration.*

**Makes 4 servings**

## Tip

Toasted sesame oil has a dark brown color and a rich, nutty flavor. It only needs to be used sparingly to add a tremendous amount of flavor.

- Preheat oven to 375°F (190°C)
- Roasting pan, lightly oiled

| | | |
|---|---|---|
| 2 | zucchini, trimmed and cut into 1-inch (2.5 cm) pieces | 2 |
| 2 | large tomatoes, halved | 2 |
| 2 | onions, quartered | 2 |
| 1 | eggplant, trimmed and cut into 1-inch (2.5 cm) pieces | 1 |
| 1 | red bell pepper, thickly sliced | 1 |
| 2 | cloves garlic | 2 |
| 1/4 cup | tamari or soy sauce | 60 mL |
| 2 tbsp | olive oil | 30 mL |
| 2 tbsp | freshly squeezed lime or lemon juice | 30 mL |
| 1 tbsp | toasted sesame oil | 15 mL |
| 8 oz | dried wide rice noodles | 250 g |

1. In prepared roasting pan, combine zucchini, tomatoes, onions, eggplant, red pepper and garlic.

2. In a bowl, whisk together tamari, olive oil, lime juice and sesame oil. Toss with vegetables in roasting pan. Bake in preheated oven, stirring once or twice, for 30 to 40 minutes or until vegetables are tender when pierced with the tip of a knife. Do not turn the oven off.

3. Meanwhile, in a bowl, cover rice noodles with hot water. Soak for 15 to 20 minutes or according to package directions, until al dente. Drain and set aside. When vegetables are cooked, toss drained noodles with roasted vegetables. Return to the oven for 10 minutes to heat through.

| Nutrients per serving | |
|---|---|
| Calories | 393 |
| Fat | 11 g |
| Carbohydrate | 70 g |
| Protein | 6 g |
| Vitamin C | 76 mg |
| Vitamin D | 0 IU |
| Vitamin E | 3 mg |
| Niacin | 3 mg |
| Folate | 93 mcg |
| Vitamin $B_6$ | 0.6 mg |
| Vitamin $B_{12}$ | 0.0 mcg |
| Zinc | 1.2 mg |
| Selenium | 6 mcg |

> ▸ **Health Tip**
>
> Rice noodles are a good example that gluten-free noodles are easy to come by.

# Rice Noodles with Spicy Spaghetti Sauce

*For spaghetti lovers trying to avoid gluten and the same old marinara sauce, this dish will come to their rescue.*

---

**Makes 6 servings**

## Tip

You can use 2 cups (500 mL) cooked kidney beans, drained and rinsed, instead of canned.

| | | |
|---|---|---|
| 1 tbsp | olive oil | 15 mL |
| 2 | onions, coarsely chopped | 2 |
| 3 | cloves garlic, finely chopped | 3 |
| 1 | red or green bell pepper, chopped | 1 |
| 1 | stalk celery, chopped | 1 |
| 1 | eggplant, coarsely chopped | 1 |
| 1 | can (28 oz/796 mL) crushed tomatoes, with juice | 1 |
| 3 tbsp | Pomegranate Molasses (see recipe, opposite) or blackstrap molasses | 45 mL |
| 1 tbsp | tamari or soy sauce | 15 mL |
| | Sea salt and freshly ground pepper | |
| 1 | can (14 to 19 oz/398 to 540 mL) red kidney beans, drained, rinsed and coarsely chopped | 1 |
| 3 tbsp | chopped fresh parsley | 45 mL |
| 1 tbsp | chopped fresh oregano | 15 mL |
| 1 tsp | fresh thyme leaves | 5 mL |
| 1 tsp | chipotle flakes (optional) | 5 mL |
| 12 oz | dried wide rice noodles | 375 g |

**1.** In a large saucepan, heat oil over medium heat. Add onions and garlic and cook, stirring occasionally, for 5 minutes or until slightly softened. Add bell pepper and celery and cook, stirring frequently, for 3 minutes. Add eggplant and cook, stirring occasionally, for about 5 minutes or until eggplant is almost tender when pierced with the tip of a knife.

**2.** Stir in tomatoes, molasses, tamari and salt and pepper to taste. Increase heat to high and bring to a boil. Partially cover, reduce heat and simmer, stirring occasionally, for 20 minutes. Stir in beans, parsley, oregano, thyme and chipotle flakes (if using). Cover and cook about 5 minutes to heat through.

| Nutrients per serving | |
|---|---|
| Calories | 390 |
| Fat | 3 g |
| Carbohydrate | 85 g |
| Protein | 8 g |
| Vitamin C | 46 mg |
| Vitamin D | 0 IU |
| Vitamin E | 1 mg |
| Niacin | 3 mg |
| Folate | 80 mcg |
| Vitamin $B_6$ | 0.5 mg |
| Vitamin $B_{12}$ | 0.0 mcg |
| Zinc | 1.2 mg |
| Selenium | 8 mcg |

## Tip

Is cutting onions bringing you to tears? Try placing them in the freezer for 10 minutes before chopping.

**3.** Meanwhile, in a bowl, cover rice noodles with hot water. Soak for 15 to 20 minutes or according to package directions, until al dente. Drain and toss with spaghetti sauce.

---

### ▶ Health Tip

A study led by Dr. Dean Ornish indicates that pomegranate juice may improve blood flow to the heart in people with coronary (or ischemic) heart disease (CHD).

---

# Pomegranate Molasses

*This slightly tart syrupy condiment is used in many Turkish and Moroccan dishes. It may be available in Middle Eastern specialty food stores, but this recipe is so easy to make and store that it can become a pantry staple.*

---

**Makes 2 cups (500 mL)**

● Canning jar

| | | |
|---|---|---|
| 4 cups | pomegranate juice | 1 L |
| 1/2 cup | organic cane sugar | 125 mL |
| 1/4 cup | freshly squeezed lemon juice | 60 mL |

**1.** In a heavy-bottomed saucepan, combine pomegranate juice, sugar and lemon juice. Bring to a gentle boil over medium-high heat, stirring until sugar is dissolved. Reduce heat and keep simmering gently for about 1 hour or until thick and syrupy. Liquid should be reduced by at least one-half. Pour the hot liquid into canning jar before cooling. Cap and then let cool completely.

**2.** Store molasses in the refrigerator for up to 2 months.

### Nutrients per 1 tbsp (15 mL)

| | |
|---|---|
| Calories | 28 |
| Fat | 0 g |
| Carbohydrate | 7 g |
| Protein | 0 g |
| Vitamin C | 1 mg |
| Vitamin D | 0 IU |
| Vitamin E | 0 mg |
| Niacin | 0 mg |
| Folate | 8 mcg |
| Vitamin $B_6$ | 0.0 mg |
| Vitamin $B_{12}$ | 0.0 mcg |
| Zinc | 0.0 mg |
| Selenium | 0 mcg |

# Baked Cranberry Tofu with Creamed Asparagus and Leeks

*Tofu's blandness and tendency to absorb its surrounding flavors is a strength here — the marinade, and then the serving of creamed asparagus and leeks on top, are mouthwatering.*

---

**Makes 4 servings**

## Tip

Sambal oelek is a condiment, used by Southeast Asians, that is made from a variety of very hot chile peppers.

- Preheat oven to 375°F (190°C)
- Rimmed baking sheet, lightly oiled

**Tofu Marinade**

| | | |
|---|---|---|
| ¼ cup | whole cranberry sauce | 60 mL |
| 2 tbsp | tamari or soy sauce | 30 mL |
| 1 tbsp | grated lime zest | 15 mL |
| | Juice of 1 lime | |
| 1 to 2 tbsp | chili paste or sambal oelek | 15 to 30 mL |
| 12 oz | extra-firm tofu | 375 g |

**Creamed Asparagus and Leeks**

| | | |
|---|---|---|
| 3 tbsp | olive oil | 45 mL |
| 3 | leeks, white and tender green parts, sliced | 3 |
| 1 | onion, halved and sliced | 1 |
| 1 tbsp | grated gingerroot | 15 mL |
| ½ cup | chopped fresh basil | 125 mL |
| 2 tbsp | chopped fresh tarragon or cilantro | 30 mL |
| 1 | can (14 oz/400 mL) coconut milk | 1 |
| 2 cups | 1-inch (2.5 cm) asparagus pieces | 500 mL |
| | Salt and freshly ground pepper | |
| 8 oz | rice noodles, cooked (optional) | 250 g |
| 4 | sprigs fresh basil or cilantro (optional) | 4 |

**1.** *Tofu Marinade:* In a bowl, combine cranberry sauce, tamari, lime zest and juice and chili paste. Slice tofu into ¾-inch (2 cm) slices and add to bowl. Set aside for 15 to 20 minutes or cover and refrigerate overnight. On prepared baking sheet, arrange slices in one layer. Spoon half of the marinade over tofu slices. Bake in preheated oven for 5 minutes. Turn, spoon remaining marinade over tofu and bake for another 5 minutes.

| Nutrients per serving | |
|---|---|
| Calories | 509 |
| Fat | 39 g |
| Carbohydrate | 28 g |
| Protein | 19 g |
| Vitamin C | 27 mg |
| Vitamin D | 0 IU |
| Vitamin E | 3 mg |
| Niacin | 2 mg |
| Folate | 125 mcg |
| Vitamin B$_6$ | 0.4 mg |
| Vitamin B$_{12}$ | 0.0 mcg |
| Zinc | 2.5 mg |
| Selenium | 17 mcg |

## Tip

Preparation time is significantly reduced if the tofu is prepared and marinated in the refrigerator the night before.

2. *Creamed Asparagus and Leeks:* In a saucepan, heat oil over medium-high heat. Add leeks and onion. Cover, reduce heat to low and sweat vegetables for 15 minutes or until soft. Add ginger, basil and tarragon and cook, stirring constantly, for 1 minute. Add coconut milk and bring to a boil over high heat. Add asparagus. Reduce heat and simmer, stirring occasionally, for 10 minutes or until tender when pierced with the tip of a knife. Season to taste with salt and pepper.

3. *To serve:* You can either spoon the creamed asparagus and leek mixture into the center of a plate or flat soup bowl or pile cooked rice noodles, if using, in the center, then top with the creamed mixture. Top with baked tofu slices. Garnish with fresh basil, if desired.

> ### ▶ Health Tip
>
> Leeks, like garlic and onions, belong to the allium family and have cardiovascular benefits.

# Spaghetti with Sun-Dried Tomatoes and Broccoli

*This truly Mediterranean dish muscles up on the broccoli for even more taste and health benefits.*

**Makes 4 servings**

## Tips

Instead of hot pepper flakes, use $\frac{1}{8}$ tsp (1 mL) cayenne pepper

Buy dry sun-dried tomatoes, not those marinated in oil.

Prepare pasta up to 2 hours ahead, leaving at room temperature. Toss before serving.

| | | |
|---|---|---|
| 8 oz | spaghetti | 250 g |
| $\frac{1}{2}$ cup | sun-dried tomatoes | 125 mL |
| 2 cups | chopped broccoli | 500 mL |
| $2\frac{1}{2}$ cups | chopped tomatoes | 625 mL |
| 2 tbsp | olive oil | 30 mL |
| $1\frac{1}{2}$ tsp | crushed garlic | 7 mL |
| Pinch | hot pepper flakes | Pinch |
| $\frac{1}{2}$ cup | chopped fresh basil (or 2 tsp/10 mL dried) | 125 mL |
| 3 tbsp | grated Parmesan cheese | 45 mL |

**1.** Cook pasta in boiling water according to package instructions or until firm to the bite. Drain and place in serving bowl.

**2.** Pour boiling water over sun-dried tomatoes. Let soak for 15 minutes. Drain, then chop. Add to pasta.

**3.** Blanch broccoli in boiling water just until barely tender. Rinse with cold water, drain and add to pasta. Add tomatoes, oil, garlic, hot pepper flakes, basil and cheese. Toss.

> ▸ **Health Tip**
>
> Tomatoes contain hydroxycinnamic acids such as caffeic acid and ferulic acid — important antioxidants.

| Nutrients per serving | |
|---|---|
| Calories | 346 |
| Fat | 10 g |
| Carbohydrate | 54 g |
| Protein | 12 g |
| Vitamin C | 58 mg |
| Vitamin D | 1 IU |
| Vitamin E | 2 mg |
| Niacin | 6 mg |
| Folate | 188 mcg |
| Vitamin $B_6$ | 0.3 mg |
| Vitamin $B_{12}$ | 0.1 mcg |
| Zinc | 1.5 mg |
| Selenium | 38 mcg |

# FISH AND SEAFOOD

# Parmesan Herb Baked Fish Fillets

*Just a touch of cayenne, basil and Parmesan cheese make these fish fillets more than just another grilled fish.*

## Makes 4 servings

## Tips

For convenience and speed, this recipe uses frozen fish fillets, but fresh fish may also be used. If you prefer a thicker fish fillet, such as salmon or halibut, increase the cooking time by about 5 minutes.

If available, substitute 1 to 2 tbsp (15 to 30 mL) chopped fresh basil for the dried basil.

Remember to use dry bread crumbs in this recipe; fresh bread crumbs will make the dish too soggy.

- Preheat oven to 400°F (200°C)
- 11- by 7-inch (28 by 18 cm) baking dish, greased

| 1 | package (1 lb/500 g) frozen fish fillets, thawed and patted dry | 1 |
| --- | --- | --- |
| ¼ cup | light mayonnaise | 60 mL |
| ¼ cup | freshly grated Parmesan cheese | 60 mL |
| 2 tbsp | chopped green onions | 30 mL |
| 1 tbsp | chopped pimiento or red bell pepper | 15 mL |
| | Cayenne pepper | |
| ½ cup | dry bread crumbs | 125 mL |
| ½ tsp | dried basil | 2 mL |
| | Freshly ground black pepper | |

1. Place fish fillets in a single layer in bottom of prepared baking dish. Set aside.

2. In a small bowl, stir together mayonnaise, Parmesan cheese, onions, pimiento and cayenne to taste. Spread mixture evenly over fish fillets.

3. In a separate bowl, combine bread crumbs, basil and pepper to taste; sprinkle over top of fish. Bake in preheated oven for 10 to 12 minutes or until fish is opaque and flakes easily with fork.

*This recipe courtesy of Marilena Rutka.*

### ▸ Health Tip

Fish is a great source of omega-3 fats. To minimize higher-mercury-content fish, try to rotate your selections.

## Nutrients per serving

| | |
| --- | --- |
| Calories | 290 |
| Fat | 18 g |
| Carbohydrate | 5 g |
| Protein | 25 g |
| Vitamin C | 8 mg |
| Vitamin D | 2 IU |
| Vitamin E | 2 mg |
| Niacin | 10 mg |
| Folate | 45 mcg |
| Vitamin $B_6$ | 0.5 mg |
| Vitamin $B_{12}$ | 1.6 mcg |
| Zinc | 0.8 mg |
| Selenium | 44 mcg |

# Salmon over White and Black Bean Salsa

*Salsas are a popular dressing for fish, and you'll see why with this salmon entrée.*

## Tip

Prepare bean mixture early in the day and keep refrigerated. Stir before serving.

- **Preheat barbecue to high or preheat oven to 425°F (220°C)**

| | | |
|---|---|---|
| 1 cup | rinsed drained canned black beans | 250 mL |
| 1 cup | rinsed drained canned white navy beans | 250 mL |
| ¾ cup | chopped tomatoes | 175 mL |
| ½ cup | chopped green bell peppers | 125 mL |
| ¼ cup | chopped red onions | 60 mL |
| ¼ cup | chopped fresh cilantro | 60 mL |
| 2 tbsp | balsamic vinegar | 30 mL |
| 2 tbsp | freshly squeezed lemon juice | 30 mL |
| 1 tbsp | olive oil | 15 mL |
| 1 tsp | minced garlic | 5 mL |
| 1 lb | salmon steaks | 500 g |

1. In a bowl, combine black beans, white beans, tomatoes, green peppers, red onions and cilantro. In a small bowl, whisk together vinegar, lemon juice, olive oil and garlic; pour over bean mixture and toss to combine.

2. Barbecue fish or bake uncovered for approximately 10 minutes for each 1-inch (2.5 cm) thickness of fish, or until fish flakes with a fork. Serve fish over bean salsa.

> ### ▶ Health Tip
>
> Salmon is a very good source of omega-3 fats, but try to stick to wild and sustainable salmon.

| Nutrients per serving | |
|---|---|
| Calories | 313 |
| Fat | 9 g |
| Carbohydrate | 25 g |
| Protein | 31 g |
| Vitamin C | 23 mg |
| Vitamin D | 493 IU |
| Vitamin E | 1 mg |
| Niacin | 10 mg |
| Folate | 99 mcg |
| Vitamin $B_6$ | 0.8 mg |
| Vitamin $B_{12}$ | 4.7 mcg |
| Zinc | 1.3 mg |
| Selenium | 37 mcg |

# Salmon Oasis

*This dish is great for a hearty weekend lunch on a busy day, when you need to be filled up and get maximum nutrition at the same time.*

**Makes 4 servings**

## Tip

Crush the bones of canned salmon for added calcium and vitamin D.

- **Preheat broiler**
- **Baking sheet, ungreased**

| | | |
|---|---|---|
| 4 | whole wheat English muffins | 4 |
| 1 | can (7½ oz/213 g) salmon, drained | 1 |
| ¼ cup | light mayonnaise | 60 mL |
| 2 tbsp | finely chopped green onion | 30 mL |
| 2 tsp | freshly squeezed lemon juice | 10 mL |
| ½ tsp | curry powder | 2 mL |
| ¼ tsp | freshly ground black pepper | 1 mL |
| 8 | green bell pepper strips | 8 |
| ¾ cup | shredded part-skim mozzarella cheese | 175 mL |
| | Paprika | |

1. Split muffins in half and toast.

2. Combine salmon, mayonnaise, green onion, lemon juice, curry powder and pepper. Spread on muffin halves; top with green pepper and cheese. Sprinkle with paprika. Place on ungreased baking sheet. Broil for about 3 minutes or just until cheese melts.

*This recipe courtesy of Ellen Craig.*

> ### ▶ Health Tip
>
> Canned salmon, although often dressed with mayonnaise, still carries the beneficial omega-3 fats the brain thrives on.

## Nutrients per serving

| | |
|---|---|
| Calories | 342 |
| Fat | 15 g |
| Carbohydrate | 30 g |
| Protein | 24 g |
| Vitamin C | 14 mg |
| Vitamin D | 426 IU |
| Vitamin E | 2 mg |
| Niacin | 6 mg |
| Folate | 39 mcg |
| Vitamin B$_6$ | 0.2 mg |
| Vitamin B$_{12}$ | 3.4 mcg |
| Zinc | 2.3 mg |
| Selenium | 48 mcg |

# Open-Face Salmon Salad Sandwich with Apple and Ginger

*Here is another use for canned salmon — which fits many budgets but still delivers the benefits of this nutritious fish.*

## Makes 4 servings

### Tip

Stir the salmon mixture gently if you like your salad flaky; stir vigorously for a smoother texture.

| Nutrients | per serving |
|---|---|
| Calories | 299 |
| Fat | 10 g |
| Carbohydrate | 37 g |
| Protein | 17 g |
| Vitamin C | 4 mg |
| Vitamin D | 248 IU |
| Vitamin E | 1 mg |
| Niacin | 6 mg |
| Folate | 56 mcg |
| Vitamin B$_6$ | 0.1 mg |
| Vitamin B$_{12}$ | 2.6 mcg |
| Zinc | 1.1 mg |
| Selenium | 35 mcg |

- Preheat broiler

| 1 | can (7½ oz/213 g) salmon, drained | 1 |
|---|---|---|
| ¼ cup | light mayonnaise | 60 mL |
| 2 tbsp | finely chopped green onion | 30 mL |
| ¼ cup | finely chopped apple | 60 mL |
| 1 tbsp | freshly squeezed lemon juice | 15 mL |
| 1 tsp | finely grated gingerroot | 5 mL |
| 2 tsp | curry powder | 10 mL |
| ½ tsp | cayenne pepper | 2 mL |
| 4 | thin whole-grain hamburger buns, split | 4 |
| 3 tbsp | ginger marmalade | 45 mL |
| 1 | apple, peeled and cut into 8 slices (optional) | 1 |
| 1 tbsp | liquid honey (optional) | 15 mL |

1. In a small bowl, combine salmon, mayonnaise, green onion, chopped apple, lemon juice, ginger, curry powder and cayenne.

2. Place hamburger buns cut side up on a baking sheet. Spread each with about 1 tsp (5 mL) ginger marmalade. Divide salmon mixture evenly on top. If desired, place 1 apple slice on top of salmon mixture and brush with honey.

3. Broil for 4 to 5 minutes or until salmon mixture is warm.

## Variation

Use canned tuna instead of salmon.

*This recipe courtesy of dietitian Mary Sue Waisman.*

### ▶ Health Tip

Ginger is an anti-inflammatory and anti-nausea agent and activates digestion even in people who are healthy.

# Tuna Salad Melt

*This is a great use of water-packed tuna, and can turn this simple fare into a delicious weekend lunch or quick dinner.*

---

**Makes 8 servings**

## Tips

The tuna mixture also makes a great filling for sandwiches, wraps and pita bread, as well as a great topping for salad greens or spinach.

If desired, substitute salmon for the tuna.

---

### ▶ Health Tip

Yogurt and cheese can deliver some of the calcium we need in a form that many people who don't tolerate cow's milk well can do just fine with.

---

### Nutrients per serving

| Calories | 196 |
|---|---|
| Fat | 3 g |
| Carbohydrate | 24 g |
| Protein | 17 g |
| Vitamin C | 7 mg |
| Vitamin D | 1 IU |
| Vitamin E | 0 mg |
| Niacin | 6 mg |
| Folate | 7 mcg |
| Vitamin B$_6$ | 0.2 mg |
| Vitamin B$_{12}$ | 1.3 mcg |
| Zinc | 0.5 mg |
| Selenium | 36 mcg |

- **Preheat broiler**
- **Large baking sheet**

| | | |
|---|---|---|
| 2 | cans (6 oz/170 g) water-packed tuna, drained | 2 |
| 1/4 cup | finely chopped celery | 60 mL |
| 1/4 cup | finely chopped sweet pickle or sweet relish | 60 mL |
| 1/4 cup | finely chopped red or green bell pepper (optional) | 60 mL |
| 1/4 cup | light mayonnaise | 60 mL |
| 2 tbsp | lower-fat plain yogurt | 30 mL |
| 1 tbsp | lemon juice or pickle juice | 15 mL |
| 1 | French stick (baguette) | 1 |
| 1/2 cup | shredded Cheddar cheese | 125 mL |

1. In a bowl, stir together tuna, celery, pickle, red pepper (if using), mayonnaise, yogurt and lemon juice. Blend well.

2. Slice French stick in half lengthwise. Cut each half into 4 equal portions, making 8 pieces; place on baking sheet. Toast under preheated broiler for 1 to 2 minutes or until golden.

3. Remove from broiler; spread tuna mixture evenly over each piece. Sprinkle with cheese. Broil for 2 to 3 minutes or until cheese is melted and golden.

## Variations

*Hot Tuna Salad Wrap:* Fill flour tortillas with tuna mixture and shredded cheese. Fold up and microwave on High for 30 to 45 seconds or until cheese is melted.

*Cold Tuna Salad Wrap:* Add any shredded or grated vegetable, such as purple cabbage, carrots, zucchini, arugula, mustard greens, kale or spinach, to the tuna mixture. Roll in a tortilla and serve.

---

*This recipe courtesy of dietitian Bev Callaghan.*

# Tuna Casserole

*A 21st-century take on a North American classic — supergrain quinoa and brown rice take the place of refined macaroni shells in a way that transforms it.*

## Makes 4 servings

## Tip

Vegan hard margarine, such as Earth Balance vegan buttery flavor sticks, has almost half as much saturated fat as regular butter and no cholesterol. Where butter is called for in a recipe, vegan hard margarine can be a heart-healthy, delicious alternative.

- Preheat oven to 350°F (180°C)
- 10- by 8-inch (25 by 20 cm) casserole dish with lid, lightly greased

| | | |
|---|---|---|
| 1 tsp | grapeseed oil | 5 mL |
| 1 cup | chopped onion | 250 mL |
| 1 cup | chopped celery | 250 mL |
| 1 tbsp | chopped fresh parsley | 15 mL |
| 1 tsp | vegan hard margarine or butter | 5 mL |
| 1 | can (6 oz/170 g) water-packed flaked tuna, drained | 1 |
| $1/2$ cup | long-grain brown rice | 125 mL |
| $1/2$ cup | quinoa, rinsed | 125 mL |
| 2 cups | fortified gluten-free non-dairy milk or lactose-free 1% milk | 500 mL |

1. In a skillet, heat oil over medium-high heat. Sauté onion, celery and parsley for 3 to 5 minutes or until onion is starting to brown. Stir in margarine. Remove from heat.

2. In prepared baking dish, combine tuna, rice, quinoa and milk. Stir in onion mixture.

3. Cover and bake in preheated oven for 45 minutes or until rice and quinoa are tender and liquid is absorbed. Uncover and bake for 5 minutes or until top is browned.

## Variation

Add $1/2$ cup (125 mL) frozen peas with the rice.

> ### ▸ Health Tip
>
> Whole grains like brown rice and quinoa combined with tuna deliver a major source of brain fuel to the body, along with a great deal of protein.

| Nutrients per serving | |
|---|---|
| Calories | 304 |
| Fat | 6 g |
| Carbohydrate | 42 g |
| Protein | 20 g |
| Vitamin C | 5 mg |
| Vitamin D | 57 IU |
| Vitamin E | 2 mg |
| Niacin | 8 mg |
| Folate | 75 mcg |
| Vitamin B$_6$ | 0.5 mg |
| Vitamin B$_{12}$ | 2.3 mcg |
| Zinc | 1.9 mg |
| Selenium | 45 mcg |

# Super-Easy Crab and Sweet Potato Sushi Rolls

*This is a great way to satisfy a sushi craving without an expensive night out — and get a nutritious meal at the same time.*

## Makes 8 servings

### Tip

Because these rolls are easy to eat with your fingers, they make great party snacks!

| | | |
|---|---|---|
| 2 cups | sushi rice | 500 mL |
| 2 tbsp | rice vinegar | 30 mL |
| 1 | sweet potato, peeled | 1 |
| 8 | sheets nori (dried seaweed) | 8 |
| 2 tbsp | light mayonnaise | 30 mL |
| 1 | avocado, cut into 16 slices | 1 |
| 1 cup | chopped cooked crabmeat or imitation crab | 250 mL |
| | Sodium-reduced soy sauce, wasabi and pickled ginger (optional) | |

1. Prepare rice according to package directions. Let cool. Stir in rice vinegar.

2. Slice sweet potato into 16 long strips, each about $\frac{1}{2}$ inch (1 cm) wide. Place in a microwave-safe dish and add a splash of water. Cover with plastic wrap, leaving one corner open for a vent, and microwave on High for 2 to 3 minutes or until just tender. Let cool.

3. Place 1 nori sheet on a work surface. Spread one-eighth of the rice in a thin layer over the bottom third of the sheet. Spread about $\frac{3}{4}$ tsp (3 mL) mayonnaise on top. Place 2 strips of sweet potato, 2 slices of avocado and one-eighth of the crab along the rice, extending the width of the nori sheet.

4. Gently lift the bottom end of the nori sheet and roll it up over the rice and filling, as you would roll a burrito. Roll slowly and tightly. When you are about 1 inch (2.5 cm) from the end, lightly moisten the remaining nori with a few drops of water and continue rolling to seal the roll. Set aside and repeat with the remaining nori sheets, rice, mayonnaise, sweet potato, avocado and crab. Slice into 2-inch (5 cm) rolls and, if desired, serve with small bowls of soy sauce, wasabi and ginger.

*This recipe courtesy of dietitian Patricia Chuey.*

### Nutrients per serving

| | |
|---|---|
| Calories | 261 |
| Fat | 5 g |
| Carbohydrate | 45 g |
| Protein | 7 g |
| Vitamin C | 5 mg |
| Vitamin D | 0 IU |
| Vitamin E | 1 mg |
| Niacin | 3 mg |
| Folate | 150 mcg |
| Vitamin B$_6$ | 0.2 mg |
| Vitamin B$_{12}$ | 0.6 mcg |
| Zinc | 1.4 mg |
| Selenium | 15 mcg |

## Tip

Keep a bowl of warm water near you as you work; you'll find it handy for cleaning your hands and knife, as the rice is very sticky.

## Variations

Replace the crab with drained canned tuna or salmon mixed with an additional 1 tbsp (15 mL) light mayonnaise.

Instead of the sweet potato and avocado, try slices of cucumber, cooked carrot, red or green bell pepper or asparagus.

> ### ▶ Health Tip
>
> Nori contains sulfur-rich starch molecules called fucoidans that have anti-inflammatory effects in the body.

# Pasta with Shrimp and Peas

*This is a simple gluten-free pasta dish that can come in handy at the end of a hectic day and still be worth looking forward to.*

**Makes 4 to 6 servings**

## Tip

If you have fresh basil and parsley on hand, use 1 tbsp (15 mL) of each in place of dried, adding them with the Romano cheese.

| | | |
|---|---|---|
| 12 oz | gluten-free penne or spiral pasta | 375 g |
| 3 tbsp | olive oil | 45 mL |
| 3 to 4 | cloves garlic, minced | 3 to 4 |
| 1 tsp | dried basil | 5 mL |
| 1 tsp | dried parsley | 5 mL |
| Pinch | cayenne pepper | Pinch |
| 8 oz | cooked peeled frozen shrimp | 250 g |
| 1 cup | frozen green peas | 250 mL |
| ¼ cup | grated Romano cheese | 60 mL |
| | Salt and freshly ground black pepper | |

1. In a large pot of boiling water, cook pasta according to package instructions until tender but firm (al dente). Drain, reserving 2 cups (500 mL) of the pasta cooking water. Return pasta to the pot.

2. In a skillet, heat oil over low heat. Sauté garlic to taste, basil, parsley and cayenne for 3 to 5 minutes or until garlic is softened and fragrant. Add shrimp and peas; sauté for about 5 minutes or until heated through.

3. Add shrimp mixture to pasta. Add enough of the reserved pasta cooking water to moisten to desired consistency, tossing gently to coat. Stir in Romano cheese and season to taste with salt and pepper.

### ▸ Health Tip

Make sure you buy organic or wild/sustainable shrimp, as some farm-raised shrimp come from unhealthy conditions and have many antibiotics added to their "pens."

### Nutrients per 1 of 6 servings

| | |
|---|---|
| Calories | 352 |
| Fat | 10 g |
| Carbohydrate | 47 g |
| Protein | 19 g |
| Vitamin C | 5 mg |
| Vitamin D | 2 IU |
| Vitamin E | 2 mg |
| Niacin | 6 mg |
| Folate | 156 mcg |
| Vitamin $B_6$ | 0.4 mg |
| Vitamin $B_{12}$ | 0.6 mcg |
| Zinc | 1.6 mg |
| Selenium | 5 mcg |

# Shrimp, Vegetables and Whole Wheat Pasta

*This is a Mediterranean dish that has many of this diet's outstanding features and is easy to make.*

| | | |
|---|---|---:|
| 4 cups | whole wheat pasta (such as fusilli or penne) | 1 L |
| 1 tbsp | olive oil | 15 mL |
| 3 | cloves garlic, minced | 3 |
| 1 | bunch broccoli, chopped | 1 |
| 1 | red bell pepper, sliced | 1 |
| 2 cups | grape tomatoes, halved | 500 mL |
| 12 oz | shrimp, peeled, deveined and halved | 375 g |
| 1 tsp | dried Italian herb seasoning | 5 mL |
| $\frac{1}{2}$ tsp | salt | 2 mL |
| $\frac{1}{2}$ tsp | freshly ground black pepper | 2 mL |

**Makes 6 servings**

## Variations

Change some of the vegetables for variety. You could try sugar snap peas, snow peas or spinach instead of the broccoli, or yellow pepper or carrot instead of the red pepper. Or use a frozen vegetable blend.

The dish does not have a lot of sauce. If you prefer a saucier dish, add a little pesto or a creamy tomato sauce. If using pesto, omit the Italian seasoning.

1. Cook pasta according to package directions until al dente (tender to the bite). Drain.

2. Meanwhile, heat a large skillet over medium-high heat. Add oil and swirl to coat pan. Sauté garlic for 1 minute, being careful not to burn it. Add broccoli, red pepper and tomatoes; sauté for 5 to 7 minutes or until vegetables are tender-crisp. Add shrimp and cook, turning once, until opaque and slightly browned, about 4 minutes. Stir in pasta, Italian seasoning, salt and pepper.

*This recipe courtesy of dietitian Beth Gould.*

## ▶ Health Tip

A whole grain, olive oil, bell peppers, broccoli and garlic in one dish add up to cardiovascular healthy eating — which is important for long-term brain health.

### Nutrients per serving

| | |
|---|---:|
| Calories | 331 |
| Fat | 4 g |
| Carbohydrate | 59 g |
| Protein | 20 g |
| Vitamin C | 59 mg |
| Vitamin D | 1 IU |
| Vitamin E | 2 mg |
| Niacin | 5 mg |
| Folate | 86 mcg |
| Vitamin B$_6$ | 0.4 mg |
| Vitamin B$_{12}$ | 0.6 mcg |
| Zinc | 2.5 mg |
| Selenium | 18 mcg |

# Peppery Shrimp with Quinoa

*Saffron gives this dish a signature flavor, and with quinoa and shrimp, it is a meal in itself.*

**Makes 4 servings**

## Tips

Saffron is expensive, but you never need a lot of it to make something really special.

To keep quinoa as fresh as possible, store it in an airtight container in the refrigerator for up to 6 months or in the freezer for up to 1 year.

| | | |
|---|---|---|
| 2 tbsp | olive oil, divided | 30 mL |
| 1 | onion, diced | 1 |
| 1 | green bell pepper, finely chopped | 1 |
| 1/4 tsp | crumbled saffron threads, dissolved in 2 tbsp (30 mL) boiling water | 1 mL |
| 1/2 cup | water or ready-to-use reduced-sodium vegetable broth | 125 mL |
| 1 | can (14 oz/398 mL) no-salt-added diced tomatoes, with juice | 1 |
| 3/4 cup | quinoa, rinsed | 175 mL |
| 12 oz | shrimp, peeled and deveined, thawed if frozen | 375 g |
| 4 | cloves garlic, minced | 4 |
| 1 tsp | finely grated lemon zest | 5 mL |
| 1/4 tsp | cayenne pepper | 1 mL |
| | Freshly ground black pepper | |
| 1/2 cup | dry white wine | 125 mL |
| 2 tbsp | freshly squeezed lemon juice | 30 mL |
| 1 cup | cooked green peas | 250 mL |
| | Salt (optional) | |

1. In a saucepan, heat 1 tbsp (15 mL) of the oil over medium heat for 30 seconds. Add onion and bell pepper and cook, stirring, until softened, about 5 minutes. Add saffron liquid, water and tomatoes and bring to a boil. Stir in quinoa. Reduce heat to low. Cover and cook until quinoa is tender, about 15 minutes. Remove from heat and let stand, covered, for 5 minutes. Fluff with a fork.

## Nutrients per serving

| | |
|---|---|
| Calories | 331 |
| Fat | 10 g |
| Carbohydrate | 37 g |
| Protein | 20 g |
| Vitamin C | 43 mg |
| Vitamin D | 2 IU |
| Vitamin E | 4 mg |
| Niacin | 4 mg |
| Folate | 115 mcg |
| Vitamin B$_6$ | 0.6 mg |
| Vitamin B$_{12}$ | 0.9 mcg |
| Zinc | 2.3 mg |
| Selenium | 29 mcg |

## Variation

*Peppery Shrimp with Millet:* Substitute an equal quantity of millet for the quinoa. For the best flavor, before using in the recipe toast the rinsed millet in a dry skillet, stirring until fragrant, about 5 minutes. Stir the millet into tomato mixture (step 1) and return to a boil. Cover and simmer over low heat for 20 minutes, then remove from heat and let stand for 10 minutes.

2. In a skillet, heat remaining 1 tbsp (15 mL) of oil over medium-high heat. Add shrimp and cook, stirring, just until they turn pink and opaque, 3 to 5 minutes. Add garlic, lemon zest, cayenne and black pepper to taste. Cook, stirring, for 1 minute. Add white wine and lemon juice and bring to a boil. Stir in peas until heated through. Season to taste with salt (if using).

3. On a deep platter, arrange quinoa in a ring around the edge, leaving the center hollow. Arrange shrimp in the center.

> ### ▶ Health Tip
>
> Green peas are a legume but not just a starch or carb source: pisumsaponins I and II and pisomosides A and B are anti-inflammatory compounds almost exclusive to peas.

# Pad Thai

*The classic and perhaps most familiar Thai dish to many North Americans. This version requires some specialty ingredients, but they give it authentic Thai flavor.*

## Tips

To get the most juice from citrus fruits, let them warm up for about 15 minutes, then roll them on the counter a few times before juicing.

For 3 tbsp (45 mL) lime juice, you'll need 2 to 3 medium limes.

| | | |
|---|---|---:|
| 8 oz | dried medium rice noodles | 250 g |
| 3 tbsp | ready-to-use chicken broth, ketchup or tomato sauce | 45 mL |
| 3 tbsp | freshly squeezed lime juice or tamarind paste | 45 mL |
| 2 tbsp | fish sauce (nam pla) | 30 mL |
| 2 tbsp | palm sugar or packed brown sugar | 30 mL |
| 1/2 tsp | hot chili sauce | 2 mL |
| 3 tbsp | vegetable oil, divided | 45 mL |
| 2 | large eggs, beaten | 2 |
| 3 | cloves garlic, chopped | 3 |
| 4 oz | shrimp, peeled, deveined and cut into small pieces | 125 g |
| 4 oz | boneless chicken or pork, cut into small pieces | 125 g |
| 2 cups | bean sprouts, divided | 500 mL |
| 2 | green onions, chopped | 2 |
| 1/4 cup | chopped peanuts | 60 mL |
| 1/4 cup | chopped fresh cilantro leaves | 60 mL |
| | Fresh red chile peppers, cut into strips (optional) | |
| 1 | lime, cut into wedges | 1 |

1. To soften noodles, place in a large bowl. Cover with very hot water and let stand for 10 to 12 minutes or until softened but still firm (pinch them to check). Rinse well with cold water and drain.

2. In a small bowl or measuring cup, combine broth, lime juice, fish sauce, sugar and chili sauce.

3. Heat a wok or large skillet over medium-high heat and add 1 tbsp (30 mL) oil. Add beaten eggs to hot pan and swirl to coat bottom of pan. Cook until starting to set, then stir to break into pieces. Remove from wok and reserve.

## Nutrients per serving

| | |
|---|---:|
| Calories | 579 |
| Fat | 25 g |
| Carbohydrate | 67 g |
| Protein | 26 g |
| Vitamin C | 16 mg |
| Vitamin D | 23 IU |
| Vitamin E | 4 mg |
| Niacin | 8 mg |
| Folate | 113 mcg |
| Vitamin B$_6$ | 0.5 mg |
| Vitamin B$_{12}$ | 0.7 mcg |
| Zinc | 2.7 mg |
| Selenium | 31 mcg |

## Tip

Make sure you buy organic or wild/ sustainable shrimp, as some farm-raised shrimp come from unhealthy conditions and have many antibiotics added to their "pens."

**4.** Add remaining oil to wok. When hot, add garlic, shrimp and chicken and stir-fry for 2 minutes, or until shrimp and chicken are just cooked. Stir in noodles and reserved sauce mixture and cook for 1 to 2 minutes, or until noodles are soft but not mushy.

**5.** Add 1 cup (250 mL) bean sprouts and cooked eggs and toss to combine.

**6.** Turn noodles onto a serving platter. Sprinkle with remaining bean sprouts, green onions, peanuts, cilantro and chiles (if using). Garnish with lime wedges.

> ### ▶ Health Tip
>
> Tamarind has traditionally been used for gastrointestinal and liver problems.

# Shrimp Risotto with Artichoke Hearts and Parmesan

*The firm, nutty texture of properly cooked Arborio rice perfectly complements the meatiness of shrimp in this classic dish.*

## Tip

If you haven't got the time or ingredients necessary to make seafood broth from scratch, you can buy it canned or in powdered form (1 tsp/5 mL in 1 cup/250 mL boiling water yields 1 cup/250 mL broth). Keep in mind, however, that these broths are often loaded with sodium. To cut back on the sodium, try using only $\frac{1}{2}$ tsp (2 mL) powder.

| | | |
|---|---|---|
| 3 cups | ready-to-use seafood or chicken broth | 750 mL |
| $\frac{1}{2}$ cup | chopped onions | 125 mL |
| 2 tsp | minced garlic | 10 mL |
| 1 cup | Arborio rice | 250 mL |
| 1 tsp | dried basil | 5 mL |
| $\frac{1}{2}$ | can (14 oz/398 mL) artichoke hearts, drained and chopped | $\frac{1}{2}$ |
| 8 oz | shrimp, peeled, deveined and chopped | 250 g |
| $\frac{1}{4}$ cup | chopped green onions | 60 mL |
| $\frac{1}{4}$ cup | freshly grated low-fat Parmesan cheese | 60 mL |
| $\frac{1}{4}$ tsp | freshly ground black pepper | 1 mL |

1. In a saucepan over medium-high heat, bring broth to a boil; reduce heat to low. In another nonstick saucepan sprayed with vegetable spray, cook onions and garlic over medium-high heat for 3 minutes or until softened. Add rice and basil; cook for 1 minute.

2. Using a ladle, add $\frac{1}{2}$ cup (125 mL) broth to rice; stir to keep rice from sticking to pan. When liquid is absorbed, add another $\frac{1}{2}$ cup (125 mL) broth. Reduce heat if necessary to maintain a slow, steady simmer. Repeat this process, ladling in hot broth and stirring constantly, for 15 minutes, reducing amount of broth added to $\frac{1}{4}$ cup (60 mL) near end of cooking time.

3. Add artichokes and shrimp; cook, adding more broth as necessary, for 3 minutes or until shrimp turn pink and rice is tender but firm. Add green onions, Parmesan cheese and pepper. Serve immediately.

> ▶ **Health Tip**
>
> Artichokes have been shown to have a cholesterol-lowering effect.

### Nutrients per serving

| | |
|---|---|
| Calories | 303 |
| Fat | 4 g |
| Carbohydrate | 49 g |
| Protein | 18 g |
| Vitamin C | 6 mg |
| Vitamin D | 2 IU |
| Vitamin E | 1 mg |
| Niacin | 6 mg |
| Folate | 171 mcg |
| Vitamin B$_6$ | 0.3 mg |
| Vitamin B$_{12}$ | 0.9 mcg |
| Zinc | 1.7 mg |
| Selenium | 25 mcg |

# POULTRY, PORK, BEEF AND LAMB

# Rosemary Chicken Breasts with Sweet Potatoes and Onions

*This dish makes good use of fragrant rosemary, added two ways.*

## Makes 4 servings

### Tips

Make extra batches of rosemary butter, shape into small logs, wrap in plastic wrap and store in the freezer. Cut into slices and use to tuck under the breast skins of whole roasting chickens or Cornish hens, or to top grilled meats.

If you purchased whole breasts with backs on, cut away backbone using poultry shears.

This recipe can easily be halved to serve 2.

### Nutrients per serving

| | |
|---|---|
| Calories | 251 |
| Fat | 9 g |
| Carbohydrate | 15 g |
| Protein | 26 g |
| Vitamin C | 5 mg |
| Vitamin D | 10 IU |
| Vitamin E | 1 mg |
| Niacin | 13 mg |
| Folate | 16 mcg |
| Vitamin B$_6$ | 1.1 mg |
| Vitamin B$_{12}$ | 0.3 mcg |
| Zinc | 0.9 mg |
| Selenium | 38 mcg |

- Preheat oven to 375°F (190°C)
- 13- by 9-inch (33 by 23 cm) baking dish, greased

| | | |
|---|---|---|
| 2 | sweet potatoes (about 1½ lbs/750 g) | 2 |
| 1 | onion | 1 |
| 1½ tsp | chopped fresh rosemary (or ½ tsp/2 mL dried rosemary, crumbled) | 7 mL |
| | Salt and freshly ground black pepper | |
| 4 | skin-on bone-in chicken breasts | 4 |

**Rosemary Butter**

| | | |
|---|---|---|
| 2 tbsp | butter | 30 mL |
| 1 | large clove garlic, minced | 1 |
| 1 tsp | grated lemon zest | 5 mL |
| 2 tsp | chopped fresh rosemary (or ¾ tsp/3 mL dried rosemary, crumbled) | 10 mL |
| ¼ tsp | salt | 1 mL |
| ¼ tsp | freshly ground black pepper | 1 mL |

1. Peel sweet potatoes and onion; cut into thin slices. Layer in prepared baking dish. Season with rosemary and salt and pepper to taste.

2. *Rosemary Butter:* In a small bowl, mash together butter, garlic, lemon zest, rosemary, salt and pepper. Divide into four portions

3. Place chicken breasts, skin side up, on work surface. Remove any fat deposits under skins. Press down on breast bone to flatten slightly. Carefully loosen the breast skins and tuck rosemary butter under skins, patting to distribute evenly.

4. Arrange chicken on top of vegetables in baking dish. Roast for 45 to 55 minutes or until vegetables are tender and chicken is nicely colored.

> ▸ **Health Tip**
>
> Rosemary contains rosmarinic acid, a compound that helps the body carry out detoxificiation reactions.

# Three-Spice Chicken with Potatoes

*Chicken thighs tend to stay moist while cooking — all the better to absorb the rich spice flavors in this dish.*

**Makes 8 servings**

## Tips

To toast coriander seeds, spread them in a dry heavy skillet. Cook over medium heat, shaking skillet occasionally to toast evenly, until seeds are a little darker and aromatic, 4 to 5 minutes. Let cool. Grind to a powder in a spice grinder.

A quick way to seed cardamoms is to put the whole pods into a spice grinder or blender jar. With a few on/off pulse motions, the skins will come loose. Remove and discard skins.

| Nutrients per serving | |
|---|---|
| Calories | 349 |
| Fat | 13 g |
| Carbohydrate | 28 g |
| Protein | 30 g |
| Vitamin C | 32 mg |
| Vitamin D | 7 IU |
| Vitamin E | 2 mg |
| Niacin | 11 mg |
| Folate | 43 mcg |
| Vitamin B$_6$ | 0.8 mg |
| Vitamin B$_{12}$ | 0.5 mcg |
| Zinc | 3.3 mg |
| Selenium | 20 mcg |

| | | |
|---|---|---|
| 6 | potatoes | 6 |
| 16 | boneless skinless chicken thighs (about 4 lbs/2 kg) | 16 |
| 1/4 cup | vegetable oil | 60 mL |
| 1/3 cup | coriander seeds, freshly toasted and powdered in spice grinder (see tip, at left) | 75 mL |
| 1/4 cup | cardamom seeds, coarsely pounded (see tip, at left) | 60 mL |
| 1 tbsp | black peppercorns, coarsely pounded | 15 mL |
| 1 1/4 tsp | salt (or to taste) | 6 mL |
| | Cherry tomatoes, halved | |

1. In a saucepan of boiling water, cook whole potatoes with skins on until tender, 20 to 25 minutes. Drain. When cool enough to handle, peel and cut into quarters. Set aside.

2. Rinse chicken and pat dry. In a large wok or saucepan with a tight-fitting lid, heat oil over medium-high heat. Add chicken.

3. Mix together coriander powder, cardamom seeds, pepper and salt. Sprinkle evenly over chicken. Reduce heat to medium. Cover and cook, shaking pan occasionally to prevent sticking. Do not stir. (There will be a fair amount of liquid from the chicken as it cooks.) After 8 to 10 minutes, when there is no more liquid, add potatoes. Brown chicken and potatoes gently. If chicken is not cooked, add 2 to 3 tbsp (30 to 45 mL) water. Cover and cook over low heat until potatoes are tender and chicken is no longer pink inside, 10 to 12 minutes.

4. *To serve:* Mound on platter and garnish with halved cherry tomatoes.

> ▶ **Health Tip**
>
> In Ayurvedic medicine, cardamom has been used for centuries to treat indigestion.

# Chicken Paprika with Noodles

*If you haven't tried chicken paprika yet (or chicken paprikash, in a Hungarian restaurant), you're missing out — this recipe will get you started.*

**Makes 4 servings**

## Tip

When ground chicken or turkey is browned in a skillet, it doesn't turn into a fine crumble like other ground meats. Overcome the problem by placing the cooked chicken in a food processor and chopping it using on-off turns to break up meat lumps.

| | | |
|---|---|---|
| 1 lb | lean ground chicken or turkey | 500 g |
| 1 tbsp | butter | 15 mL |
| 1 | onion, chopped | 1 |
| 8 oz | mushrooms, sliced | 250 g |
| 1 tbsp | paprika | 15 mL |
| 2 tbsp | all-purpose flour | 30 mL |
| 1⅓ cups | ready-to-use chicken broth | 325 mL |
| ½ cup | sour cream | 125 mL |
| 2 tbsp | chopped fresh dill or parsley | 30 mL |
| | Salt and freshly ground black pepper | |
| 8 oz | fettuccine or broad egg noodles | 250 g |

1. In a large nonstick skillet over medium-high heat, cook chicken, breaking up with a wooden spoon, for 5 minutes or until no longer pink. Transfer to a bowl.

2. Melt butter in skillet. Add onion, mushrooms and paprika; cook, stirring often, for 3 minutes or until vegetables are softened.

3. Sprinkle with flour; stir in broth and return chicken to skillet. Bring to a boil; cook, stirring, until thickened. Reduce heat, cover and simmer for 5 minutes. Remove from heat and stir in sour cream (it may curdle if added over the heat) and dill; season with salt and pepper to taste.

4. Meanwhile, cook pasta in a large pot of boiling salted water until tender but firm. Drain well. Return to pot and toss with chicken mixture. Serve immediately.

## ▸ Health Tip

Paprika comes from members of the capsicum species, but most varieties used or sold as the spice are not very hot (though some can be). It is loaded with carotenoids such as lutein and zeaxanthin.

### Nutrients per serving

| | |
|---|---|
| Calories | 501 |
| Fat | 17 g |
| Carbohydrate | 56 g |
| Protein | 32 g |
| Vitamin C | 2 mg |
| Vitamin D | 7 IU |
| Vitamin E | 1 mg |
| Niacin | 16 mg |
| Folate | 178 mcg |
| Vitamin B$_6$ | 0.8 mg |
| Vitamin B$_{12}$ | 0.9 mcg |
| Zinc | 3.2 mg |
| Selenium | 50 mcg |

# Red Curry Chicken with Snap Peas and Cashews

*This dish is a delicious and spicy way to satisfy a craving for Thai curry.*

## Tips

If lime leaves aren't available, substitute $\frac{1}{2}$ tsp (2 mL) finely grated lime zest and add with the lime juice in step 2.

The cashews give the best texture to the sauce if pulsed in a food processor to a coarse meal (without processing too much into butter). You may need to do more than $\frac{1}{4}$ cup (60 mL), depending on the size of your food processor. Extra ground nuts can be frozen for future use.

| 1 tbsp | vegetable oil | 15 mL |
| 1 | red or yellow bell pepper, thinly sliced | 1 |
| 1 cup | sugar snap peas or frozen green peas | 250 mL |
| 2 | wild lime leaves (see tip, at left) | 2 |
| $\frac{1}{4}$ cup | salted roasted cashews, ground or finely chopped (see tip, at left) | 60 mL |
| 1 tbsp | packed brown sugar or palm sugar | 15 mL |
| 1 | can (14 oz/400 mL) coconut milk | 1 |
| $\frac{1}{4}$ cup | water | 60 mL |
| 1 tbsp | Thai red curry paste | 15 mL |
| 1 lb | boneless skinless chicken breast or thighs, cut into thin strips | 500 g |
| 2 tbsp | freshly squeezed lime juice | 30 mL |
| | Salt | |
| | Salted roasted cashews | |
| | Chopped fresh mint and/or Thai basil | |
| | Lime wedges | |

1. In a large skillet, heat oil over medium heat. Add red pepper, peas and lime leaves; cook, stirring, until pepper is starting to soften, about 1 minute. Add ground cashews, brown sugar, coconut milk, water and curry paste; bring to a boil, stirring until blended. Reduce heat and boil gently, stirring often, until slightly thickened, about 2 minutes.

2. Stir in chicken and return to a simmer, stirring. Reduce heat and simmer gently, stirring often, until chicken is no longer pink inside and peas are tender-crisp, about 5 minutes. Discard lime leaves, if desired. Stir in lime juice and season to taste with salt. Serve sprinkled with cashews, mint and/or basil and garnished with lime wedges to squeeze over top.

## Nutrients per serving

| | |
|---|---|
| Calories | 328 |
| Fat | 29 g |
| Carbohydrate | 16 g |
| Protein | 5 g |
| Vitamin C | 47 mg |
| Vitamin D | 0 IU |
| Vitamin E | 1 mg |
| Niacin | 2 mg |
| Folate | 52 mcg |
| Vitamin $B_6$ | 0.2 mg |
| Vitamin $B_{12}$ | 0.0 mcg |
| Zinc | 1.4 mg |
| Selenium | 2 mcg |

### ▸ Health Tip

Coconut oil provides a useful vehicle for absorption of the beneficial compounds in the curry paste, as does the addition of black pepper in the paste itself.

# Tandoori Chicken

*Tandoori is a wonderful way to roast chicken, and the spices and yogurt are the real stars of this dish.*

## Tip

If you have time, let the chicken marinate in the refrigerator for several hours or overnight to intensify the flavors.

---

▶ **Health Tip**

Curry paste contains turmeric and therefore curcuminoids, which are anti-inflammatory in the body.

---

### Nutrients per serving

| | |
|---|---|
| Calories | 206 |
| Fat | 5 g |
| Carbohydrate | 9 g |
| Protein | 30 g |
| Vitamin C | 5 mg |
| Vitamin D | 7 IU |
| Vitamin E | 1 mg |
| Niacin | 13 mg |
| Folate | 18 mcg |
| Vitamin B$_6$ | 1.0 mg |
| Vitamin B$_{12}$ | 0.8 mcg |
| Zinc | 1.6 mg |
| Selenium | 41 mcg |

- Food processor
- Rimmed baking sheet, with greased rack (if using oven)

### Tandoori Marinade

| | | |
|---|---|---|
| ½ cup | plain yogurt | 125 mL |
| 1 tbsp | tomato paste | 15 mL |
| 2 | green onions, coarsely chopped | 2 |
| 2 | cloves garlic, quartered | 2 |
| 1 | 1½-inch (4 cm) piece gingerroot, coarsely chopped | 1 |
| 2 tsp | mild curry paste | 10 mL |
| 1 tsp | garam masala | 5 mL |
| 1 tsp | ground coriander | 5 mL |
| ½ tsp | ground cumin | 2 mL |
| ¼ tsp | salt | 1 mL |
| ¼ tsp | cayenne pepper | 1 mL |
| 4 | bone-in skinless chicken breasts | 4 |
| 2 tbsp | chopped fresh cilantro or parsley | 30 mL |
| | Cucumber Raita (see recipe, opposite) | |

1. *Marinade:* In food processor, purée yogurt, tomato paste, green onions, garlic, ginger, curry paste, garam masala, coriander, cumin, salt and cayenne until smooth.

2. Arrange chicken in a shallow dish; coat with yogurt mixture. Cover and refrigerate for at least 1 hour or for up to 1 day.

### Grill Method

3. Preheat greased barbecue grill to medium-high. Remove chicken from marinade, discarding marinade. Place chicken, bone side up, on grill; cook for 15 minutes. Turn and cook for 10 to 15 minutes or until no longer pink in center. Garnish with cilantro. Serve with Cucumber Raita.

### Oven Method

3. Preheat oven to 350°F (180°C). Remove chicken from marinade, discarding marinade. Place chicken on rack on baking sheet; roast for 50 to 55 minutes or until no longer pink in center. Garnish with cilantro. Serve with Cucumber Raita.

# Cucumber Raita

*Raita is a yogurt-based side dish served as a cool, refreshing accompaniment to cut the heat in Indian dishes.*

## Tip

Use yogurt with 2% or more milk fat; nonfat yogurt has too thin a consistency for this recipe.

| | | |
|---|---|---:|
| 1 cup | plain yogurt | 250 mL |
| 1 | small clove garlic | 1 |
| ¼ tsp | salt | 1 mL |
| ¼ tsp | ground cumin | 1 mL |
| ¼ cup | grated seeded peeled cucumber | 60 mL |
| 2 tbsp | chopped fresh cilantro (or 1 tbsp/15 mL chopped fresh mint) | 30 mL |

1. In a bowl, combine yogurt, garlic, salt and cumin.
2. Place cucumber in a sieve and squeeze out moisture. Shortly before serving, stir cucumber into yogurt mixture. Sprinkle with cilantro.

### Nutrients per 2 tbsp (30 mL)

| | |
|---|---:|
| Calories | 17 |
| Fat | 0 g |
| Carbohydrate | 2 g |
| Protein | 1 g |
| Vitamin C | 0 mg |
| Vitamin D | 0 IU |
| Vitamin E | 0 mg |
| Niacin | 0 mg |
| Folate | 3 mcg |
| Vitamin B$_6$ | 0.0 mg |
| Vitamin B$_{12}$ | 0.1 mcg |
| Zinc | 0.2 mg |
| Selenium | 1 mcg |

# Bengali Chicken Stew

*This stew tastes great and has numerous herbs and spices that activate digestion.*

**Makes 6 to 8 servings**

## Tip

Panchphoran is a mix of equal proportions of five aromatic seeds: mustard, cumin, fennel, fenugreek and nigella. It can be premixed and stored indefinitely.

| | | |
|---|---|---|
| 12 | bone-in skinless chicken thighs | 12 |
| 3½ tbsp | vegetable oil, divided | 52 mL |
| 1 tbsp | panchphoran (see tip, at left) | 15 mL |
| 2 | bay leaves | 2 |
| 1 tbsp | minced gingerroot | 15 mL |
| 1 tbsp | minced garlic | 15 mL |
| 3 | plum (Roma) tomatoes, cut into 1-inch (2.5 cm) wedges | 3 |
| 1 tbsp | ground coriander | 15 mL |
| 1 tbsp | ground cumin | 15 mL |
| 2 tsp | ground turmeric | 10 mL |
| 2 tsp | salt | 10 mL |
| 8 oz | all-purpose potatoes, peeled and cut into chunks (about 2) | 250 g |
| 6 to 8 | large cauliflower florets | 6 to 8 |

1. Rinse chicken and pat dry. In a large saucepan, heat 2 tbsp (30 mL) oil over medium heat. Brown chicken, in two batches, 6 to 8 minutes per batch. Remove with tongs and set aside. Remove from heat. Scrape up any bits and pieces that may be stuck to the pan and add to chicken.

2. Add remaining oil to pan and heat over medium-high heat. Add panchphoran. When the seeds stop popping, in a few seconds, reduce heat to medium. Immediately add bay leaves, ginger, garlic and tomatoes and stir to mix. Add coriander, cumin and turmeric and sauté for 1 minute.

3. Add 4 cups (1 L) water. Increase heat to medium-high. Add chicken, making sure all pieces are submerged. Add salt. Cover and bring to a boil. Reduce heat to low and simmer for 35 minutes.

4. Add potatoes and cauliflower. Cook, stirring occasionally, until vegetables are tender and chicken is no longer pink inside, 12 to 14 minutes.

## ▶ Health Tip

Both the cauliflower and the mustard seed (from panchphoran) in this dish are sources of isothiocyanates, powerful cancer-preventive and detoxification compounds.

## Nutrients per 1 of 8 servings

| | |
|---|---|
| Calories | 225 |
| Fat | 11 g |
| Carbohydrate | 9 g |
| Protein | 22 g |
| Vitamin C | 12 mg |
| Vitamin D | 5 IU |
| Vitamin E | 2 mg |
| Niacin | 7 mg |
| Folate | 25 mcg |
| Vitamin B$_6$ | 0.5 mg |
| Vitamin B$_{12}$ | 0.4 mcg |
| Zinc | 2.2 mg |
| Selenium | 16 mcg |

# Curried Chicken Salad Wraps

*Chicken salad has never been so lively — it's amazing what a bit of curry can do.*

**Makes 10 wraps**

## Tips

Stuff this chicken mixture into mini pita breads for a tasty appetizer. It also makes a great sandwich filling for pumpernickel bread.

If you don't have any cooked chicken on hand, pick up a cooked chicken at the grocery store. One cooked deli chicken yields about 3 cups (750 mL) cubed cooked chicken.

You can substitute cooked turkey for the chicken — a great way to use up Christmas or Thanksgiving leftovers.

| | | |
|---|---|---|
| 3 cups | cubed cooked chicken | 750 mL |
| 1 cup | chopped celery | 250 mL |
| 1 cup | halved seedless red or green grapes | 250 mL |
| 1/2 cup | toasted slivered almonds | 125 mL |
| 1 tbsp | freshly squeezed lemon juice | 15 mL |
| 3/4 tsp | curry powder | 3 mL |
| 2/3 cup | light mayonnaise | 150 mL |
| | Salt and freshly ground black pepper | |
| 10 | lettuce leaves | 10 |
| 10 | large (10-inch/25 cm) flour tortillas | 10 |

1. In a large bowl, stir together chicken, celery, grapes, almonds, lemon juice, curry powder and mayonnaise. Season to taste with salt and pepper.

2. Place 1 lettuce leaf on each tortilla. Divide chicken mixture evenly along center of each lettuce leaf. Fold up bottom and roll up tortilla.

*This recipe courtesy of Cheryl Wren.*

> ▸ **Health Tip**
>
> Curcuminoids from the turmeric in the curry are very beneficial (anti-inflammatory), and a food with fatty acids in it — mayonnaise in this case — is excellent for their absorption, as is the ground pepper.

| Nutrients per wrap | |
|---|---|
| Calories | 403 |
| Fat | 15 g |
| Carbohydrate | 46 g |
| Protein | 21 g |
| Vitamin C | 5 mg |
| Vitamin D | 3 IU |
| Vitamin E | 2 mg |
| Niacin | 9 mg |
| Folate | 107 mcg |
| Vitamin $B_6$ | 0.3 mg |
| Vitamin $B_{12}$ | 0.1 mcg |
| Zinc | 1.2 mg |
| Selenium | 29 mcg |

# Turkey Cutlets in Gingery Lemon Gravy with Cranberry Rice

*This dish combines two foods — cranberry and turkey — that many of us have great associations with, but it does so in a way that is unique, gluten-free and chock full of valuable phytonutrients.*

## Makes 4 servings

## Tips

If you prefer a bit of heat, use hot rather than sweet paprika when dredging the turkey.

One medium orange yields about 1½ tbsp (22 mL) zest and ⅓ to ½ cup (75 to 125 mL) juice.

### Cranberry Rice

| | | |
|---|---|---|
| 1¼ cups | water or ready-to-use reduced-sodium chicken broth | 300 mL |
| 1 tsp | grated orange zest | 5 mL |
| 2 tbsp | freshly squeezed orange juice | 30 mL |
| ¾ cup | long-grain brown rice, rinsed and drained | 175 mL |
| ⅓ cup | dried cranberries | 75 mL |

### Turkey Cutlets

| | | |
|---|---|---|
| 2 tbsp | sorghum flour | 30 mL |
| 1 tbsp | cornstarch | 15 mL |
| 1 tsp | paprika | 5 mL |
| ½ tsp | freshly ground black pepper | 2 mL |
| 4 | turkey cutlets (about 12 oz/375 g total) | 4 |
| 2 tbsp | olive oil, divided | 30 mL |
| 1 tbsp | butter, divided | 15 mL |
| 2 | cloves garlic, minced | 2 |
| 1 tbsp | minced gingerroot | 15 mL |
| 1 cup | ready-to-use reduced-sodium chicken broth | 250 mL |
| 1 tbsp | freshly squeezed lemon juice | 15 mL |

1. *Cranberry Rice:* In a heavy saucepan with a tight-fitting lid over medium heat, bring water and orange juice to a boil. Stir in rice and return to a boil. Reduce heat to low. Cover and simmer until rice is tender and water has been absorbed, about 50 minutes. Remove from heat and fluff with a fork. Stir in cranberries and orange zest and keep warm.

2. *Turkey Cutlets:* On a plate or in a plastic bag, combine sorghum flour, cornstarch, paprika and pepper. Add turkey and toss until well coated with mixture. Reserve any excess.

## Nutrients per serving

| | |
|---|---|
| Calories | 385 |
| Fat | 13 g |
| Carbohydrate | 43 g |
| Protein | 25 g |
| Vitamin C | 7 mg |
| Vitamin D | 2 IU |
| Vitamin E | 2 mg |
| Niacin | 8 mg |
| Folate | 18 mcg |
| Vitamin B$_6$ | 0.7 mg |
| Vitamin B$_{12}$ | 0.5 mcg |
| Zinc | 2.2 mg |
| Selenium | 29 mcg |

## Variation

*Chicken Cutlets in Gingery Lemon Gravy with Cranberry Rice:* Substitute an equal quantity of chicken cutlets for the turkey.

**3.** In a large skillet, heat 1 tbsp (15 mL) of the oil and $1\frac{1}{2}$ tsp (7 mL) of the butter over medium-high heat until butter has melted. Add 2 cutlets and cook until browned, about 2 minutes. Turn and cook until no longer pink inside, about 2 minutes more. Transfer to a warm platter and keep warm. Repeat with remaining cutlets, oil and butter. Reduce heat to medium.

**4.** Add garlic and ginger to pan and cook, stirring, for 1 minute. Add reserved flour mixture and cook, stirring, for 1 minute. Add broth, lemon juice and any turkey juices that have accumulated on the platter and cook, stirring, until thickened, about 2 minutes. Pour over cutlets. Serve on a bed of Cranberry Rice.

---

### ▶ Health Tips

Cranberries are packed with brain-protecting antioxidants.

In addition to being protein-rich, turkey is also a good source of important B vitamins — niacin, $B_6$ and $B_{12}$ — as well as zinc, an immune system protector that can be challenging to obtain from dietary sources. The body can utilize the zinc in turkey and other meats more readily than that from non-meat sources.

# Turkey Apple Meatloaf

*This meatloaf is lower in fat than the traditional version — but not light on flavor.*

## Tip

Make extra turkey mixture and form into burger patties. After cooking, freeze in freezer bags for quick healthy lunches. Reheat burgers in the microwave on High for about 1 minute.

An extra meatloaf can be sliced to use in sandwiches or frozen for another day.

- Preheat oven to 350°F (180°C)
- 9- by 5-inch (23 by 12.5 cm) loaf pan, lightly greased

| | | |
|---|---|---|
| 2 | cloves garlic, minced | 2 |
| 1 | large egg | 1 |
| 1 | tart apple (such as Mutsu or Granny Smith), finely chopped | 1 |
| 1 lb | lean ground turkey | 500 g |
| ½ cup | chopped onion | 125 mL |
| ⅓ cup | oat bran | 75 mL |
| ⅓ cup | ground flax seeds (flaxseed meal) | 75 mL |
| 3 tbsp | prepared yellow mustard | 45 mL |
| 1 tbsp | ketchup | 15 mL |
| 1 tsp | salt | 5 mL |

1. In a large bowl, combine garlic, egg, apple, turkey, onion, oat bran, flaxseed, mustard, ketchup and salt. Pack into prepared loaf pan.

2. Bake in preheated oven for 45 to 60 minutes or until a meat thermometer inserted in the center registers an internal temperature of 175°F (80°C).

## Variation

*Turkey Apple Burgers:* This mixture can also be used to make burgers, which can be cooked on a barbecue or grill or in the oven. They're excellent served on a whole wheat bun with sliced tomato and a spoonful of low-fat cucumber dressing.

*This recipe courtesy of dietitian Gillian Proctor.*

### ▶ Health Tip

Ground flax seeds and oat bran provide plenty of fiber, and flaxmeal itself provides a great source of omega-3 fats.

### Nutrients per serving

| | |
|---|---|
| Calories | 200 |
| Fat | 10 g |
| Carbohydrate | 12 g |
| Protein | 19 g |
| Vitamin C | 3 mg |
| Vitamin D | 17 IU |
| Vitamin E | 0 mg |
| Niacin | 5 mg |
| Folate | 22 mcg |
| Vitamin B$_6$ | 0.5 mg |
| Vitamin B$_{12}$ | 0.8 mcg |
| Zinc | 2.4 mg |
| Selenium | 26 mcg |

# Barbecued Lemongrass Pork

*This fragrant, spiced take on pork will add some variety to your table.*

**Makes 4 servings**

## Tip

If you're watching your sodium intake, look for reduced-sodium soy sauce, now readily available at grocery stores.

| | | |
|---|---|---|
| 3 tbsp | coconut milk | 45 mL |
| 3 tbsp | finely chopped lemongrass (white part only) | 45 mL |
| 2 | cloves garlic, minced | 2 |
| 1 | green onion, finely chopped | 1 |
| 2 tbsp | fish sauce (nam pla) | 30 mL |
| 1 tbsp | soy sauce | 15 mL |
| 1 tbsp | granulated sugar | 15 mL |
| 2 tsp | sesame oil | 10 mL |
| $\frac{1}{2}$ tsp | coarsely chopped fresh red chile peppers | 2 mL |
| $\frac{1}{2}$ tsp | freshly ground black pepper | 2 mL |
| 1 | pork tenderloin (about 12 oz/375 g), trimmed and cut crosswise into $\frac{1}{2}$-inch (1 cm) slices | 1 |

1. In a bowl, combine coconut milk, lemongrass, garlic, green onion, fish sauce, soy sauce, sugar, sesame oil, chiles and pepper.

2. Arrange pork slices in a shallow dish. Pour marinade over meat and turn pork to coat all sides. Cover and marinate, refrigerated, for several hours.

3. Grill pork for 4 to 6 minutes per side, or until no longer pink.

---

▸ **Health Tip**

Lemongrass is full of essential oils that have numerous effects (antioxidant and anti-inflammatory) in the body.

---

### Nutrients per serving

| | |
|---|---|
| Calories | 168 |
| Fat | 8 g |
| Carbohydrate | 6 g |
| Protein | 19 g |
| Vitamin C | 1 mg |
| Vitamin D | 9 IU |
| Vitamin E | 0 mg |
| Niacin | 6 mg |
| Folate | 11 mcg |
| Vitamin B$_6$ | 0.7 mg |
| Vitamin B$_{12}$ | 0.5 mcg |
| Zinc | 1.8 mg |
| Selenium | 27 mcg |

# Saucy Swiss Steak

*Swiss steak evokes a memory of warm kitchens, hot ovens and comfort food on a cold winter's day. But you can enjoy this dish anytime.*

**Makes 8 servings**

## Tip

This dish can be partially prepared the night before. Complete step 2, heating 1 tbsp (15 mL) oil in pan before softening onions, carrots and celery. Cover and refrigerate mixture overnight. The next morning, brown steak (step 1), or skip this step and place steak directly in stoneware. Continue cooking as directed. Alternatively, cook steak overnight and refrigerate. When ready to serve, bring to a boil in a large skillet and simmer for 10 minutes, until meat is heated through and sauce is bubbling.

### Nutrients per serving

| | |
|---|---|
| Calories | 224 |
| Fat | 8 g |
| Carbohydrate | 11 g |
| Protein | 26 g |
| Vitamin C | 14 mg |
| Vitamin D | 0 IU |
| Vitamin E | 2 mg |
| Niacin | 8 mg |
| Folate | 21 mcg |
| Vitamin $B_6$ | 0.9 mg |
| Vitamin $B_{12}$ | 4.9 mcg |
| Zinc | 4.7 mg |
| Selenium | 37 mcg |

- **Slow cooker**

| | | |
|---|---|---|
| 1 tbsp | vegetable oil | 15 mL |
| 2 lbs | round steak or simmering steak | 1 kg |
| 2 | onions, finely chopped | 2 |
| ¼ cup | thinly sliced carrots | 60 mL |
| ¼ cup | thinly sliced celery | 1 |
| ½ tsp | salt | 2 mL |
| ¼ tsp | freshly ground black pepper | 1 mL |
| 2 tbsp | all-purpose flour | 30 mL |
| 1 | can (28 oz/796 mL) tomatoes, drained and chopped, ½ cup (125 mL) juice reserved | 1 |
| 1 tbsp | Worcestershire sauce | 15 mL |
| 1 | bay leaf | 1 |

1. In a skillet, heat oil over medium-high heat. Add steak, in pieces, if necessary, and brown on both sides. Transfer to slow cooker stoneware.

2. Reduce heat to medium-low. Add onion, carrots, celery, salt and pepper to pan. Cover and cook until vegetables are softened, about 8 minutes. Sprinkle flour over vegetables and cook for 1 minute, stirring. Add tomatoes, reserved juice and Worcestershire sauce. Bring to a boil, stirring until slightly thickened. Add bay leaf.

3. Pour tomato mixture over steak and cook on Low for 8 to 10 hours or on High for 4 to 5 hours, until meat is tender. Discard bay leaf.

> ▶ **Health Tip**
>
> Although it's not necessary to eat beef every day, it's an excellent source of heme iron, which is easily absorbed and helps maintain normal hemoglobin levels in the body — especially important for elderly people and those with a history of anemia.

# African Beef Stew

*This dish combines a full complement of vegetables and plenty of seasonings with the beef.*

## Tips

*Slow Cooker Method:* Combine all ingredients in slow cooker. Cover and cook on Low for 6 to 8 hours or until beef is fork-tender.

If you prefer your vegetables sautéed in oil, add 1 tbsp (15 mL) vegetable oil to the saucepan and heat over medium heat before adding the vegetables. But keep in mind that doing this will affect the nutrient analysis, since you are adding fat to the recipe.

- Preheat oven to 350°F (180°C)
- 12-cup (3 L) Dutch oven or casserole dish with cover

| | | |
|---|---|---|
| 2 lbs | lean stewing beef, cubed | 1 kg |
| 5 | stalks celery, diced | 5 |
| 2 | onions, finely chopped | 2 |
| 1 | green bell pepper, finely chopped | 1 |
| 1 | red bell pepper, finely chopped | 1 |
| 1 cup | diced zucchini | 250 mL |
| 1/4 cup | lightly packed brown sugar | 60 mL |
| 1/4 cup | white vinegar or cider vinegar | 60 mL |
| 1/2 tsp | Worcestershire sauce | 2 mL |
| | Hot pepper sauce | |
| | Salt and freshly ground black pepper | |

1. In Dutch oven, combine beef, celery, onions, green pepper, red pepper, zucchini, brown sugar, vinegar, Worcestershire sauce, hot pepper sauce to taste, and salt and pepper to taste.

2. Cook in preheated oven for 3 hours or until beef is fork-tender. Season to taste with hot pepper sauce, salt and pepper.

*This recipe courtesy of dietitian Claude Gamache.*

### ▶ Health Tip

Ingredients in Worcestershire sauce, such as molasses, contain vitamins $B_1$ and $B_6$, which are important for brain function.

## Nutrients per serving

| | |
|---|---|
| Calories | 280 |
| Fat | 9 g |
| Carbohydrate | 15 g |
| Protein | 34 g |
| Vitamin C | 48 mg |
| Vitamin D | 0 IU |
| Vitamin E | 1 mg |
| Niacin | 10 mg |
| Folate | 41 mcg |
| Vitamin $B_6$ | 1.3 mg |
| Vitamin $B_{12}$ | 6.6 mcg |
| Zinc | 6.2 mg |
| Selenium | 49 mcg |

# Beef with Broccoli

*This classic stir-fry has the right seasonings, including the oyster sauce, to bring out the best in beef.*

### Makes 4 to 6 servings

## Tip

When preparing food for stir-frying, cut into small pieces of approximately equal size so that they will cook through rapidly and in the same period of time. Have sauce and ingredients prepared and easily accessible before starting to cook.

| | | |
|---|---|---|
| 1 lb | sirloin steak, cut into thin strips | 500 g |
| ¼ cup | soy sauce | 60 mL |
| 2 tbsp | cornstarch, divided | 30 mL |
| 1 | clove garlic, minced | 1 |
| 1 | thin slice gingerroot, minced | 1 |
| 2 tbsp | safflower oil, divided | 30 mL |
| 2 | onions, cut into wedges | 2 |
| 3 | large carrots, sliced into coins | 3 |
| 1 | head broccoli, cut into florets | 1 |
| 1¼ cups | water, divided | 300 mL |
| 1 tbsp | oyster sauce | 15 mL |
| 1 tsp | granulated sugar | 5 mL |

1. Place steak in a medium bowl. In a separate bowl, combine soy sauce, 1 tbsp (15 mL) of the cornstarch, garlic and ginger; pour over steak.

2. In a wok or nonstick skillet, heat 1 tbsp (15 mL) of the oil over high heat. Add beef and stir-fry until browned. Set aside.

3. In wok, heat remaining oil over high heat. Add onions and stir-fry for 1 minute. Add carrots, broccoli and 1 cup (250 mL) of the water; cover and steam for 4 minutes.

4. Combine remaining water, oyster sauce, remaining cornstarch and sugar. Stir sauce into wok; cook until smooth and thickened. Return meat to wok. Reheat to serving temperature.

*This recipe courtesy of M. Kathy Dyck.*

## ▸ Health Tip

Broccoli has important cancer- and aging-preventive compounds, and this dish is a way to get a full serving.

## Nutrients per 1 of 6 servings

| | |
|---|---|
| Calories | 216 |
| Fat | 8 g |
| Carbohydrate | 17 g |
| Protein | 21 g |
| Vitamin C | 94 mg |
| Vitamin D | 2 IU |
| Vitamin E | 3 mg |
| Niacin | 6 mg |
| Folate | 87 mcg |
| Vitamin B$_6$ | 0.8 mg |
| Vitamin B$_{12}$ | 0.7 mcg |
| Zinc | 3.6 mg |
| Selenium | 26 mcg |

# Orange Ginger Beef

*This dish balances the heaviness of beef with an array of aromatic spices, including fresh cilantro.*

## Tips

Eye of round is a lean cut of beef. Marinating it before cooking maximizes its tenderness.

Be sure not to crowd the beef while sautéing it, or it will steam instead of browning. You may need to brown it in three batches if you have a smaller skillet.

| | | |
|---|---|---|
| 2 tbsp | minced gingerroot | 30 mL |
| 1 tbsp | minced garlic | 15 mL |
| 1 tsp | freshly ground black pepper | 5 mL |
| 2 tbsp | canola oil, divided | 30 mL |
| 1 tbsp | hoisin sauce | 15 mL |
| 1 lb | beef eye of round marinating steak, cut into 3- by $\frac{1}{2}$-inch (7.5 by 1 cm) strips | 500 g |
| 1 tbsp | cornstarch | 15 mL |
| 1 tbsp | grated orange zest | 15 mL |
| $\frac{3}{4}$ cup | orange juice | 175 mL |
| 2 cups | quartered mushrooms | 500 mL |
| 2 tbsp | chopped fresh cilantro | 30 mL |

1. In a shallow bowl, combine ginger, garlic, pepper, 1 tbsp (15 mL) of the oil and hoisin sauce. Add beef and stir to coat well. Cover and refrigerate for at least 4 hours or up to 12 hours.

2. Drain marinade from beef, discarding marinade. Pat beef strips dry with paper towels. Heat a large nonstick skillet over medium heat. Add half the beef and sauté for 3 to 4 minutes or until lightly browned. Transfer to a bowl and set aside. Repeat with the remaining beef.

3. In a small bowl, whisk together cornstarch and orange juice.

4. Add the remaining oil to skillet and sauté mushrooms for 3 to 4 minutes or until lightly browned. Return beef and accumulated juices to skillet. Stir in cornstarch mixture and cook, stirring, for about 3 minutes or until sauce is thickened. Serve garnished with orange zest and cilantro.

## Variation

Use trimmed snow peas instead of mushrooms.

*This recipe courtesy of dietitian Jennifer Garus.*

| Nutrients per serving | |
|---|---|
| Calories | 289 |
| Fat | 14 g |
| Carbohydrate | 13 g |
| Protein | 26 g |
| Vitamin C | 26 mg |
| Vitamin D | 2 IU |
| Vitamin E | 1 mg |
| Niacin | 10 mg |
| Folate | 38 mcg |
| Vitamin B$_6$ | 0.9 mg |
| Vitamin B$_{12}$ | 4.9 mcg |
| Zinc | 4.7 mg |
| Selenium | 38 mcg |

### ▸ Health Tip

Cilantro contains helpful compounds called bioflavonoids.

# Shepherd's Pie with Creamy Corn Filling

*Shepherd's pie is an old-time favorite for many people. This version leaves behind the bland and brings out the flavor with black pepper, paprika and garlic.*

**Makes 6 servings**

## Tip

This dish can be partially prepared the night before it is cooked. Make mashed potatoes, cover and refrigerate. Complete steps 1 and 2, chilling cooked meat and onion mixture separately. Refrigerate overnight. The next morning, continue cooking as directed in step 3.

### Nutrients per serving

| | |
|---|---|
| Calories | 366 |
| Fat | 14 g |
| Carbohydrate | 38 g |
| Protein | 23 g |
| Vitamin C | 21 mg |
| Vitamin D | 19 IU |
| Vitamin E | 1 mg |
| Niacin | 7 mg |
| Folate | 65 mcg |
| Vitamin B$_6$ | 0.6 mg |
| Vitamin B$_{12}$ | 1.9 mcg |
| Zinc | 4.8 mg |
| Selenium | 18 mcg |

- **Slow cooker**

| | | |
|---|---|---|
| 1 tbsp | vegetable oil | 15 mL |
| 1 lb | lean ground beef | 500 g |
| 2 | onions, finely chopped | 2 |
| 4 | cloves garlic, minced | 4 |
| 2 tsp | paprika | 10 mL |
| 1 tsp | salt (optional) | 5 mL |
| 1/2 tsp | cracked black peppercorns | 2 mL |
| 2 tbsp | all-purpose flour | 30 mL |
| 1 cup | condensed beef broth (undiluted) | 250 mL |
| 2 tbsp | tomato paste | 30 mL |
| 1 | can (19 oz/540 mL) cream-style corn | 1 |
| 4 cups | mashed potatoes, seasoned with 1 tbsp (15 mL) butter, 1/2 tsp (2 mL) salt (optional) and 1/4 tsp (1 mL) freshly ground black pepper | 1 L |
| 1/4 cup | shredded Cheddar cheese | 60 mL |

1. In a skillet, heat oil over medium-high heat. Add beef and cook, breaking up with the back of a spoon, until meat is no longer pink. Using a slotted spoon, transfer to slow cooker stoneware. Drain off liquid.

2. Reduce heat to medium. Add onions to pan and cook until softened. Add garlic, paprika, salt (if using) and pepper and cook, stirring, for 1 minute. Sprinkle flour over mixture, stir and cook for 1 minute. Add beef broth and tomato paste, stir to combine and cook, stirring, until thickened.

3. Transfer mixture to slow cooker stoneware. Spread corn evenly over mixture and top with mashed potatoes. Sprinkle cheese on top, cover and cook on Low for 4 to 6 hours or on High for 3 to 4 hours, until hot and bubbly.

> ▶ **Health Tip**
>
> Beef is very high in iron and the B vitamins, important for many reactions in the body, including energy use in the brain.

# Beef and Quinoa Power Burgers

*This burger adds some classic seasonings and the kick of quinoa.*

## Tips

Be careful to mix the beef mixture as little as possible; over-mixing can make the burgers tough.

Whenever possible, use whole-grain or multigrain hamburger buns.

## Variation

Substitute lean ground turkey or extra-lean ground pork for the beef.

| | | |
|---|---|---|
| ⅔ cup | quinoa, rinsed | 150 mL |
| 1 cup | water | 250 mL |
| ⅓ cup | barbecue sauce | 75 mL |
| 1 lb | extra-lean ground beef | 500 g |
| ½ cup | finely chopped green onions | 125 mL |
| 2 tsp | ground cumin | 10 mL |
| ½ tsp | fine sea salt | 2 mL |
| ¼ tsp | freshly cracked black pepper | 1 mL |
| 2 tsp | olive oil | 10 mL |
| 4 | hamburger buns (gluten-free, if needed), split and toasted | 4 |

### Suggested Accompaniments

Thinly sliced cheese (such as sharp Cheddar or Gruyère) or crumbled goat cheese

Large tomato slices

Baby spinach, arugula or tender watercress sprigs

Additional barbecue sauce

1. In a medium saucepan, combine quinoa, water and barbecue sauce. Bring to a boil over medium-high heat. Reduce heat to low, cover and simmer for 12 to 15 minutes or until liquid is absorbed. Remove from heat and let cool to room temperature.

2. In a large bowl, combine quinoa, beef, green onions, cumin, salt and pepper. Form into four ¾-inch (2 cm) thick patties.

3. In a large, deep skillet, heat oil over medium-high heat. Add patties and cook for 4 minutes. Turn and cook for 4 to 5 minutes or until no longer pink inside.

4. Transfer patties to toasted buns. Top with any of the suggested accompaniments, as desired.

### ▸ Health Tip

Gluten-free buns vary in their composition. Look for those that have brown rice flour or teff and not just tapioca starch or rice starch, as these can be very high on the glycemic index.

### Nutrients per serving

| | |
|---|---|
| Calories | 441 |
| Fat | 12 g |
| Carbohydrate | 49 g |
| Protein | 33 g |
| Vitamin C | 3 mg |
| Vitamin D | 3 IU |
| Vitamin E | 2 mg |
| Niacin | 9 mg |
| Folate | 106 mcg |
| Vitamin $B_6$ | 0.6 mg |
| Vitamin $B_{12}$ | 2.6 mcg |
| Zinc | 7.0 mg |
| Selenium | 31 mcg |

# Peppery Meatloaf with Quinoa

*With both ground beef and Italian sausage, this definitely qualifies as a meaty main dish, but the addition of quinoa and various spices and herbs take it out the realm of the ordinary daily special and into the 21st-century kitchen.*

## Tip

To enhance the pleasantly nutty flavor of the quinoa, toast it in a dry skillet (or the saucepan you are using for cooking) for about 4 minutes over medium heat, stirring constantly until fragrant.

- **Preheat oven to 350°F (180°C)**
- **9- by 5-inch (23 by 12.5 cm) loaf pan**
- **Instant-read thermometer**

| | | |
|---|---|---|
| ¾ cup | water | 175 mL |
| ½ cup | ready-to-use reduced-sodium beef broth or water | 125 mL |
| ¾ cup | quinoa, rinsed (see tip, at left) | 175 mL |
| 1 lb | extra-lean ground beef | 500 g |
| 8 oz | Italian sausage, removed from casings and crumbled (see tip, at left) | 250 mL |
| 1 | onion, finely chopped | 1 |
| 1 | red bell pepper, finely chopped | 1 |
| ½ cup | finely chopped fresh parsley | 125 mL |
| 2 | large eggs, beaten | 2 |
| 1 cup | reduced-sodium tomato sauce, divided | 250 mL |
| 1 tbsp | sweet paprika | 15 mL |
| 1 tbsp | ground cumin | 15 mL |
| 1 tsp | ground coriander | 5 mL |
| ½ tsp | salt | 2 mL |
| ¼ tsp | cayenne pepper | 1 mL |

1. In a saucepan, bring water and beef broth to a boil. Gradually stir in quinoa. Return to a boil. Cover and simmer over low heat for 15 minutes. Remove from heat, cover and set aside for 5 minutes. Fluff with a fork before using.

| Nutrients per serving | |
|---|---|
| Calories | 221 |
| Fat | 8 g |
| Carbohydrate | 15 g |
| Protein | 22 g |
| Vitamin C | 27 mg |
| Vitamin D | 12 IU |
| Vitamin E | 2 mg |
| Niacin | 4 mg |
| Folate | 57 mcg |
| Vitamin B$_6$ | 0.5 mg |
| Vitamin B$_{12}$ | 1.7 mcg |
| Zinc | 4.2 mg |
| Selenium | 18 mcg |

## Tip

Is cutting onions bringing you to tears? Try placing them in the freezer for 10 minutes before chopping.

**2.** In a large bowl, combine ground beef, sausage, onion, bell pepper, parsley, eggs, all but 2 tbsp (30 mL) of the tomato sauce, paprika, cumin, coriander, salt, cayenne and quinoa. Using your hands, mix until well blended. Transfer to loaf pan and spread remaining 2 tbsp (30 mL) of tomato sauce over top. Bake in preheated oven until temperature reaches 165°F (75°C) on a thermometer, about 1 hour.

## Variation

Substitute millet for the quinoa. For the best flavor, before using, toast it in a dry skillet, stirring until fragrant, about 5 minutes. Complete step 1, simmering the millet over low heat for 20 minutes, then remove from the heat and let stand for 10 minutes.

> ### ▶ Health Tip
>
> Spices help stimulate digestion — including the production of stomach acid and salivation in the mouth — which is very important when it comes to digesting a big serving of protein (beef, sausage, eggs, quinoa) like the one in this dish.

# Lamb Tagine with Chickpeas and Apricots

*Lamb is a staple for some people and a rare treat for others. This sweet and spicy version brings out lamb's best and adds wonderful phytonutrients in the process.*

## Makes 6 servings

## Tips

Buy a 3-lb (1.5 kg) leg of lamb or shoulder roast to get $1\frac{1}{2}$ lbs (750 g) boneless lamb.

*Slow Cooker Method:* Follow step 1 and transfer lamb to slow cooker. Follow step 2, then stir in tomatoes and broth; bring to a boil. Transfer to slow cooker. Cover and cook on Low for 6 hours or on High for 3 hours, until almost tender. Add chickpeas, apricots and honey. Cover and cook on Low for 1 hour or on High for 30 minutes.

### Nutrients per serving

| | |
|---|---|
| Calories | 419 |
| Fat | 11 g |
| Carbohydrate | 52 g |
| Protein | 31 g |
| Vitamin C | 14 mg |
| Vitamin D | 0 IU |
| Vitamin E | 2 mg |
| Niacin | 9 mg |
| Folate | 106 mcg |
| Vitamin B$_6$ | 0.8 mg |
| Vitamin B$_{12}$ | 3.0 mcg |
| Zinc | 5.8 mg |
| Selenium | 30 mcg |

| | | |
|---|---|---|
| 2 tbsp | olive oil (approx.) | 30 mL |
| $1\frac{1}{2}$ lbs | lean boneless lamb, cut into 1-inch (2.5 cm) cubes | 750 g |
| 5 | carrots, peeled and thickly sliced | 5 |
| 1 | large onion, chopped | 1 |
| 3 | cloves garlic, finely chopped | 3 |
| 1 tsp | each ground ginger, cumin, cinnamon and turmeric | 5 mL |
| $\frac{1}{2}$ tsp | salt | 2 mL |
| $\frac{1}{2}$ tsp | freshly ground black pepper | 2 mL |
| 1 | can (14 oz/398 mL) diced tomatoes, with juice | 1 |
| 1 cup | ready-to-use chicken broth (approx.) | 250 mL |
| 1 | can (19 oz/540 mL) chickpeas, drained and rinsed | 1 |
| $\frac{1}{2}$ cup | dried apricots or figs, roughly chopped | 125 mL |
| $\frac{1}{4}$ cup | liquid honey | 60 mL |

1. In a Dutch oven, heat 1 tbsp (15 mL) oil over medium-high heat. Brown lamb, in batches, adding more oil as needed. Transfer to a plate as meat browns.

2. Reduce heat to medium. Add carrots, onion, garlic, ginger, cumin, cinnamon, turmeric, salt and pepper to pan; cook, stirring, for about 5 minutes or until onion is softened.

3. Add tomatoes, broth and lamb, along with any accumulated juices; bring to a boil. Reduce heat to medium-low, cover and simmer for $1\frac{1}{2}$ hours or until lamb is just tender.

4. Add chickpeas, apricots and honey. Add more broth, if necessary. Cover and simmer for 30 minutes or until lamb is very tender.

> ### ▸ Health Tip
>
> Honey has cancer prevention properties and contains a powerful antioxidant, caffeic acid phenethyl ester.

# SIDE DISHES

# Orange Broccoli with Red Pepper

*Forget the salty cheese sauce — this fruit and vegetable combination beautifully complements broccoli.*

## Tip

While North American tastes are generally restricted to broccoli florets, Asian cooking also uses broccoli stalks extensively. So don't throw them away — trim the woody bottoms and peel the stalks using a paring knife; then cut the tender, mild interior into slices or strips.

| | | |
|---|---|---|
| 1 tsp | grated orange zest | 5 mL |
| $1/3$ cup | orange juice | 75 mL |
| $1/2$ tsp | cornstarch | 2 mL |
| 1 tbsp | olive oil | 15 mL |
| 4 cups | small broccoli florets and stalks, cut into $1\frac{1}{2}$- by $1/2$-inch (4 by 1 cm) lengths | 1 L |
| 1 | red bell pepper, cut into 2- by $1/2$-inch (5 by 1 cm) strips | 1 |
| 1 | clove garlic, minced | 1 |
| $1/4$ tsp | salt | 1 mL |
| $1/4$ tsp | freshly ground black pepper | 1 mL |

1. In a glass measuring cup, stir together orange juice and cornstarch until smooth; reserve.

2. Heat oil in a large nonstick skillet over high heat. Add broccoli, red pepper and garlic; cook, stirring, for 2 minutes.

3. Add orange juice mixture; cover and cook 1 to 2 minutes or until vegetables are tender-crisp. Sprinkle with orange zest; season with salt and pepper. Serve immediately.

> ### ▶ Health Tip
>
> Broccoli and peppers are a winning combination, providing excellent sources of vitamins A and C and folate.

## Nutrients per serving

| | |
|---|---|
| Calories | 78 |
| Fat | 4 g |
| Carbohydrate | 10 g |
| Protein | 3 g |
| Vitamin C | 113 mg |
| Vitamin D | 0 IU |
| Vitamin E | 2 mg |
| Niacin | 1 mg |
| Folate | 70 mcg |
| Vitamin B$_6$ | 0.2 mg |
| Vitamin B$_{12}$ | 0.0 mcg |
| Zinc | 0.4 mg |
| Selenium | 2 mcg |

# Creamy Broccoli Curry

*This dish surrounds broccoli with a selection of spices and herbs, then adds yogurt to create a creamy sauce.*

---

## Tip

Serve with rice or an Indian bread.

| | | |
|---|---|---|
| • **Blender** | | |
| 2 tbsp | vegetable oil | 30 mL |
| 1 cup | chopped onion | 250 mL |
| 1 tbsp | minced green chile peppers (see tip, page 328) | 15 mL |
| 1 tsp | minced gingerroot | 5 mL |
| 1 tsp | minced garlic | 5 mL |
| 3 cups | finely chopped broccoli | 750 mL |
| 1 tsp | ground coriander | 5 mL |
| $\frac{1}{2}$ tsp | cayenne pepper | 2 mL |
| $\frac{1}{2}$ tsp | ground turmeric | 2 mL |
| $\frac{1}{3}$ to $\frac{1}{2}$ cup | milk or water (optional) | 75 to 125 mL |
| 1 cup | plain nonfat yogurt | 250 mL |
| 2 tbsp | chickpea flour (besan) | 30 mL |
| 1 tsp | salt (or to taste) | 5 mL |

1. In a saucepan, heat oil over medium-high heat. Sauté onion until beginning to turn golden, 6 to 8 minutes.

2. Reduce heat to medium. Stir in chiles, ginger and garlic and sauté for 2 minutes. Add broccoli, coriander, cayenne and turmeric. Mix well and sauté for 3 to 4 minutes. Remove from heat and let cool slightly.

3. In blender, purée mixture, adding a little milk or water if necessary for blending. Return to saucepan.

4. Whisk together yogurt, chickpea flour, 1 cup (250 mL) water and salt, making sure to remove all lumps. Pour into broccoli purée. Reduce heat to medium-low. Mix well and bring to a gentle boil. Cook, uncovered, until curry thickens, 6 to 8 minutes.

> ▸ **Health Tip**
>
> The combination of herbs and the broccoli in this dish make a detoxification support cocktail.

## Nutrients per serving

| | |
|---|---|
| Calories | 73 |
| Fat | 4 g |
| Carbohydrate | 7 g |
| Protein | 3 g |
| Vitamin C | 32 mg |
| Vitamin D | 0 IU |
| Vitamin E | 1 mg |
| Niacin | 0 mg |
| Folate | 28 mcg |
| Vitamin B$_6$ | 0.1 mg |
| Vitamin B$_{12}$ | 0.2 mcg |
| Zinc | 0.5 mg |
| Selenium | 2 mcg |

# Green Beans and Carrots with Aromatic Spices

*This dish has some heat, but for those who like some spice in their daily fare, it's a great way to bring a new twist to green beans and carrots.*

## Tip

The important thing in Indian cooking is to use a chile with spirit. Fresh cayenne peppers, or any similar ones, would work very well. If using fresh Thai peppers, now readily available in North America, use only half the amount called for in the recipe. In a pinch, jalapeños could also be used.

| | | |
|---|---|---|
| 2 tbsp | vegetable oil | 30 mL |
| 1 tsp | mustard seeds | 5 mL |
| 1 tsp | cumin seeds | 5 mL |
| 1 tbsp | minced garlic | 15 mL |
| 1 tbsp | minced green chile peppers (see tip, at left) | 15 mL |
| 1/4 cup | coarsely crushed roasted peanuts | 60 mL |
| 1/4 cup | grated unsweetened fresh or frozen coconut, divided | 60 mL |
| 1/2 tsp | ground turmeric | 2 mL |
| 1/2 tsp | cayenne pepper | 2 mL |
| 8 oz | green beans, cut into 2-inch (5 cm) sections | 250 g |
| 8 oz | carrots (2 to 3), peeled and sliced diagonally 1/4 inch (0.5 cm) thick | 250 g |
| 1 tsp | salt (or to taste) | 5 mL |

1. In a large skillet with a tight-fitting lid, heat oil over high heat until a couple of mustard seeds thrown in start to sputter. Add remaining mustard seeds and cover quickly.

2. When seeds stop popping in a few seconds, uncover, reduce heat to medium and add cumin seeds. Sauté for 30 seconds. Add garlic, chiles, peanuts and 3 tbsp (45 mL) of the coconut. Reduce heat slightly to prevent burning and stir-fry for 2 minutes. Add turmeric and cayenne. Sauté for 1 minute longer (add 1 1/2 tsp/7 mL water if necessary). Do not allow masala to burn.

3. Stir in beans and carrots. Add salt and mix well. Sprinkle with 1 tbsp (15 mL) water. Cover and cook over medium heat for 5 minutes. Reduce heat to low and stir. Cook, covered, until vegetables are tender, 5 to 8 minutes.

4. Garnish with remaining coconut to serve.

> ▶ **Health Tip**
>
> Chile and cayenne peppers are species of capsicum, which has circulatory and digestive support benefits.

### Nutrients per 1 of 8 servings

| | |
|---|---|
| Calories | 94 |
| Fat | 7 g |
| Carbohydrate | 7 g |
| Protein | 2 g |
| Vitamin C | 6 mg |
| Vitamin D | 0 IU |
| Vitamin E | 1 mg |
| Niacin | 1 mg |
| Folate | 21 mcg |
| Vitamin $B_6$ | 0.1 mg |
| Vitamin $B_{12}$ | 0.0 mcg |
| Zinc | 0.5 mg |
| Selenium | 1 mcg |

# Simple Stir-Fried Kale

*This easy-to-prepare dish uses some basic Asian — and Middle East — flavors to enliven one of our most nutritious greens.*

**Makes 4 servings**

## Tips

Tahini is often used in Middle Eastern cooking and is an ingredient in hummus. It is made from ground sesame seeds and adds a nutty flavor to dishes.

Leave out the hot pepper sauce if your family does not like spice.

| | | |
|---|---|---|
| 1 tbsp | vegetable oil | 15 mL |
| 1 tsp | sesame oil | 5 mL |
| 4 cups | julienned kale (tough center rib removed first) | 1 L |
| 2 | leeks (white and light green parts only), julienned | 2 |
| 1 tbsp | tahini | 15 mL |
| 2 tsp | hot pepper sauce | 10 mL |
| 2 tsp | soy sauce | 10 mL |
| | Freshly ground white or black pepper | |

1. In a wok or large skillet, heat vegetable oil and sesame oil over high heat. Add kale and leeks; stir-fry for 3 to 5 minutes or until limp.

2. Combine tahini, hot pepper sauce and soy sauce; pour over vegetables. Season to taste with pepper. Serve warm.

*This recipe courtesy of dietitian Gerry Kasten.*

---

### ▶ Health Tip

Sesame oil and tahini provide lots of the antioxidant compound sesamol.

---

## Nutrients per serving

| | |
|---|---|
| Calories | 126 |
| Fat | 7 g |
| Carbohydrate | 14 g |
| Protein | 4 g |
| Vitamin C | 88 mg |
| Vitamin D | 0 IU |
| Vitamin E | 1 mg |
| Niacin | 1 mg |
| Folate | 52 mcg |
| Vitamin $B_6$ | 0.3 mg |
| Vitamin $B_{12}$ | 0.0 mcg |
| Zinc | 0.5 mg |
| Selenium | 2 mcg |

# New Orleans Braised Onions

*This dish takes its time, but since slow cookers allow you to do other tasks, the end result is well worth it.*

**Makes 10 servings**

## Tips

Onions are high in natural sugars, which long, slow simmering brings out, as does the orange juice in this recipe.

If you halve this recipe, use a $1\frac{1}{2}$- to $3\frac{1}{2}$-quart slow cooker, checking to make sure the whole onions will fit.

• **Minimum 5-quart slow cooker**

| | | |
|---|---|---|
| 2 to 3 | large Spanish onions | 2 to 3 |
| 6 to 9 | whole cloves | 6 to 9 |
| $\frac{1}{2}$ tsp | salt | 2 mL |
| $\frac{1}{2}$ tsp | cracked black peppercorns | 2 mL |
| Pinch | dried thyme | Pinch |
| | Grated zest and juice of 1 orange | |
| $\frac{1}{2}$ cup | ready-to-use vegetable broth | 125 mL |
| | Finely chopped fresh parsley (optional) | |
| | Hot pepper sauce (optional) | |

1. Stud onions with cloves. Place in slow cooker stoneware and sprinkle with salt, peppercorns, thyme and orange zest. Pour orange juice and vegetable broth over onions, cover and cook on Low for 8 hours or on High for 4 hours, until onions are tender.

2. Using a slotted spoon, transfer onions to a serving dish and keep warm in a 250°F (120°C) oven. Transfer liquid to a saucepan over medium heat. Cook until reduced by half.

3. When ready to serve, cut onions into quarters. Place on a deep platter and cover with sauce. Sprinkle with parsley, if desired, and pass the hot pepper sauce, if desired.

> ▸ **Health Tip**
>
> As the beneficial flavonoids in onions tend to be located in the outer layers, peel off as little as possible of the edible portion when removing the paper-like layer.

## Nutrients per serving

| | |
|---|---|
| Calories | 13 |
| Fat | 0 g |
| Carbohydrate | 3 g |
| Protein | 0 g |
| Vitamin C | 2 mg |
| Vitamin D | 0 IU |
| Vitamin E | 0 mg |
| Niacin | 0 mg |
| Folate | 6 mcg |
| Vitamin B$_6$ | 0.0 mg |
| Vitamin B$_{12}$ | 0.0 mcg |
| Zinc | 0.1 mg |
| Selenium | 0 mcg |

# Roasted Bell Peppers

*The garlic on these peppers brings out a flavor that will have your guests asking for seconds.*

## Tips

These multipurpose peppers are always great to have on hand, as they can be used in a number of recipes. Use a variety of colored peppers, such as yellow, red, orange and green, to add vibrancy to pasta sauces and salads or to use in one of the variations.

If some of the skin adheres to the flesh after the peppers have cooled, use your fingers to peel it off. Marinating peppers in balsamic vinegar extends their shelf life.

### Nutrients per 1 of 4 servings

| | |
|---|---|
| Calories | 97 |
| Fat | 7 g |
| Carbohydrate | 7 g |
| Protein | 1 g |
| Vitamin C | 114 mg |
| Vitamin D | 0 IU |
| Vitamin E | 3 mg |
| Niacin | 1 mg |
| Folate | 42 mcg |
| Vitamin B$_6$ | 0.3 mg |
| Vitamin B$_{12}$ | 0.0 mcg |
| Zinc | 0.3 mg |
| Selenium | 1 mcg |

- Preheat oven to 350°F (180°C)
- 13- by 9-inch (33 by 23 cm) baking dish, greased

| | | |
|---|---|---|
| 3 | bell peppers, seeds and ribs removed, peppers quartered | 3 |
| 2 tbsp | garlic-infused oil | 25 mL |
| 1 tbsp | garlic powder | 15 mL |
| | Salt and freshly ground black pepper | |

1. Place peppers in prepared baking dish. Brush both sides of each pepper piece with garlic oil and sprinkle with garlic powder and salt and pepper to taste. Bake in preheated oven for 45 to 50 minutes or until very soft and wrinkled.

2. Transfer to a bowl, cover with a plate and let cool to room temperature. The skins will naturally separate from the flesh of the pepper (see tip, at left). Store in an airtight container and refrigerate for up to 4 days.

## Variations

*Balsamic Marinated Peppers:* Cut peeled roasted peppers into quarters. Add ½ cup (125 mL) balsamic vinegar and toss to coat. Cover and refrigerate for 8 hours or for up to 1 week.

*Garlic Marinated Peppers:* Toss peeled roasted peppers with 2 cloves garlic, thinly sliced, and ¼ cup (60 mL) extra virgin olive oil. Marinate for several hours or overnight, then remove the garlic. Add sea salt and freshly ground black pepper to taste and serve immediately.

### ▸ Health Tip

*Allium sativa* — garlic — has numerous beneficial effects on cardiovascular health.

# Stuffed Zucchini

*This is a great side when entertaining, or just because it's something that you were craving.*

**Makes 4 servings**

## Tip

For convenience, look for vegetable broth in Tetra Paks. Once opened, these can be stored in the refrigerator for up to 1 week.

• **Preheat oven to 350°F (180°C)**

| | | |
|---|---|---|
| ¾ cup | ready-to-use reduced-sodium vegetable broth | 175 mL |
| 2 | small zucchini, halved lengthwise | 2 |
| 2 | green onions, chopped | 2 |
| 2 | cloves garlic, minced | 2 |
| 1 | tomato, diced | 1 |
| ½ tsp | dried basil | 2 mL |
| ½ tsp | dried thyme | 2 mL |
| ¼ tsp | hot pepper sauce | 1 mL |
| ¾ cup | shredded Cheddar cheese | 175 mL |

1. In a large skillet over medium-high heat, bring broth to a boil. Reduce heat to medium and add zucchini halves, skin side up. Cook for 2 to 3 minutes or until tender. Remove zucchini and let cool. Discard excess liquid.

2. Using a spoon, scoop out zucchini flesh, leaving a shell. Chop zucchini flesh. In a large bowl, combine zucchini flesh, green onions, garlic, tomato, basil, thyme and hot pepper sauce. Fill zucchini shells with mixture and top with cheese. Place filled shells on a baking sheet.

3. Bake in preheated oven for 10 minutes or until heated through and cheese is melted.

*This recipe courtesy of Laurie Evans.*

> ### ▶ Health Tip
>
> Zucchini is rich in fiber, as well as magnesium and potassium.

## Nutrients per serving

| Calories | 107 |
|---|---|
| Fat | 7 g |
| Carbohydrate | 5 g |
| Protein | 6 g |
| Vitamin C | 16 mg |
| Vitamin D | 5 IU |
| Vitamin E | 0 mg |
| Niacin | 1 mg |
| Folate | 25 mcg |
| Vitamin B$_6$ | 0.2 mg |
| Vitamin B$_{12}$ | 0.2 mcg |
| Zinc | 0.9 mg |
| Selenium | 3 mcg |

# Mandarin Rice and Walnut–Stuffed Acorn Squash

*This hearty stuffed squash has a list of super-healthy ingredients.*

> ▶ **Health Tip**
>
> Unsweetened canned mandarin oranges deliver the vitamin C of the oranges without the sugary syrup typically associated with this fruit.

- **Preheat oven to 375°F (190°C)**
- **13- by 9-inch (33 by 23 cm) glass baking dish**

| | | |
|---|---|---|
| 1 | acorn squash, halved lengthwise, seeds and pulp removed | 1 |
| 2 tsp | olive oil | 10 mL |
| 2 tsp | pure maple syrup | 10 mL |

**Stuffing**

| | | |
|---|---|---|
| 1/4 cup | dried figs, diced | 60 mL |
| 1 | can (10 oz/284 mL) unsweetened mandarin oranges, with juice | 1 |
| 1 tbsp | olive oil | 15 mL |
| 2 | shallots, chopped | 2 |
| 1 tsp | grated gingerroot | 5 mL |
| 2 tsp | garam masala | 10 mL |
| 1/4 cup | toasted walnuts | 60 mL |
| 2 tbsp | golden raisins (sultanas) | 30 mL |
| 1 cup | cooked long-grain brown rice | 250 mL |
| 2 tbsp | chopped fresh cilantro | 30 mL |
| | Salt and freshly ground black pepper | |

1. Place squash in baking dish cut side up and drizzle inside of each half with 1 tsp (5 mL) of the oil and 1 tsp (5 mL) of the maple syrup. Add 1/2 inch (1 cm) water and bake in preheated oven for 45 minutes.

2. *Stuffing:* In a small bowl, combine figs and oranges with juice. Set aside.

3. Place a skillet over medium heat and let pan get hot. Add oil and tip pan to coat. Add shallots, ginger and garam masala and cook, stirring occasionally, until shallots are softened, 2 to 3 minutes. Stir in walnuts, raisins, rice and cilantro. Remove from heat and season with salt and pepper to taste. Mix in fig and orange mixture.

4. Transfer par-cooked squash to a cutting board and when cool enough to handle stuff each half with rice mixture, mounding high without compacting. Return squash to baking dish, cover loosely with foil and bake until squash is tender and stuffing is slightly crunchy on top, 10 to 15 minutes. Let cool slightly before serving.

**Nutrients** per 1 of 8 servings

| | |
|---|---|
| Calories | 230 |
| Fat | 11 g |
| Carbohydrate | 33 g |
| Protein | 3 g |
| Vitamin C | 20 mg |
| Vitamin D | 0 IU |
| Vitamin E | 1 mg |
| Niacin | 2 mg |
| Folate | 17 mcg |
| Vitamin B$_6$ | 0.2 mg |
| Vitamin B$_{12}$ | 0.0 mcg |
| Zinc | 0.8 mg |
| Selenium | 6 mcg |

# Spaghetti Squash with Mushrooms

*Spaghetti squash is known for its pasta-like texture, but it cooks like other squashes and goes well with the pasta-style sauce given here.*

## Makes 6 servings

## Tips

Spaghetti squash is easily recognized by its oblong shape and pale to bright yellow skin. It bakes and microwaves quite easily. To keep the strands intact, be sure to cut squash in half lengthwise.

Serve this dish over brown rice for a light meal.

- **Preheat oven to 350°F (180°C)**

| | | |
|---|---|---|
| 1 | spaghetti squash (about 3½ lbs/1.5 kg) | 1 |
| 2 tbsp | butter or margarine | 30 mL |
| 2 cups | sliced mushrooms | 500 mL |
| 1 | green onion, sliced | 1 |
| 1 | small stalk celery, chopped | 1 |
| 2 cups | chopped tomatoes (about 4 small) | 500 mL |
| 2 tbsp | all-purpose flour | 30 mL |
| 1 cup | milk | 250 mL |
| ½ cup | shredded Cheddar cheese | 125 mL |
| 1 tsp | dried oregano | 5 mL |
| ½ tsp | garlic powder | 2 mL |
| ½ tsp | salt | 2 mL |
| ¼ tsp | freshly ground black pepper | 1 mL |
| | Grated Parmesan cheese | |

1. Cut squash in half lengthwise. Bake cut side down on a baking sheet in preheated oven for 25 to 30 minutes or boil, cut side down and covered, in 2 inches (5 cm) of water for about 20 minutes.

2. In a skillet over medium-high heat, cook mushrooms, green onion, celery and tomatoes in butter for about 5 minutes or until tender. Stir in flour; gradually add milk. Cook, stirring constantly, until thickened. Stir in Cheddar cheese and seasonings until cheese is melted.

3. Pour sauce over squash; sprinkle with Parmesan cheese and serve.

*This recipe courtesy of Marlyn Ambrose-Chase.*

### ▸ Health Tip

In addition to having good nutritional value, squash is a good source of dietary fiber in a useful and easy-to-tolerate form.

## Nutrients per serving

| | |
|---|---|
| Calories | 181 |
| Fat | 7 g |
| Carbohydrate | 27 g |
| Protein | 7 g |
| Vitamin C | 14 mg |
| Vitamin D | 24 IU |
| Vitamin E | 1 mg |
| Niacin | 5 mg |
| Folate | 64 mcg |
| Vitamin B$_6$ | 0.4 mg |
| Vitamin B$_{12}$ | 0.3 mcg |
| Zinc | 1.1 mg |
| Selenium | 4 mcg |

# Exotic Spiced Roasties

*Leave the oily French fries and "potato products" behind and sail away to this spiced desert island. Great as a side or a snack.*

**Makes 4 to 6 servings**

## Tips

The spice combo in this recipe lends an Indian flavor to food. It can be used as a dry rub on boneless chicken or pork chops before grilling or searing.

Sea salt has a much cleaner, crisper taste and a greater mineral content than refined table salt.

- Preheat oven to 400°F (200°C)
- Rimmed baking sheet, lightly brushed with olive oil

### Spice Mixture

| | | |
|---|---|---|
| 1 tbsp | ground cardamom | 15 mL |
| 1 tbsp | cayenne pepper | 15 mL |
| 1 tbsp | ground coriander | 15 mL |
| 1 tbsp | ground cumin | 15 mL |
| 1 tbsp | paprika | 15 mL |
| 1 tsp | ground cinnamon | 5 mL |
| 1 tsp | ground cloves | 5 mL |
| 1 tsp | freshly ground black pepper | 5 mL |
| 1 tsp | ground nutmeg | 5 mL |
| 1 tsp | ground turmeric | 5 mL |
| 1 tsp | salt | 5 mL |
| 1 tsp | granulated sugar | 5 mL |

### Potatoes

| | | |
|---|---|---|
| 2 lbs | small waxy new potatoes, lightly scrubbed and thoroughly dried | 1 kg |
| 1/4 cup | olive oil | 60 mL |

1. *Spice Mixture:* In a small bowl, combine all ingredients. Mix well. Transfer to a glass jar with a tight-fitting lid and store in a cool, dark place for up to 2 weeks. (Makes about 1/2 cup/125 mL.)

2. *Potatoes:* Using a fork, prick each potato a few times and transfer to a large bowl. Add oil and 1 to 2 tbsp (15 to 30 mL) of the spice mixture. Toss to coat.

3. Arrange in a single layer on prepared baking sheet. Roast in preheated oven, turning once or twice, for 45 minutes to 1 hour or until tender. Serve immediately.

> ▶ **Health Tip**
>
> This dish is an excellent source of vitamin C and potassium, and a good source of fiber. Leaving the skin on the potatoes increases the fiber content.

### Nutrients per 1 of 6 servings

| | |
|---|---|
| Calories | 219 |
| Fat | 10 g |
| Carbohydrate | 31 g |
| Protein | 4 g |
| Vitamin C | 31 mg |
| Vitamin D | 0 IU |
| Vitamin E | 2 mg |
| Niacin | 2 mg |
| Folate | 27 mcg |
| Vitamin $B_6$ | 0.5 mg |
| Vitamin $B_{12}$ | 0.0 mcg |
| Zinc | 0.6 mg |
| Selenium | 1 mcg |

# Saffron Mash

*This is a heart-healthy mashed potato blend that goes all out on flavor.*

## Tips

To crush garlic, use the broad side of a chef's knife to crush each clove. Then remove the skin and discard.

Saffron is expensive, but you never need a lot of it to make something really special.

Make sure to warm the olive oil and add it gradually to the mashed potato mixture. It may seem like a lot, but it is the quality of the extra virgin olive oil that makes these potatoes what they are.

| ½ cup | whole milk | 125 mL |
| 2 | cloves garlic, crushed (see tip, at left) | 2 |
| 2 | sprigs fresh thyme | 2 |
| 2 | generous pinches saffron | 2 |
| 2 lbs | floury or all-purpose potatoes, peeled and quartered | 1 kg |
| 1 tsp | salt | 5 mL |
| ½ to 1 cup | extra virgin olive oil, warmed | 125 to 250 mL |

1. In a small saucepan, combine milk, garlic and thyme and bring to a boil. Remove from heat, cover and set aside for 10 minutes to infuse flavors. Using a fine-mesh sieve, strain into a bowl and sprinkle with saffron. Set aside.

2. Place potatoes in a large saucepan and add cold water to barely cover. Add salt, cover loosely and bring to a boil over high heat. Reduce heat and cook for 20 minutes or until potatoes are tender all the way through when prodded with the tip of a paring knife. Drain, leaving potatoes in the saucepan. Return to very low heat and shake the pot back and forth to remove any trace of moisture (this is an important step — the drier the cooked potato, the lighter and fluffier your mash will be).

3. With saucepan still over heat, add milk mixture and, using a potato masher, mash in thoroughly. Add the olive oil, ¼ cup (60 mL) at a time, in a thin stream; mash until potato mixture starts to get fluffy and looks glossy and rich (you may not need to use all the oil). Bang masher against the rim of the saucepan so any sticking potato mixture falls into the pot. Tilt saucepan slightly and, using a flat whisk, wooden spoon or large fork, briskly stir potato mixture to incorporate air into the mash, until smooth, creamy and fluffy. (You may decide that it needs a little more oil if you haven't used it all; if so, stir it in now.) Serve immediately.

### ▶ Health Tip

Olive oil is a dietary fat that is heart-friendly and is a cornerstone of the Mediterranean diet.

**Nutrients** per 1 of
6 servings

| Calories | 278 |
| --- | --- |
| Fat | 19 g |
| Carbohydrate | 25 g |
| Protein | 3 g |
| Vitamin C | 31 mg |
| Vitamin D | 10 IU |
| Vitamin E | 3 mg |
| Niacin | 2 mg |
| Folate | 28 mcg |
| Vitamin B$_6$ | 0.3 mg |
| Vitamin B$_{12}$ | 0.1 mcg |
| Zinc | 0.5 mg |
| Selenium | 1 mcg |

# Perfect Steamed Rice

*Here is a simple recipe for that perfect complement to curries and other spiced dishes.*

## Makes 8 servings

## Tips

True basmati rice comes from the foothills of the Himalayas. There is rice available in the bulk bins of some supermarkets that is marked basmati, but it is usually from California and will not work in this recipe. Be sure to use only Indian or Pakistani basmati rice.

Rice should always be transferred to a platter, never a bowl, as the weight of the freshly steamed rice causes the rice on the bottom to get mushy.

- Large saucepan with tight-fitting lid

| | | |
|---|---|---|
| 2 cups | Indian basmati rice (see tip, at left) | 500 mL |
| 1 tbsp | oil | 15 mL |
| 2 tsp | salt (or to taste) | 10 mL |

1. Place rice in a bowl with plenty of cold water and swish vigorously with fingers. Drain. Repeat process 4 or 5 times until water is fairly clear. Cover with 3 to 4 inches (7.5 to 10 cm) cold water and soak for at least 15 minutes or up to 2 hours.

2. In a large saucepan, heat oil over medium-high heat. Drain rice and add to saucepan. Stir to coat rice. Add $3\frac{1}{2}$ cups (875 mL) cold water and salt.

3. Cover with a tight-fitting lid and bring to a boil over high heat. Reduce heat as low as possible and cook, covered, without peeking, for 25 minutes.

4. Remove from heat and set lid slightly ajar to allow steam to escape. Let rest for 5 minutes. Gently fluff with fork and carefully spoon onto platter to serve.

> ▶ **Health Tip**
>
> Rice is often considered a hypoallergenic food — that is, many people with food allergies do not react to rice in the way they react to wheat, dairy, soy and other foods.

## Nutrients per serving

| | |
|---|---|
| Calories | 156 |
| Fat | 3 g |
| Carbohydrate | 31 g |
| Protein | 3 g |
| Vitamin C | 0 mg |
| Vitamin D | 0 IU |
| Vitamin E | 0 mg |
| Niacin | 2 mg |
| Folate | 119 mcg |
| Vitamin $B_6$ | 0.2 mg |
| Vitamin $B_{12}$ | 0.0 mcg |
| Zinc | 0.5 mg |
| Selenium | 9 mcg |

# Home-Style Skillet Rice with Tomato Crust

*Skillet dishes are popular these days. Here is one with great natural seasonings where you can control the added salt.*

## Makes 6 servings

## Tip

Lundberg sells a variety of brown rice mixes, all of which would work well in this recipe. Their Jubilee blend, which includes Wehani and Black Japonica, is particularly nice in this dish.

### Nutrients per serving

| Calories | 253 |
|---|---|
| Fat | 8 g |
| Carbohydrate | 33 g |
| Protein | 13 g |
| Vitamin C | 39 mg |
| Vitamin D | 14 IU |
| Vitamin E | 2 mg |
| Niacin | 3 mg |
| Folate | 42 mcg |
| Vitamin B$_6$ | 0.5 mg |
| Vitamin B$_{12}$ | 0.5 mcg |
| Zinc | 1.8 mg |
| Selenium | 10 mcg |

- **Preheat oven to 350°F (180°C)**

| | | |
|---|---|---|
| 3 cups | cooked red or brown rice, or brown and wild rice mixture (see tip, at left) | 750 mL |
| 1 tbsp | olive oil | 15 mL |
| 8 oz | hot or mild Italian sausage, removed from casings | 250 g |
| 1 | onion, finely chopped | 1 |
| 4 | stalks celery, diced | 4 |
| 2 | green bell peppers, finely chopped | 2 |
| 4 | cloves garlic, minced | 4 |
| 1 tbsp | chili powder | 15 mL |
| 2 tsp | caraway seeds | 10 mL |
| 1 tsp | dried oregano | 5 mL |
| 1/2 tsp | salt (or to taste) | 2 mL |
| | Freshly ground black pepper | |
| 1 1/2 cups | reduced-sodium tomato sauce | 375 mL |
| 2 | large eggs, beaten | 2 |
| 8 oz | sliced mozzarella cheese (optional) | 250 g |

1. In a cast-iron or other ovenproof skillet, heat oil over medium heat for 30 seconds. Add sausage, onion, celery and bell peppers and cook, stirring and breaking up sausage with a spoon, until vegetables are very tender and sausage is no longer pink, about 7 minutes. Add garlic, chili powder, caraway seeds, oregano, salt and black pepper to taste and cook, stirring, for 1 minute. Add cooked rice and cook, stirring, until heated through. Remove from heat.

2. In a bowl, beat tomato sauce and eggs until blended. Spread evenly over rice in skillet. Lay sliced mozzarella (if using) evenly over top. Place skillet in preheated oven and bake until top is crusty and cheese (if using) is melted, about 15 minutes.

> ▸ ## Health Tip
>
> Caraway is a natural digestive aid.

# Baked Risotto with Spinach

*Risotto maximizes the texture and taste of short-grain rice and can reflect the other ingredients added to it — in this case spinach, leeks, cheese and a hint of nutmeg.*

## Makes 8 servings

## Tips

To clean leeks, trim dark green tops. Cut down center almost to root end and chop. Rinse in a sink full of cold water to remove sand; scoop up leeks and place in colander to drain or use a salad spinner.

Make risotto up to 1 day ahead. Cover and refrigerate. Increase baking time by 10 minutes.

### Nutrients per serving

| | |
|---|---|
| Calories | 385 |
| Fat | 11 g |
| Carbohydrate | 59 g |
| Protein | 14 g |
| Vitamin C | 23 mg |
| Vitamin D | 7 IU |
| Vitamin E | 2 mg |
| Niacin | 6 mg |
| Folate | 298 mcg |
| Vitamin B$_6$ | 0.3 mg |
| Vitamin B$_{12}$ | 0.4 mcg |
| Zinc | 1.6 mg |
| Selenium | 12 mcg |

- Preheat oven to 350°F (180°C)
- 13- by 9-inch (33 by 23 cm) baking dish, greased

| | | |
|---|---|---|
| 2 | packages (each 10 oz/300 g) fresh spinach | 2 |
| 2 tbsp | butter, divided | 30 mL |
| 2 | leeks (white and light green parts only), cut in half lengthwise, then sliced crosswise | 2 |
| ½ tsp | salt | 2 mL |
| ¼ tsp | freshly ground black pepper | 1 mL |
| ¼ tsp | freshly grated nutmeg | 1 mL |
| 2½ cups | short-grain rice (such as Arborio) | 625 mL |
| 3 | cloves garlic, finely chopped | 3 |
| 7 cups | hot ready-to-use chicken or vegetable broth | 1.75 L |
| 4 oz | herb-and-garlic-flavored cream cheese or herb-flavored goat cheese | 125 g |
| ½ cup | freshly grated Parmesan cheese | 125 mL |

1. Rinse spinach; remove tough ends. Place in Dutch oven with just the water clinging to leaves; cook over medium-high heat, stirring, until just wilted. Drain well and squeeze dry; finely chop.

2. In a large nonstick skillet, melt 1 tbsp (15 mL) butter over medium heat; cook leeks, stirring, for 3 minutes or until softened. Add spinach, salt, pepper and nutmeg; cook, stirring, for 5 minutes or until vegetables are tender.

3. In a Dutch oven, heat remaining butter over medium heat; cook rice and garlic, stirring, for 2 minutes. Add 5 cups (1.25 L) hot broth; bring to a boil. Reduce heat to medium-low, cover and simmer for 15 minutes or until rice is almost tender and most of liquid is absorbed.

4. Stir in remaining broth and cream cheese until blended; add spinach mixture. Spread in prepared baking dish. Sprinkle with Parmesan. Bake in preheated oven for 25 to 30 minutes or until center is piping hot and top is light golden.

---

▶ **Health Tip**

Garlic can have a positive impact on LDL cholesterol.

# Couscous with Currants and Carrots

*Couscous is wonderfully light and nourishing, and seems to have an endless capacity to absorb the flavors of stock, a little olive oil and whatever spices, herbs, dried fruits or other ingredients you mix with it.*

## Makes 6 servings

## Tips

Store unpeeled gingerroot in the freezer for up to 3 months. You can grate it from frozen for dishes that will be cooked.

Use whole wheat couscous to boost the whole grains in your menu.

| | | |
|---|---|---:|
| 2 cups | ready-to-use chicken broth | 500 mL |
| 1 | carrot, diced | 1 |
| 1/4 cup | olive oil | 60 mL |
| 1 tbsp | grated gingerroot | 15 mL |
| 1/4 tsp | ground turmeric | 1 mL |
| 1/4 tsp | ground cinnamon | 1 mL |
| 1/4 tsp | ground cumin | 1 mL |
| 1 cup | couscous | 250 mL |
| 1/2 cup | currants | 125 mL |

1. In a medium saucepan over medium-high heat, bring broth to a boil. Add carrot, oil, ginger, turmeric, cinnamon and cumin. Boil until carrot is tender-crisp, about 4 minutes.

2. Remove from heat and stir in couscous and currants. Cover and let stand for 10 minutes, until couscous is softened and has absorbed most of the water. Fluff with a fork.

*This recipe courtesy of dietitian Corilee Watters.*

> ▸ **Health Tip**
>
> Currants are a great source of the polyphenolic and other antioxidant molecules that we have discussed in this book as important for tissue protection, in the brain and beyond.

### Nutrients per serving

| | |
|---|---|
| Calories | 213 |
| Fat | 10 g |
| Carbohydrate | 26 g |
| Protein | 6 g |
| Vitamin C | 18 mg |
| Vitamin D | 0 IU |
| Vitamin E | 1 mg |
| Niacin | 2 mg |
| Folate | 8 mcg |
| Vitamin $B_6$ | 0.1 mg |
| Vitamin $B_{12}$ | 0.1 mcg |
| Zinc | 0.4 mg |
| Selenium | 0 mcg |

# DESSERTS

# Rhubarb Strawberry Cobbler

*Here is a delicious, gluten-free baked dessert that brings on the fruit and the flavor.*

## Makes 8 servings

### Tips

You'll need a long shallow baking dish rather than a deep square one to accommodate the topping in a single layer.

You can make cobblers with an endless variety of fruits. You'll need about 8 cups (2 L) of cubed fruit (roughly $\frac{1}{2}$-inch/1 cm cubes). Orange flavoring is good with rhubarb, but lemon zest and lemon juice work well with most other combinations.

- Preheat oven to 375°F (190°C)
- 8-cup (2 L) baking dish (see tip, at left), greased

### Fruit

| | | |
|---|---|---|
| 1$\frac{1}{4}$ cups | granulated sugar | 300 mL |
| 1 tbsp | tapioca flour | 15 mL |
| 1 tsp | ground cinnamon | 5 mL |
| 4 cups | halved hulled strawberries | 1 L |
| 4 cups | chopped rhubarb ($\frac{1}{2}$-inch/1 cm cubes) | 1 L |
| 1 tbsp | finely grated orange zest | 15 mL |

### Topping

| | | |
|---|---|---|
| $\frac{2}{3}$ cup | sorghum flour | 150 mL |
| $\frac{2}{3}$ cup | coconut flour | 150 mL |
| 3 tbsp | tapioca flour | 45 mL |
| 2 tbsp | granulated sugar (approx.) | 30 mL |
| 1 tsp | gluten-free baking powder | 5 mL |
| 1 tsp | xanthan gum | 5 mL |
| 1 tsp | finely grated orange zest | 5 mL |
| $\frac{1}{2}$ tsp | salt | 2 mL |
| $\frac{1}{2}$ cup | cold butter, cut into 1-inch (2.5 mL) cubes | 125 mL |
| 1$\frac{1}{4}$ cups | buttermilk + 1 tbsp (15 mL) for brushing | 300 mL |

1. *Fruit:* In a large bowl, combine sugar, tapioca flour and cinnamon. Mix well. Add strawberries, rhubarb and orange zest and toss well. Transfer to prepared baking dish.

2. *Topping:* In a bowl, combine sorghum, coconut and tapioca flours, sugar, baking powder, xanthan gum, orange zest and salt. Using your fingers or a pastry blender, cut in butter until mixture resembles coarse crumbs. Drizzle with buttermilk and stir with a fork until a batter forms. Divide dough into 8 equal parts and flatten each into a rough circle. Place on top of fruit mixture. Brush tops with remaining buttermilk and sprinkle with sugar. Place dish on a baking sheet and bake in preheated oven until fruit is hot and bubbly and top is golden, about 45 minutes. Let cool for at least 10 minutes. Serve warm.

### ▸ Health Tip

Strawberries are a brain superfood.

### Nutrients per serving

| | |
|---|---|
| Calories | 395 |
| Fat | 17 g |
| Carbohydrate | 60 g |
| Protein | 5 g |
| Vitamin C | 52 mg |
| Vitamin D | 9 IU |
| Vitamin E | 1 mg |
| Niacin | 1 mg |
| Folate | 26 mcg |
| Vitamin B$_6$ | 0.1 mg |
| Vitamin B$_{12}$ | 0.2 mcg |
| Zinc | 0.4 mg |
| Selenium | 4 mcg |

# Pumpkin Pie

*This is a classic, not only for Thanksgiving but year-round.*

## Tip

*To make pumpkin purée:* Cut pumpkin into halves, quarters or chunks and remove seeds. Place in a 12- to 16-cup (3 to 4 L) casserole dish. Add 1/2 cup (125 mL) water. Microwave, covered, on High for 15 to 30 minutes or until tender when tested in several places. Let stand until cool enough to handle. Scoop out pulp and mash or purée in a blender or food processor. Place purée in a fine-mesh strainer for several hours to drain excess moisture. Freeze in airtight containers for up to 3 months.

### Nutrients per serving

| | |
|---|---|
| Calories | 274 |
| Fat | 10 g |
| Carbohydrate | 43 g |
| Protein | 4 g |
| Vitamin C | 3 mg |
| Vitamin D | 13 IU |
| Vitamin E | 1 mg |
| Niacin | 1 mg |
| Folate | 26 mcg |
| Vitamin $B_6$ | 0.1 mg |
| Vitamin $B_{12}$ | 0.2 mcg |
| Zinc | 0.6 mg |
| Selenium | 6 mcg |

- **9-inch (23 cm) pie plate, lightly greased**

| | Pastry for a single-crust 9-inch (23 cm) pie | |
|---|---|---|
| 2 | large eggs | 2 |
| 1 cup | packed brown sugar | 250 mL |
| 2 cups | pumpkin purée (not pie filling) | 500 mL |
| 1 cup | half-and-half (10%) cream | 250 mL |
| 1½ tsp | ground cinnamon | 7 mL |
| ½ tsp | ground allspice | 2 mL |
| ½ tsp | freshly grated nutmeg | 2 mL |
| ¼ tsp | ground cloves | 1 mL |
| ¼ tsp | salt | 1 mL |

1. On a lightly floured surface, roll out pastry into a 12-inch (30 cm) round. Roll pastry loosely around rolling pin; unroll into pie plate. Trim edge, leaving a ½-inch (1 cm) overhang; turn pastry edge under and flute edge. Refrigerate for 30 minutes to chill.

2. Preheat oven to 425°F (220°C).

3. In a bowl, beat eggs with brown sugar. Stir in pumpkin purée, cream, cinnamon, allspice, nutmeg, cloves and salt until spices are well combined.

4. Pour filling into pie shell; bake on middle rack in preheated oven for 15 minutes, then reduce temperature to 350°F (180°C). Bake for 35 to 40 minutes or until tip of knife inserted in center comes out clean. Place on a wire rack to cool; refrigerate.

▸ ## Health Tip

Pumpkins are a great source of carotenoids, including beta-carotene.

# Chocolate Cherry Drops

*This is a succulent and sweet dessert that gives new meaning to the phrase "it's hard to have only one"!*

## Tips

To toast almonds: Preheat oven to 350°F (180°C). Spread nuts on a baking sheet lined with foil or parchment. Bake for 5 to 7 minutes or until light brown and fragrant.

Lightly dust chocolates with confectioners' sugar just before serving, if desired, for a fancier presentation.

Store the chocolates in a covered airtight container in a cool place for up to 2 days.

- **Baking sheet, lined with parchment paper**

| | | |
|---|---|---|
| 10 oz | bittersweet chocolate, chopped | 300 g |
| ¾ cup | whole almonds, toasted (see tip, at left) | 175 mL |
| ½ cup | dried sour cherries | 125 mL |

1. In a microwave-safe bowl, microwave chocolate, uncovered, on Medium (50%) for 1 to 2 minutes, stirring every 30 seconds, or until chocolate is soft and almost melted. Stir until completely melted and smooth.

2. Stir in toasted almonds and dried cherries. Drop by teaspoons (5 mL) onto prepared baking sheet.

3. Refrigerate chocolates until firm to the touch.

## Variation

Substitute chopped dried apricots for the cherries or toasted hazelnuts for the almonds.

> ▶ **Health Tip**
>
> Cherries are a great source of vitamin C and other nutrients.

## Nutrients per drop

| | |
|---|---|
| Calories | 98 |
| Fat | 8 g |
| Carbohydrate | 9 g |
| Protein | 2 g |
| Vitamin C | 0 mg |
| Vitamin D | 0 IU |
| Vitamin E | 1 mg |
| Niacin | 0 mg |
| Folate | 2 mcg |
| Vitamin B$_6$ | 0.0 mg |
| Vitamin B$_{12}$ | 0.0 mcg |
| Zinc | 0.2 mg |
| Selenium | 0 mcg |

# Blueberry Lemon Bundt

*This is a sweet dessert in the classic sense, balanced with lemon zest and the brightness of blueberries for a scrumptious finish to any meal.*

**Makes
20 servings**

## Tips

Take heart if blueberry season has passed — frozen ones also yield excellent results.

Store the cooled cake at room temperature in a cake keeper, or loosely wrapped in foil or plastic wrap, for up to 3 days. Alternatively, wrap the cooled cake in plastic wrap, then foil, completely enclosing cake, and freeze for up to 6 months. Let cake thaw at room temperature for 4 to 6 hours before serving.

- Preheat oven to 350°F (180°C)
- 10-inch (25 cm) Bundt pan, sprayed with nonstick baking spray with flour

| | | |
|---|---|---:|
| 2½ cups | all-purpose flour | 625 mL |
| 2 cups | granulated sugar | 500 mL |
| 2 tsp | baking powder | 10 mL |
| ½ tsp | salt | 2 mL |
| 4 | large eggs, at room temperature | 4 |
| 1 cup | unsalted butter, softened | 250 mL |
| 1 cup | sour cream | 250 mL |
| 1 tbsp | finely grated lemon zest | 15 mL |
| 1 tsp | vanilla extract | 5 mL |
| 2 cups | fresh or frozen (unthawed) blueberries, divided | 500 mL |
| 2 tbsp | confectioners' (icing) sugar | 30 mL |

1. In a large bowl, whisk together flour, sugar, baking powder and salt.

2. Add eggs, butter, sour cream, lemon zest and vanilla to flour mixture. Using an electric mixer on medium speed, beat for 1 minute, until blended. Scrape sides and bottom of bowl with a spatula. Beat on high speed for 2 minutes. Gently stir in half the blueberries.

3. Spread batter evenly in prepared pan. Sprinkle the remaining berries evenly over batter.

4. Bake in preheated oven for about 60 minutes or until a piece of uncooked spaghetti inserted in the center comes out with a few moist crumbs attached. Let cool in pan on a wire rack for 20 minutes, then invert cake onto rack to cool. Just before serving, dust with confectioners' sugar.

### ▶ Health Tip

Blueberries are one of those superfoods containing molecules protective to the brain, heart, eyes and more.

## Nutrients per serving

| | |
|---|---:|
| Calories | 260 |
| Fat | 12 g |
| Carbohydrate | 36 g |
| Protein | 4 g |
| Vitamin C | 2 mg |
| Vitamin D | 16 IU |
| Vitamin E | 1 mg |
| Niacin | 1 mg |
| Folate | 36 mcg |
| Vitamin $B_6$ | 0.0 mg |
| Vitamin $B_{12}$ | 0.2 mcg |
| Zinc | 0.3 mg |
| Selenium | 4 mcg |

# Perfect Chocolate Bundt

*Here is a chocolate lover's take on Bundt cake.*

**Makes
16 servings**

## Tip

Store the glazed cake at room temperature in a cake keeper, or loosely wrapped in foil or plastic wrap, for up to 3 days. Alternatively, wrap the cooled, unglazed cake in plastic wrap, then foil, completely enclosing cake, and freeze for up to 6 months. Let cake thaw at room temperature for 4 to 6 hours before glazing and serving.

### Nutrients per serving

| | |
|---|---|
| Calories | 426 |
| Fat | 22 g |
| Carbohydrate | 58 g |
| Protein | 6 g |
| Vitamin C | 0 mg |
| Vitamin D | 22 IU |
| Vitamin E | 1 mg |
| Niacin | 1 mg |
| Folate | 39 mcg |
| Vitamin B$_6$ | 0.1 mg |
| Vitamin B$_{12}$ | 0.2 mcg |
| Zinc | 1.1 mg |
| Selenium | 7 mcg |

- 10-inch (25 cm) Bundt pan, sprayed with nonstick baking spray with flour

| | | |
|---|---|---|
| 1 cup | semisweet chocolate chips | 250 mL |
| ¾ cup | unsweetened cocoa powder (not Dutch process) | 175 mL |
| 1 tsp | instant espresso powder | 5 mL |
| ¾ cup | boiling water | 175 mL |
| 2 cups | packed light brown sugar | 500 mL |
| 1 tsp | baking soda | 5 mL |
| 1 tsp | salt | 5 mL |
| 5 | large eggs, at room temperature | 5 |
| 1 cup | sour cream (see tip, at right) | 250 mL |
| ¾ cup | unsalted butter, softened | 175 mL |
| 1 tbsp | vanilla extract | 15 mL |
| 1¾ cups | all-purpose flour | 425 mL |
| | Chocolate Ganache Glaze (see recipe, opposite) | |

1. In a large bowl, combine chocolate chips, cocoa powder and espresso powder. Add boiling water and whisk until chocolate is melted and mixture is smooth. Let cool for 20 minutes.

2. Meanwhile, preheat oven to 350°F (180°C).

3. Add brown sugar, baking soda, salt, eggs, sour cream, butter and vanilla to cocoa mixture. Using an electric mixer on high speed, beat for 2 minutes, until blended and fluffy. Add flour and beat on medium speed for 1 minute. Scrape sides and bottom of bowl with a spatula. Beat on high speed for 1 minute.

4. Spread batter evenly in prepared pan.

5. Bake in preheated oven for about 60 minutes or until a piece of uncooked spaghetti inserted in the center comes out with a few moist crumbs attached. Let cool in pan on a wire rack for 10 minutes, then invert cake onto rack to cool completely. Spoon glaze over top of cooled cake, letting it drizzle down the sides.

## Tip

Use full-fat (not reduced-fat) sour cream. Reduced-fat sour cream will alter the taste and texture of the cake.

## Variation

*Mexican Chocolate Bundt*: Add $1\frac{1}{2}$ tsp (7 mL) ground cinnamon and $\frac{1}{4}$ tsp (1 mL) cayenne pepper with the brown sugar. Omit the glaze and dust the cooled cake with 2 tbsp (30 mL) confectioners' (icing) sugar.

> ▶ **Health Tip**
>
> Unsweetened chocolate and cocoa powder that have not been Dutch processed have the higher concentration of flavonols that are the key to this food's health benefits.

# Chocolate Ganache Glaze

| Makes about 1 cup (250 mL) | | |
|---|---|---|

| $\frac{1}{3}$ cup | heavy or whipping (35%) cream | 75 mL |
|---|---|---|
| 1 tbsp | light (white or golden) corn syrup | 15 mL |
| $1\frac{1}{4}$ cups | semisweet chocolate chips | 300 mL |
| $\frac{1}{2}$ tsp | vanilla extract | 2 mL |

1. In a small saucepan, bring cream and corn syrup to a simmer over medium heat.

2. Place chocolate chips in a large heatproof bowl and pour in hot cream mixture. Let stand for 3 minutes or until chocolate chips are melted. Add vanilla and whisk until smooth. Let cool for 10 minutes, until slightly thickened.

### Nutrients per 1 tbsp (15 mL)

| | |
|---|---|
| Calories | 80 |
| Fat | 6 g |
| Carbohydrate | 9 g |
| Protein | 1 g |
| Vitamin C | 0 mg |
| Vitamin D | 1 IU |
| Vitamin E | 0 mg |
| Niacin | 0 mg |
| Folate | 2 mcg |
| Vitamin $B_6$ | 0.0 mg |
| Vitamin $B_{12}$ | 0.0 mcg |
| Zinc | 0.2 mg |
| Selenium | 1 mcg |

# Chocolate Ganache Stout Cake

*This recipe incorporates dark beer (stout) along with a generous amount of intense unsweetened chocolate for a moist, hearty cake.*

---

### Makes
### 16 servings

## Tip

Store the frosted cake in the refrigerator in a cake keeper, or loosely wrapped in foil or waxed paper, for up to 3 days. Alternatively, wrap the cooled, unfrosted cake layers individually in plastic wrap, then foil, and freeze for up to 6 months. Let cake layers thaw at room temperature for 2 to 3 hours before frosting and serving.

### Nutrients per serving

| | |
|---|---|
| Calories | 622 |
| Fat | 31 g |
| Carbohydrate | 86 g |
| Protein | 5 g |
| Vitamin C | 0 mg |
| Vitamin D | 22 IU |
| Vitamin E | 1 mg |
| Niacin | 1 mg |
| Folate | 38 mcg |
| Vitamin B$_6$ | 0.1 mg |
| Vitamin B$_{12}$ | 0.2 mcg |
| Zinc | 0.7 mg |
| Selenium | 4 mcg |

- **Preheat oven to 350°F (180°C)**
- **Three 9-inch (23 cm) round metal baking pans, sprayed with nonstick baking spray with flour**

| | | |
|---|---|---|
| ¾ cup | unsweetened cocoa powder (not Dutch process) | 175 mL |
| 1 cup | stout or other dark beer | 250 mL |
| 1 cup | unsalted butter, cut into small pieces | 250 mL |
| 2 cups | all-purpose flour | 500 mL |
| 2 cups | packed light brown sugar | 500 mL |
| 1½ tsp | baking soda | 7 mL |
| ¾ tsp | salt | 3 mL |
| 2 | large eggs, at room temperature | 2 |
| ⅔ cup | sour cream | 150 mL |
| 2 tsp | vanilla extract | 10 mL |
| | Chocolate Ganache (see recipe, opposite) | |

1. In a large microwave-safe bowl, combine cocoa powder, beer and butter. Microwave on High for 1 to 2 minutes, until butter is melted. Whisk until smooth and let cool for 15 minutes.

2. Add flour, brown sugar, baking soda, salt, eggs, sour cream and vanilla to cocoa mixture. Using an electric mixer, beat on medium speed for 1 minute, until blended. Scrape sides and bottom of bowl with a spatula. Beat on high speed for 1 minute.

3. Spread batter evenly in prepared pans, dividing equally.

4. Bake in preheated oven for 23 to 28 minutes or until a toothpick inserted in the center comes out with a few moist crumbs attached. Let cool in pans on a wire rack for 10 minutes. Run a knife around edge of pans, then invert cakes onto rack to cool completely.

5. Place one cake layer, flat side up, on a cake plate or platter. Spread ¾ cup (175 mL) of the ganache evenly over bottom layer. Top with the second cake layer, flat side up. Spread evenly with ¾ cup (175 mL) of the ganache. Top with the third cake layer, flat side down. Spread the remaining ganache over top and sides of cake. Refrigerate for at least 1 hour before serving.

# Chocolate Ganache

**Makes 2¾ cups (675 mL)**

## Tip

If ganache becomes too thick, let stand at room temperature until slightly softened.

| | | |
|---|---|---|
| 1¾ cups | heavy or whipping (35%) cream | 425 mL |
| 2⅓ cups | bittersweet or semisweet chocolate chips | 575 mL |

1. In a small saucepan, bring cream to a simmer over medium heat.

2. Place chocolate chips in a large heatproof bowl and pour in hot cream. Let stand for 3 minutes or until chocolate chips are melted, then whisk until smooth. Loosely cover bowl with plastic wrap and refrigerate, stirring occasionally, for about 4 hours or until thickened but spreadable.

> ▶ **Health Tip**
>
> Plan the use of fancy desserts — they can liven up a weekday or accent a special meal, but they always ought to be a minor component of our total caloric intake across a week and even a day.

## Nutrients per 1 tbsp (15 mL)

| | |
|---|---|
| Calories | 74 |
| Fat | 6 g |
| Carbohydrate | 6 g |
| Protein | 1 g |
| Vitamin C | 0 mg |
| Vitamin D | 3 IU |
| Vitamin E | 0 mg |
| Niacin | 0 mg |
| Folate | 2 mcg |
| Vitamin B$_6$ | 0.0 mg |
| Vitamin B$_{12}$ | 0.0 mcg |
| Zinc | 0.2 mg |
| Selenium | 0 mcg |

# Cinnamon Cake with Whipped Mocha Frosting

*Here is a delicious, cinnamon-based cake with an energizing mocha frosting to boot.*

**Makes 16 servings**

## Tips

If using a stand mixer, decrease the high-speed beating time by 1 minute.

Store the frosted cake in the refrigerator in a cake keeper, or loosely wrapped in foil or waxed paper, for up to 3 days. Alternatively, wrap the cooled, unfrosted cake layers individually in plastic wrap, then foil, and freeze for up to 6 months. Let cake layers thaw at room temperature for 2 to 3 hours before frosting and serving.

### Nutrients per serving

| | |
|---|---|
| Calories | 447 |
| Fat | 26 g |
| Carbohydrate | 49 g |
| Protein | 5 g |
| Vitamin C | 0 mg |
| Vitamin D | 34 IU |
| Vitamin E | 1 mg |
| Niacin | 1 mg |
| Folate | 38 mcg |
| Vitamin $B_6$ | 0.0 mg |
| Vitamin $B_{12}$ | 0.3 mcg |
| Zinc | 0.5 mg |
| Selenium | 5 mcg |

- **Preheat oven to 350°F (180°C)**
- **Two 9-inch (23 cm) round metal baking pans, sprayed with nonstick baking spray with flour**

| | | |
|---|---|---|
| 2 cups | all-purpose flour | 500 mL |
| 2 cups | granulated sugar | 500 mL |
| 2 tsp | ground cinnamon | 10 mL |
| 1 tsp | baking soda | 5 mL |
| 1 tsp | baking powder | 5 mL |
| ½ tsp | salt | 2 mL |
| 4 | large eggs, at room temperature | 4 |
| 1 cup | unsalted butter, softened | 250 mL |
| 1 cup | sour cream | 250 mL |
| 2 tsp | vanilla extract | 10 mL |
| ½ cup | milk | 125 mL |
| | Whipped Mocha Frosting (see recipe, opposite) | |

1. In a large bowl, whisk together flour, sugar, cinnamon, baking soda, baking powder and salt.

2. Add eggs, butter, sour cream and vanilla to flour mixture. Using an electric mixer on medium-low speed, beat for 1 minute, until blended. Scrape sides and bottom of bowl with a spatula. Beat on high speed for 2 minutes. Add milk and beat on low speed for 15 to 30 seconds, until just blended.

3. Spread batter evenly in prepared pans, dividing equally.

4. Bake in preheated oven for 27 to 32 minutes or until a toothpick inserted in the center comes out with a few moist crumbs attached. Let cool in pans on a wire rack for 10 minutes. Run a knife around edge of pans, then invert cakes onto rack to cool completely.

5. Place one cake layer, flat side up, on a cake plate or platter. Spread ¾ cup (175 mL) of the frosting evenly over bottom layer. Top with the second cake layer, flat side down. Spread the remaining frosting over top and sides of cake. Refrigerate for at least 1 hour before serving.

# Whipped Mocha Frosting

**Makes 4 cups
(1 L)**

## Tip

Select natural cocoa powder, which has a deep, true chocolate flavor.

| | | |
|---|---|---|
| 1 cup | confectioners' (icing) sugar | 250 mL |
| $\frac{1}{2}$ cup | unsweetened cocoa powder (not Dutch process) | 125 mL |
| $\frac{1}{8}$ tsp | salt | 0.5 mL |
| $\frac{1}{4}$ cup | milk | 60 mL |
| 2 tsp | instant espresso powder | 10 mL |
| 2 tsp | vanilla extract | 10 mL |
| 2 cups | heavy or whipping (35%) cream | 500 mL |

1. In a large bowl, whisk together confectioners' sugar, cocoa powder, salt, milk, espresso and vanilla until blended and smooth. Cover and refrigerate for 1 hour.

2. Add cream to chilled cocoa mixture. Using an electric mixer on medium-high speed, beat, stopping to scrape the bowl occasionally, until stiff peaks form. Use immediately.

> ▸ **Health Tip**
>
> Cinnamon has been shown to have a regulating effect on blood sugar — which is beneficial when incorporated into a sweet dessert like this one.

## Nutrients per 1 tbsp (15 mL)

| | |
|---|---|
| Calories | 138 |
| Fat | 11 g |
| Carbohydrate | 10 g |
| Protein | 1 g |
| Vitamin C | 0 mg |
| Vitamin D | 9 IU |
| Vitamin E | 0 mg |
| Niacin | 0 mg |
| Folate | 1 mcg |
| Vitamin $B_6$ | 0.0 mg |
| Vitamin $B_{12}$ | 0.1 mcg |
| Zinc | 0.1 mg |
| Selenium | 0 mcg |

# Chocolate Chile Cupcakes

*Chocolate and chile blend wonderfully here. If you're looking for a cupcake with a zing, this is the one.*

---

**Makes
12 cupcakes**

## Tip

These are best served the day that they're made.

- **Preheat oven to 350°F (180°C)**
- **12-cup muffin pan, lined with paper liners**

| | | |
|---|---|---|
| 1¼ cups | all-purpose flour | 300 mL |
| ½ cup | unsweetened cocoa powder, sifted | 125 mL |
| 1 tbsp | ancho chile powder (or 1 tsp/5 mL chipotle chile powder) | 15 mL |
| 2 tsp | finely ground espresso or French-roast coffee | 10 mL |
| ¾ tsp | baking soda | 4 mL |
| ¼ tsp | salt | 1 mL |
| 1 cup | granulated sugar | 250 mL |
| ⅓ cup | vegetable oil | 75 mL |
| 1 | large egg | 1 |
| 1 tsp | vanilla extract | 5 mL |
| ¾ cup | buttermilk | 175 mL |
| 1 tbsp | instant coffee granules | 15 mL |
| ½ cup | semisweet chocolate chips | 125 mL |
| | Chocolate Fudge Frosting (see recipe, opposite) | |

1. In a small bowl, mix together flour, cocoa powder, chile powder, ground coffee, baking soda and salt.

2. In a large bowl, whisk together sugar, oil, egg and vanilla until smooth. In a separate bowl, stir together buttermilk and instant coffee.

3. Alternately whisk flour mixture and buttermilk mixture into oil mixture, making three additions of flour mixture and two of buttermilk mixture, beating until smooth. Mix in chocolate chips.

4. Scoop batter into prepared muffin cups. Bake for 22 to 27 minutes or until tops of cupcakes spring back when lightly touched. Let cool in pan on rack for 10 minutes. Remove from pan and let cool completely on rack. Top cooled cupcakes with frosting.

| Nutrients per cupcake | |
|---|---|
| Calories | 397 |
| Fat | 18 g |
| Carbohydrate | 55 g |
| Protein | 5 g |
| Vitamin C | 0 mg |
| Vitamin D | 9 IU |
| Vitamin E | 1 mg |
| Niacin | 1 mg |
| Folate | 29 mcg |
| Vitamin B$_6$ | 0.1 mg |
| Vitamin B$_{12}$ | 0.1 mcg |
| Zinc | 0.3 mg |
| Selenium | 2 mcg |

# Chocolate Fudge Frosting

## Tip

Extra frosting will keep in an airtight container in the refrigerator for several days. Let soften and stir until smooth before spreading.

- **Food processor**

| | | |
|---|---|---|
| 1½ cups | confectioners' (icing) sugar | 375 mL |
| ¾ cup | unsweetened cocoa powder, sifted | 175 mL |
| ½ cup | unsalted butter, at room temperature | 125 mL |
| 2 tbsp | chocolate cream liqueur | 30 mL |
| 1 tbsp | strong brewed coffee or milk | 15 mL |
| Pinch | salt | Pinch |

**1.** In food processor, process confectioners' sugar, cocoa powder, butter, chocolate liqueur, coffee and salt until smooth, scraping down sides as necessary.

**2.** Spread frosting on cooled cupcakes.

## Variations

If you prefer your frosting a little less sweet, you can reduce the confectioners' sugar by ½ cup (125 mL).

To make this frosting vegan, substitute margarine for the butter and replace the chocolate cream liqueur with chocolate liqueur or rum.

### ▶ Health Tip

The beneficial compounds in chocolate can interrupt some of the chemical processes that drive atherosclerosis — a degenerative process that ages arteries.

**Nutrients** per 1 tbsp (15 mL)

| | |
|---|---|
| Calories | 75 |
| Fat | 4 g |
| Carbohydrate | 9 g |
| Protein | 1 g |
| Vitamin C | 0 mg |
| Vitamin D | 3 IU |
| Vitamin E | 0 mg |
| Niacin | 0 mg |
| Folate | 0 mcg |
| Vitamin $B_6$ | 0.0 mg |
| Vitamin $B_{12}$ | 0.0 mcg |
| Zinc | 0.0 mg |
| Selenium | 0 mcg |

# Peanut Butter and Chocolate Rice Crisp Bars

*These rice treats are perfect for those who love the marriage of chocolate and peanut butter.*

**Makes 12 bars**

## Tip

Be sure to use unsalted, unsweetened peanut butter for this recipe.

- 8-inch (20 cm) square baking pan, lightly greased

| | | |
|---|---|---|
| 1 cup | natural peanut butter | 250 mL |
| 1 cup | semisweet chocolate chips | 250 mL |
| $\frac{1}{2}$ cup | agave nectar | 125 mL |
| $\frac{1}{4}$ tsp | salt | 1 mL |
| 4 cups | brown rice crisp cereal | 1 L |
| 1 tsp | vanilla extract | 5 mL |

1. In a large saucepan over low heat, combine peanut butter, chocolate chips, agave nectar and salt. Cook, stirring, until melted and smooth.

2. Remove from heat and stir in cereal and vanilla until cereal is well coated. Press evenly into prepared baking pan. Refrigerate for 20 minutes or until firm. Cut into bars.

## Variation

Substitute cashew butter or hazelnut butter for the peanut butter.

> ▶ **Health Tip**
>
> By using brown rice crisp cereal, we incorporate some fiber into this dish. Peanut butter, while high in fat, adds some protein. This all works to lower the glycemic index of this rich dessert.

| Nutrients per bar | |
|---|---|
| Calories | 244 |
| Fat | 16 g |
| Carbohydrate | 25 g |
| Protein | 6 g |
| Vitamin C | 2 mg |
| Vitamin D | 0 IU |
| Vitamin E | 1 mg |
| Niacin | 3 mg |
| Folate | 12 mcg |
| Vitamin B$_6$ | 0.1 mg |
| Vitamin B$_{12}$ | 0.0 mcg |
| Zinc | 1.0 mg |
| Selenium | 11 mcg |

# Old-Fashioned Dark Chocolate Pudding

*What could be more comforting than a classic chocolate pudding? This recipe won't disappoint.*

## Tip

You will find it easiest to cook this pudding in a heavy-bottomed nonstick saucepan.

| | | |
|---|---|---|
| ½ cup | unsweetened cocoa powder, sifted | 125 mL |
| ⅓ cup | cornstarch | 75 mL |
| ¼ tsp | salt | 1 mL |
| 2 cups | milk | 500 mL |
| 2 cups | half-and-half (10%) cream | 500 mL |
| ¾ cup | granulated sugar | 175 mL |
| 1 cup | semisweet chocolate chips | 250 mL |
| 2 tsp | vanilla extract, divided | 10 mL |
| 1 cup | heavy or whipping (35%) cream | 250 mL |
| 2 tbsp | confectioners' (icing) sugar | 30 mL |

1. In a small bowl, combine cocoa powder, cornstarch and salt.

2. In a large saucepan over medium-high heat, heat milk, half-and-half and sugar until sugar is dissolved. Quickly whisk in cocoa powder mixture until completely dissolved with no lumps. Reduce heat to medium and cook, stirring constantly, until thickened. Continue cooking and stirring for 2 minutes longer or until thickened. Remove from heat. Stir in chocolate chips and 1 tsp (5 mL) of the vanilla. Pour pudding into large bowl or six individual dishes.

3. Press a sheet of plastic wrap directly on surface of pudding to prevent a skin from forming. Let cool for 20 minutes. Refrigerate for several hours or until chilled, or overnight.

4. Meanwhile, in a small bowl, using electric mixer, whip together cream, confectioners' sugar and remaining vanilla until soft peaks form.

5. Remove plastic wrap. Serve pudding with whipped cream.

> ▸ **Health Tip**
>
> The flavonols from chocolate increase blood flow to the heart and the brain.

## Nutrients per serving

| | |
|---|---|
| Calories | 565 |
| Fat | 34 g |
| Carbohydrate | 65 g |
| Protein | 9 g |
| Vitamin C | 1 mg |
| Vitamin D | 56 IU |
| Vitamin E | 1 mg |
| Niacin | 0 mg |
| Folate | 14 mcg |
| Vitamin $B_6$ | 0.1 mg |
| Vitamin $B_{12}$ | 0.7 mcg |
| Zinc | 1.8 mg |
| Selenium | 7 mcg |

# Dark Chocolate Mousse

*Mousse may sound like a sophisticated recipe that only accomplished French pastry chefs can master, but in fact an excellent dessert mousse can be easily made in your kitchen.*

**Makes 8 servings**

## Tips

Superfine sugar dissolves very quickly in liquid. It is sometimes labeled "instant dissolving fruit powdered sugar." If you can't find it, make your own by processing granulated sugar in a food processor until very finely ground.

Garnish mousse with fresh raspberries and sprigs of mint.

| | | |
|---|---|---|
| 8 oz | bittersweet chocolate, chopped | 250 g |
| 2½ cups | heavy or whipping (35%) cream, divided | 625 mL |
| 3 tbsp | superfine sugar (see tip, at left) | 45 mL |
| 2 tsp | vanilla extract | 10 mL |

**1.** In a microwave-safe bowl, combine chocolate and $\frac{1}{2}$ cup (125 mL) cream. Microwave on High for 60 seconds or until cream is hot and chocolate is soft and almost melted. Stir until completely melted and smooth. Let cool slightly.

**2.** In a medium bowl, using electric mixer, whip remaining cream, sugar and vanilla until stiff peaks form. With a rubber spatula, fold melted chocolate mixture into whipped cream mixture.

**3.** Scoop mousse into small cups. Chill for several hours before serving.

## Variation

Substitute 1 tbsp (15 mL) orange-flavored liqueur for the vanilla extract.

> ▶ **Health Tip**
>
> The fats in chocolate are either heart-healthy or heart-neutral, but that's only true of chocolate that has not been mixed with other ingredients, such as caramel or hydrogenated fats.

| Nutrients per serving | |
|---|---|
| Calories | 422 |
| Fat | 43 g |
| Carbohydrate | 15 g |
| Protein | 5 g |
| Vitamin C | 0 mg |
| Vitamin D | 20 IU |
| Vitamin E | 1 mg |
| Niacin | 0 mg |
| Folate | 11 mcg |
| Vitamin B$_6$ | 0.0 mg |
| Vitamin B$_{12}$ | 0.1 mcg |
| Zinc | 2.9 mg |
| Selenium | 3 mcg |

# BEVERAGES

# Super Antioxidant Smoothie

*This simple smoothie provides a wide range of antioxidants and plenty of sweetness to balance and carry the spinach.*

## Tip

Almond milk is available in a variety of flavors, but be sure to choose plain almond milk for this recipe.

• **Blender**

| | | |
|---|---|---|
| 1 cup | loosely packed baby spinach | 250 mL |
| 1 cup | frozen cherries, blueberries or blackberries | 250 mL |
| 1 cup | plain almond milk | 250 mL |

**1.** In blender, purée spinach, cherries and almond milk until smooth. Pour into two glasses and serve immediately.

> ▸ ## Health Tip
>
> In addition to being high in protein, almond milk is an excellent source of vitamin E, an important antioxidant that plays a role in supporting normal heart and brain function, as well as in promoting a healthy complexion.

**Nutrients** per serving

| | |
|---|---|
| Calories | 69 |
| Fat | 1 g |
| Carbohydrate | 14 g |
| Protein | 1 g |
| Vitamin C | 5 mg |
| Vitamin D | 50 IU |
| Vitamin E | 6 mg |
| Niacin | 1 mg |
| Folate | 29 mcg |
| Vitamin B$_6$ | 0.0 mg |
| Vitamin B$_{12}$ | 0.0 mcg |
| Zinc | 0.6 mg |
| Selenium | 0 mcg |

# C-Blitz

*This dynamic juice makes an effective eye-opener or a refreshing drink throughout the day.*

## Tip

To keep parsley fresh, wrap it in several layers of paper towels and place in a plastic bag. Store in the warmest part of your refrigerator — in the butter keeper, for example, or the side door.

- **Juicer**

| | | |
|---|---|---|
| 1 | grapefruit, cut to fit tube | 1 |
| 2 | oranges | 2 |
| 6 | sprigs fresh parsley | 6 |
| 3 | kiwifruit | 3 |

1. Using juicer, process grapefruit, oranges, parsley and kiwis. Whisk and pour into one large or two smaller glasses.

> ## ▶ Health Tip
>
> Parsley packs a whopping amount of vitamin C and is one of the few fresh herbs widely available throughout the year.

## Nutrients per serving

| | |
|---|---|
| Calories | 171 |
| Fat | 1 g |
| Carbohydrate | 43 g |
| Protein | 3 g |
| Vitamin C | 217 mg |
| Vitamin D | 0 IU |
| Vitamin E | 2 mg |
| Niacin | 1 mg |
| Folate | 85 mcg |
| Vitamin $B_6$ | 0.2 mg |
| Vitamin $B_{12}$ | 0.0 mcg |
| Zinc | 0.4 mg |
| Selenium | 1 mcg |

# Cherry Juice

*This cherry-based juice incorporates two other fruits and digestion-friendly fennel.*

**Makes 1 serving**

## Tip

Whole ripe cherries are best used immediately, but will keep in the refrigerator for up to 2 days.

- Juicer

| | | |
|---|---|---|
| 1 cup | pitted cherries | 250 mL |
| $\frac{1}{4}$ | bulb fresh fennel | $\frac{1}{4}$ |
| 1 cup | grapes | 250 mL |
| $\frac{1}{2}$ | lime | $\frac{1}{2}$ |

**1.** Using juicer, process cherries, fennel, grapes and lime. Whisk and pour into a glass.

### ▸ Health Tip

Cherries contain numerous antioxidants that can help protect body tissues, including the brain.

| Nutrients per serving | |
|---|---|
| Calories | 187 |
| Fat | 1 g |
| Carbohydrate | 48 g |
| Protein | 3 g |
| Vitamin C | 32 mg |
| Vitamin D | 0 IU |
| Vitamin E | 0 mg |
| Niacin | 1 mg |
| Folate | 26 mcg |
| Vitamin $B_6$ | 0.2 mg |
| Vitamin $B_{12}$ | 0.0 mcg |
| Zinc | 0.3 mg |
| Selenium | 1 mcg |

# Cran-Apple

*Carrots and apples provide the sweetness to balance the tartness of cranberries — a perfect match made in your juicer.*

## Tip

Fresh cranberries can be stored in the crisper drawer of your refrigerator for up to 3 weeks.

- **Juicer**

| ¾ cup | whole cranberries, fresh or frozen | 175 mL |
|-------|-----------------------------------|--------|
| 3 | carrots | 3 |
| 2 | apples | 2 |

1. Using juicer, process cranberries, carrots and apples. Whisk and pour into a glass.

> ▸ **Health Tip**
>
> Cranberries are a great anti-aging food.

| Nutrients per serving | |
|---|---|
| Calories | 299 |
| Fat | 1 g |
| Carbohydrate | 77 g |
| Protein | 3 g |
| Vitamin C | 38 mg |
| Vitamin D | 0 IU |
| Vitamin E | 3 mg |
| Niacin | 1 mg |
| Folate | 46 mcg |
| Vitamin B$_6$ | 0.4 mg |
| Vitamin B$_{12}$ | 0.0 mcg |
| Zinc | 0.7 mg |
| Selenium | 0 mcg |

# Orange Zinger

*This juice will liven up the palate and give you lots of vitamin C.*

## Tip

Although citrus fruits will keep for at least a couple of weeks if kept moist in the refrigerator, they are best when used within 1 week.

- **Juicer**

| | | |
|---|---|---|
| 1 | orange | 1 |
| 3 | carrots | 3 |
| 1 | ½-inch (1 cm) piece gingerroot | 1 |
| 1 | apple | 1 |

**1.** Using juicer, process orange, carrots, ginger and apple. Whisk and pour into a glass.

---

▸ **Health Tip**

Ginger is anti-inflammatory to the stomach, and vitamin C is great for stress and the health of the stomach.

---

**Nutrients** per serving

| | |
|---|---|
| Calories | 233 |
| Fat | 1 g |
| Carbohydrate | 58 g |
| Protein | 3 g |
| Vitamin C | 89 mg |
| Vitamin D | 0 IU |
| Vitamin E | 2 mg |
| Niacin | 2 mg |
| Folate | 80 mcg |
| Vitamin $B_6$ | 0.4 mg |
| Vitamin $B_{12}$ | 0.0 mcg |
| Zinc | 0.6 mg |
| Selenium | 1 mcg |

# Slippery Beet

*This is a straight-ahead beet juice, with the power of garlic along for the ride.*

## Tip

Store unwashed beets in a plastic bag in the refrigerator for up to 10 days. Wash just before juicing.

- **Juicer**

| | | |
|---|---|---|
| 2 | beets | 2 |
| 1 | clove garlic | 1 |
| 1 | apple | 1 |
| 1 tbsp | powdered slippery elm (optional) | 15 mL |

1. Using juicer, process beets, garlic and apple. Whisk together with slippery elm (if using) and pour into a glass.

> ▶ **Health Tip**
>
> The choline content of beets makes them a good support for the liver, while the addition of slippery elm make this juice an even better detox drink.

## Nutrients per serving

| | |
|---|---|
| Calories | 85 |
| Fat | 0 g |
| Carbohydrate | 21 g |
| Protein | 2 g |
| Vitamin C | 9 mg |
| Vitamin D | 0 IU |
| Vitamin E | 0 mg |
| Niacin | 0 mg |
| Folate | 92 mcg |
| Vitamin B$_6$ | 0.1 mg |
| Vitamin B$_{12}$ | 0.0 mcg |
| Zinc | 0.3 mg |
| Selenium | 1 mcg |

# Spiced Carrot

*Carrot juice is popular these days, not least because it's one of the sweetest. This version brings in cinnamon and some spicy heat from ginger and cayenne.*

## Tip

Store carrots in a vented plastic bag in the crisper drawer of your refrigerator for up to 2 weeks.

- **Juicer**

| | | |
|---|---|---|
| 3 | carrots | 3 |
| 1 | spear broccoli | 1 |
| 1/2 cup | fresh spinach | 125 mL |
| 1 | 1/2-inch (1 cm) piece gingerroot | 1 |
| 1/2 tsp | ground cinnamon | 2 mL |
| 1/8 tsp | cayenne pepper (or to taste) | 0.5 mL |

1. Using juicer, process carrots, broccoli, spinach and ginger. Whisk together with cinnamon and cayenne and pour into a glass.

> ▸ **Health Tip**
>
> Broccoli and cayenne both have cancer-preventing properties.

## Nutrients per serving

| | |
|---|---|
| Calories | 95 |
| Fat | 1 g |
| Carbohydrate | 22 g |
| Protein | 3 g |
| Vitamin C | 43 mg |
| Vitamin D | 0 IU |
| Vitamin E | 2 mg |
| Niacin | 2 mg |
| Folate | 84 mcg |
| Vitamin $B_6$ | 0.4 mg |
| Vitamin $B_{12}$ | 0.0 mcg |
| Zinc | 0.7 mg |
| Selenium | 1 mcg |

# Dandelion Slam Dunk

*Dandelion greens are becoming increasingly well known as a salad ingredient or just cooked. In this recipe, you can juice them along with some other healthy ingredients.*

**Makes 1 serving**

## Tip

Look for fresh dandelion leaves from spring through fall at some supermarkets, farmers' markets and health food stores.

- **Juicer**

| | | |
|---|---|---|
| ½ cup | fresh dandelion leaves | 125 mL |
| ¼ | cabbage, cut to fit tube | ¼ |
| 2 | apples | 2 |
| 1 | 1-inch (2.5 cm) piece fresh dandelion root | 1 |

1. Using juicer, process dandelion leaves, cabbage, apples and dandelion root. Whisk and pour into a glass.

> ### ▶ Health Tip
>
> Dandelion root supports liver function and the leaves are known to increase kidney activity; hence this juice is a good supporter of natural detoxification pathways.

## Nutrients per serving

| | |
|---|---|
| Calories | 260 |
| Fat | 1 g |
| Carbohydrate | 66 g |
| Protein | 5 g |
| Vitamin C | 142 mg |
| Vitamin D | 0 IU |
| Vitamin E | 2 mg |
| Niacin | 1 mg |
| Folate | 148 mcg |
| Vitamin B$_6$ | 0.4 mg |
| Vitamin B$_{12}$ | 0.0 mcg |
| Zinc | 0.7 mg |
| Selenium | 2 mcg |

# Cruciferous Chiller

*This juice is like an injection of detoxification-inducing compounds and a great example of how juicing can concentrate the benefits of raw foods.*

## Tip

Store cauliflower and broccoli in vented plastic bags in the crisper drawer of your refrigerator. Broccoli will keep for up to 3 days; cauliflower for up to 1 week.

- **Juicer**

| | | |
|---|---|---|
| 4 | cauliflower florets | 4 |
| 4 | broccoli florets | 4 |
| 1 cup | torn kale, spinach or bok choy leaves | 250 mL |
| ½ | Vidalia onion | ½ |
| | Ice (optional) | |

1. Using juicer, process cauliflower, broccoli, kale and onion. Whisk and pour over ice (if using).

> ▶ **Health Tip**
>
> Sulfur-based compounds from cauliflower and broccoli are key to detoxification pathways.

| Nutrients per serving | |
|---|---|
| Calories | 73 |
| Fat | 1 g |
| Carbohydrate | 15 g |
| Protein | 5 g |
| Vitamin C | 149 mg |
| Vitamin D | 0 IU |
| Vitamin E | 0 mg |
| Niacin | 149 mg |
| Folate | 87 mcg |
| Vitamin B$_6$ | 0.4 mg |
| Vitamin B$_{12}$ | 0.0 mcg |
| Zinc | 0.7 mg |
| Selenium | 2 mcg |

# Cell Support Juice

*This is a nutritive boost with plenty of sweetness from apples.*

## Tip

Look for whole or cut dried alfalfa leaves at health food stores.

- Juicer

| | | |
|---|---|---|
| 3 | apples | 3 |
| 1 | handful fresh parsley | 1 |
| 1 | handful fresh alfalfa tops or 1 tbsp (15 mL) dried | 1 |

**1.** Using juicer, process apples, parsley and, if using, fresh alfalfa. Whisk together and pour into a large glass. If using dried alfalfa, whisk into juice.

> ▶ **Health Tip**
>
> Alfalfa used to be given to convalescents who needed to put on weight. This plant has some "phytoestrogen" attributes as well, somewhat akin to soy.

## Nutrients per serving

| | |
|---|---|
| Calories | 291 |
| Fat | 1 g |
| Carbohydrate | 77 g |
| Protein | 2 g |
| Vitamin C | 46 mg |
| Vitamin D | 0 IU |
| Vitamin E | 1 mg |
| Niacin | 1 mg |
| Folate | 42 mcg |
| Vitamin B$_6$ | 0.2 mg |
| Vitamin B$_{12}$ | 0.0 mcg |
| Zinc | 0.5 mg |
| Selenium | 0 mcg |

# Green Energy

*This green energy drink can be a midafternoon pick-me-up or a later in the day serving of veggies.*

## Tip

Reduce the amount of soy milk to ¼ cup (60 mL) if using frozen spinach.

- **Blender**

| | | |
|---|---|---|
| 2 cups | spinach, fresh or frozen | 500 mL |
| ½ cup | soy milk (see tip, at left) | 125 mL |
| ¼ cup | apricot milk or soy milk | 60 mL |
| 3 tbsp | chopped wheat or barley grass | 45 mL |
| 1 tbsp | pumpkin seeds | 15 mL |
| 1 tsp | ginkgo (optional) | 5 mL |

**1.** In blender, process spinach, soy milk, apricot milk, grass, pumpkin seeds and ginkgo (if using) until smooth. Pour into a glass.

> ▶ **Health Tip**
>
> Getting the maximum number of servings of vegetables per day depends on taking opportunities to eat them — using a vegetable-based (and low-sodium) drink is a great way to up your veggie intake.

| **Nutrients** per serving | |
|---|---|
| Calories | 257 |
| Fat | 7 g |
| Carbohydrate | 38 g |
| Protein | 13 g |
| Vitamin C | 17 mg |
| Vitamin D | 78 IU |
| Vitamin E | 2 mg |
| Niacin | 3 mg |
| Folate | 144 mcg |
| Vitamin B$_6$ | 0.3 mg |
| Vitamin B$_{12}$ | 1.6 mcg |
| Zinc | 2.3 mg |
| Selenium | 18 mcg |

# Resources

## Alzheimer's Disease

**Alzheimer's Association**
www.alz.org

**Alzheimer Society of Canada**
www.alzheimer.ca/en

## Naturopathic Medicine

**American Association of Naturopathic Physicians**
www.naturopathic.org

**Canadian Association of Naturopathic Doctors**
www.cand.ca

## Neuroplasticity and Brain Health

**Sharp Brains**
sharpbrains.com

## Parkinson's Disease

**National Parkinson Foundation**
www.parkinson.org

**Parkinson Society Canada**
www.parkinson.ca

## Sleep

**American Sleep Association**
www.sleepassociation.org

## Traumatic Brain Injury

**Brain Injury Association of America**
www.biausa.org

**Library and Archives Canada Cataloguing in Publication**

Smith, Fraser, 1968-, author
    Keep your brain young : a health & diet program for your brain, including 150 recipes /
Dr. Fraser Smith, BA, ND with Dr. Ellie Aghdassi, PhD, RD.

Includes index.
ISBN 978-0-7788-0472-7 (pbk.)

1. Brain—Diseases—Prevention—Popular works.
2. Brain—Diseases—Nutritional aspects—Popular works.
3. Brain—Diseases—Diet therapy—Recipes. 4. Cookbooks.
I. Aghdassi, Ellie, 1966-, author II. Title.

RC386.2.S65 2014          616.805          C2013-908542-4

# References

## Articles

Adan A. Cognitive performance and dehydration. *J Am Coll Nutr*, 2012 Apr; 31(2): 71–78.

Amieva H, Meillon C, Helmer C, et al. Ginkgo biloba extract and long-term cognitive decline: A 20-year follow-up population-based study. *PLoS One*, 2013; 8(1): e52755.

Birch EE, Garfield S, Castañeda Y, et al. Visual acuity and cognitive outcomes at 4 years of age in a double-blind, randomized trial of long-chain polyunsaturated fatty acid-supplemented infant formula. *Early Hum Dev*, 2007 May; 83(5): 279–84.

Bongiovanni B, Ferri A, Brusco A, et al. Adverse effects of 2,4-dichlorophenoxyacetic acid on rat cerebellar granule cell cultures were attenuated by amphetamine. *Neurotox Res*, 2011 May; 19(4): 544–55.

Bourre JM. Effects of nutrients (in food) on the structure and function of the nervous system: Update on dietary requirements for brain. Part 1: Micronutrients. *J Nutr Health Aging*, 2006 Sep–Oct; 10(5): 377–85.

Briones TL, Darwish H. Vitamin D mitigates age-related cognitive decline through the modulation of pro-inflammatory state and decrease in amyloid burden. *J Neuroinflammation*, 2012 Oct 25; 9: 244.

Buell JS, Dawson-Hughes B. Vitamin D and neurocognitive dysfunction: Preventing "D"ecline? *Mol Aspects Med*, 2008 Dec; 29(6): 415–22.

Conklin SM, Gianaros PJ, Brown SM, et al. Long-chain omega-3 fatty acid intake is associated positively with corticolimbic gray matter volume in healthy adults. *Neurosci Lett*, 2007 Jun 29; 421(3): 209–12.

Cramer SC, Sur M, Dobkin BH, et al. Harnessing neuroplasticity for clinical applications. *Brain*, 2011 Jun; 134(Pt 6): 1591–609.

Daulatzai MA. Neurotoxic saboteurs: Straws that break the hippo's (hippocampus) back drive cognitive impairment and Alzheimer's disease. *Neurotox Res*, 2013 Oct; 24(3): 407–59.

Epel E, Daubenmier J, Moskowitz JT, et al. Can meditation slow rate of cellular aging? Cognitive stress, mindfulness, and telomeres. *Ann N Y Acad Sci*, 2009 Aug; 1172: 34–53.

Ganio MS, Armstrong LE, Casa DJ, et al. Mild dehydration impairs cognitive performance and mood of men. *Br J Nutr*, 2011 Nov; 106(10): 1535–43.

Grimm MO, Rothhaar TL, Grösgen S, et al. Trans fatty acids enhance amyloidogenic processing of the Alzheimer amyloid precursor protein (APP). *J Nutr Biochem*, 2012 Oct; 23(10): 1214–23.

Hayden KM, Norton MC, Darcey D, et al; Cache County Study Investigators. Occupational exposure to pesticides increases the risk of incident AD: The Cache County study. *Neurology*, 2010 May 11; 74(19): 1524–30.

Islam Z, Harkema JR, Pestka JJ. Satratoxin G from the black mold *Stachybotrys chartarum* evokes olfactory sensory neuron loss and inflammation in the murine nose and brain. *Environ Health Perspect*, 2006 Jul; 114(7): 1099–107.

Johnson EJ. A possible role for lutein and zeaxanthin in cognitive function in the elderly. *Am J Clin Nutr*, 2012 Nov; 96(5): 1161S–65S.

Kennedy DO, Scholey AB. The psychopharmacology of European herbs with cognition-enhancing properties. *Curr Pharm Des*, 2006; 12(35): 4613–23.

Kesse-Guyot E, Fezeu L, Jeandel C, et al. French adults' cognitive performance after daily supplementation with antioxidant vitamins and minerals at nutritional doses: A post hoc analysis of the Supplementation in Vitamins and Mineral Antioxidants (SU.VI.MAX) trial. *Am J Clin Nutr*, 2011 Sep; 94(3): 892–99.

Li C, Ford ES, Zhao G, et al. Serum $\alpha$-carotene concentrations and risk of death among US adults: The Third National Health and Nutrition Examination Survey Follow-up Study. *Arch Intern Med*, 2011 Mar 28; 171(6): 507–15.

Lim AS, Kowgier M, Yu L, et al. Sleep fragmentation and the risk of incident Alzheimer's disease and cognitive decline in older persons. *Sleep*, 2013 Jul 1; 36(7): 1027–32.

Liu J, Atamna H, Kuratsune H, Ames BN. Delaying brain mitochondrial decay and aging with mitochondrial antioxidants and metabolites. *Ann N Y Acad Sci*, 2002 Apr; 959: 133–66.

Liu J, Killilea DW, Ames BN. Age-associated mitochondrial oxidative decay: Improvement of carnitine acetyltransferase substrate-binding affinity and activity in brain by feeding old rats acetyl-L-carnitine and/or R-alpha-lipoic acid. *Proc Natl Acad Sci U S A*, 2002 Feb 19; 99(4): 1876–81. Erratum in: *Proc Natl Acad Sci U S A*, 2002 May 14; 99(10): 7184.

Mahncke HW, Bronstone A, Merzenich MM. Brain plasticity and functional losses in the aged: Scientific bases for a novel intervention. *Prog Brain Res*, 2006; 157: 81–109.

Mandel SA, Amit T, Weinreb O, Youdim MB. Understanding the broad-spectrum neuroprotective action profile of green tea polyphenols in aging and neurodegenerative diseases. *J Alzheimers Dis*, 2011; 25(2): 187–208.

McDaniel MA, Maier SF, Einstein GO. "Brain-specific" nutrients: A memory cure? *Nutrition*, 2003 Nov–Dec; 19(11–12): 957–75.

Mechan AO, Fowler A, Seifert N, et al. Monoamine reuptake inhibition and mood-enhancing potential of a specified oregano extract. *Br J Nutr*, 2011 Apr; 105(8): 1150–63.

Morgan A, Stevens J. Does *Bacopa monnieri* improve memory performance in older persons? Results of a randomized, placebo-controlled, double-blind trial. *J Altern Complement Med*, 2010 Jul; 16(7): 753–59.

Naismith SL, Mowszowski L, Diamond K, Lewis SJ. Improving memory in Parkinson's disease: A healthy brain ageing cognitive training program. *Mov Disord*, 2013 Jul; 28(8): 1097–103.

Norton MC, Smith KR, Østbye T, et al; Cache County Investigators. Greater risk of dementia when spouse has dementia? The Cache County study. *J Am Geriatr Soc*, 2010 May; 58(5): 895–900. Erratum in: *J Am Geriatr Soc*, 2012 May; 60(5): 1000.

Patel S, Singh V, Kumar A, et al. Status of antioxidant defense system and expression of toxicant responsive genes in striatum of maneb- and paraquat-induced Parkinson's disease phenotype in mouse: Mechanism of neurodegeneration. *Brain Res*, 2006 Apr 7; 1081(1): 9–18.

Pengelly A, Snow J, Mills SY, et al. Short-term study on the effects of rosemary on cognitive function in an elderly population. *J Med Food*, 2012 Jan; 15(1): 10–17.

Perry E, Howes MJ. Medicinal plants and dementia therapy: Herbal hopes for brain aging? *CNS Neurosci Ther*, 2011 Dec; 17(6): 683–98.

Peterson DW, George RC, Scaramozzino F, et al. Cinnamon extract inhibits tau aggregation associated with Alzheimer's disease in vitro. *J Alzheimers Dis*, 2009; 17(3): 585–97.

Pludowski P, Holick MF, Pilz S, et al. Vitamin D effects on musculoskeletal health, immunity, autoimmunity, cardiovascular disease, cancer, fertility, pregnancy, dementia and mortality — a review of recent evidence. *Autoimmun Rev*, 2013 Aug; 12(10): 976–89.

Rafii MS, Walsh S, Little JT, et al. Alzheimer's Disease Cooperative Study: A phase II trial of huperzine A in mild to moderate Alzheimer disease. *Neurology*, 2011 Apr 19; 76(16): 1389–94.

Rinwa P, Kumar A. Quercetin along with piperine prevents cognitive dysfunction, oxidative stress and neuro-inflammation associated with mouse model of chronic unpredictable stress. *Arch Pharm Res*, 2013 Jul 16. [Epub ahead of print.]

Ritz P, Berrut G. The importance of good hydration for day-to-day health. *Nutr Rev*, 2005 Jun; 63(6 Pt 2): S6–13.

Roodenrys S, Booth D, Bulzomi S, et al. Chronic effects of brahmi (*Bacopa monnieri*) on human memory. *Neuropsychopharmacology*, 2002 Aug; 27(2): 279–81.

Simopoulos AP. Genetic variants in the metabolism of omega-6 and omega-3 fatty acids: Their role in the determination of nutritional requirements and chronic disease risk. *Exp Biol Med* (Maywood), 2010 Jul; 235(7): 785–95.

Singhal NK, Chauhan AK, Jain SK, et al. Silymarin- and melatonin-mediated changes in the expression of selected genes in pesticides-induced Parkinsonism. *Mol Cell Biochem*, 2013 Dec; 384(1–2): 47–58.

Virmani A, Pinto L, Binienda Z, Ali S. Food, nutrigenomics, and neurodegeneration-neuroprotection by what you eat! *Mol Neurobiol*, 2013 Oct; 48(2): 353–62.

Wang A, Costello S, Cockburn M, et al. Parkinson's disease risk from ambient exposure to pesticides. *Eur J Epidemiol*, 2011 Jul; 26(7): 547–55.

Witte AV, Kerti L, Hermannstädter HM, et al. Long-chain omega-3 fatty acids improve brain function and structure in older adults. *Cereb Cortex*, 2013 Jun 24. [Epub ahead of print.]

Zaganas I, Kapetanaki S, Mastorodemos V, et al. Linking pesticide exposure and dementia: What is the evidence? *Toxicology*, 2013 May 10; 307: 3–11.

Zeidan F, Johnson SK, Diamond BJ, et al. Mindfulness meditation improves cognition: Evidence of brief mental training. *Conscious Cogn*, 2010 Jun; 19(2): 597–605.

## Books

Davis W. *Wheat Belly: Lose the Wheat, Lose the Weight, and Find Your Way Back to Health*. New York: Rodale, 2011.

Doidge N. *The Brain That Changes Itself: Stories of Personal Triumph from the Frontiers of Brain Science*. London: Penguin Books, 2007.

Pollan M. *In Defense of Food: An Eater's Manifesto*. London: Penguin Books, 2008.

Ratey JJ. *Spark: The Revolutionary New Science of Exercise and the Brain*. New York: Little, Brown and Company, 2008.

Smith F. *Introduction to the Principles and Practices of Naturopathic Medicine*, 1st ed. Kingston, Ontario: CCNM Press, 2008.

Zeff JL, Snider P, Myers SP, DeGrandpre Z. A hierarchy of healing: The therapeutic order. In Pizzorno JE, Murray MT, eds. *A Textbook of Natural Medicine*, 4th ed. St. Louis, MO: Churchill Livingston, 2013: 18–33.

## Websites and Web Pages

Alzheimer's Association: www.alz.org.

Brain Injury Association of America. Diagnosing brain injury: www.biausa.org/brain-injury-diagnosis.htm.

WEIL: Andrew Weil, M.D. Dr. Weil's anti-inflammatory diet: www.drweil.com/drw/u/ART02012/anti-inflammatory-diet.

Oldways: Health Through Heritage. Mediterranean diet & pyramid: oldwayspt.org/resources/heritage-pyramids/mediterranean-diet-pyramid?gclid=CLOc1q_JxbsCFepaMgod2TwAUg

American Sleep Association: www.sleepassociation.org.

# Contributing Authors

**Alexandra Anca and Theresa Santandrea-Cull**
*Complete Gluten-Free Diet and Nutrition Guide*
Recipes from this book are found on pages 196, 206, 207, 230, 240, 249, 253, 293, 296 and 354.

**Byron Ayanoglu with contributions from Algis Kemezys**
*125 Best Vegetarian Recipes*
Recipes from this book are found on pages 216, 245, 247 and 251.

**Byron Ayanoglu and Jennifer MacKenzie**
*Complete Curry Cookbook*
Recipes from this book are found on pages 226, 271, 272 and 307.

**Johanna Burkhard**
*500 Best Comfort Food Recipes*
Recipes from this book are found on pages 191, 194, 214, 304, 306, 308, 324, 339 and 343.

**Johanna Burkhard**
*The Comfort Food Cookbook*
Recipes from this book are found on pages 252 and 326.

**Pat Crocker**
*The Juicing Bible*
Recipes from this book are found on pages 359, 360, 361, 362, 363, 364, 365, 366, 367 and 368.

**Pat Crocker**
*The Vegan Cook's Bible*
Recipes from this book are found on pages 211, 224, 231, 243, 260, 256, 281, 282 and 284.

**Dietitians of Canada**
*Cook!*
Recipes from this book are found on pages 183, 209, 213, 255, 291, 294 and 319.

**Dietitians of Canada**
*Cook Great Food*
Recipes from this book are found on pages 238, 264, 266, 269, 288, 290, 292, 311, 318 and 334.

**Dietitians of Canada**
*Simply Great Food*
Recipes from this book are found on pages 254, 280, 297, 314, 317, 329, 332 and 340.

**Maxine Effenson-Chuck and Beth Gurney**
*125 Best Vegan Recipes*
Recipes from this book are found on pages 212, 276 and 331.

**Judith Finlayson**
*150 Best Slow Cooker Recipes*
A recipe from this book is found on page 316.

**Judith Finlayson**
*The Complete Gluten-Free Whole Grains Cookbook*
Recipes from this book are found on pages 184, 223, 275, 298, 312, 322, 338 and 342.

**Judith Finlayson**
*The Vegetarian Slow Cooker*
A recipe from this book is found on page 330.

**Julie Hasson**
*300 Best Chocolate Recipes*
Recipes from this book are found on pages 199, 344, 352, 355 and 356.

**Lynn Roblin, Nutrition Editor**
*500 Best Healthy Recipes*
Recipes from this book are found on pages 241, 242, 244, 250, 286 and 289.

**Deb Roussou**
*350 Best Vegan Recipes*
Recipes from this book are found on pages 190, 192, 198, 219, 222, 261, 262, 278 and 333.

**Camilla V. Saulsbury**
*5 Easy Steps to Healthy Cooking*
Recipes from this book are found on pages 180, 181, 185, 186, 197, 208, 210, 246, 248 and 358.

**Camilla V. Saulsbury**
*500 Best Quinoa Recipes*
Recipes from this book are found on pages 182, 187, 188, 189, 268, 270, 218 and 321.

**Camilla V. Saulsbury**
*750 Best Muffin Recipes*
Recipes from this book are found on pages 202, 203 and 204.

**Camilla V. Saulsbury**
*Piece of Cake!*
Recipes from this book are found on pages 345, 346, 348 and 350.

**Kathleen Sloan-McIntosh**
*300 Best Potato Recipes*
Recipes from this book are found on pages 335 and 336.

**Carla Snyder and Meredith Deeds**
*300 Sensational Soups*
Recipes from this book are found on pages 220, 228, 232, 234 and 236.

**Linda Stephen**
*Complete Book of Thai Cooking*
Recipes from this book are found on pages 300 and 315.

**Suneeta Vaswani**
*Complete Book of Indian Cooking*
Recipes from this book are found on pages 273, 274, 310 and 337.

**Suneeta Vaswani**
*Easy Indian Cooking*
Recipes from this book are found on pages 305, 327 and 328.

**Katherine E. Younker, Editor**
*America's Complete Diabetes Cookbook*
Recipes from this book are found on pages 258, 302 and 320.

# Index

## A

Abilify (aripiprazole), 96
acetaminophen, 47, 51
acetylcholines, 14, 153
acetyl-L-carnitine (ALC), 153
acrodermatitis enteropathica, 91
acupuncture, 103–4, 108
adrenal glands, 56
adrenaline (epinephrine), 56, 58–59
African Beef Stew, 317
AGEs (advanced glycation end products), 35, 58, 135
AI (adequate intake), 67
almond milk
    Super Antioxidant Smoothie, 358
    Walnut Flax Waffles, 197
almonds. *See also* almond milk
    Chocolate Cherry Drops, 344
    Curried Chicken Salad Wraps, 311
    Green Macaroni and Cheese, 280
alpha-carotene, 141
alprazolam, 100
aluminum toxicity, 27, 53
Alzheimer's disease, 24–30. *See also* dementia
    assessment scale, 28–29
    case study, 12, 22, 37, 64, 94
    diagnosis, 27–29
    herbal remedies for, 101–3
    incidence, 6
    location, 23
    medications for, 95–96
    physical therapies for, 103–5
    symptoms, 24, 28
amantadine, 99
Ambien, 100
AMDR (acceptable macronutrient distribution range), 67
amino acids, 14
amygdala, 17
amyloidosis, 25
amyotrophic lateral sclerosis (ALS), 23, 33–34, 99
anemia
    macrocytic, 75
    sickle-cell, 78
anthocyanins, 152
anticholinergics, 98, 99
anticoagulants, 82

antidepressants, 95, 98
antihistamines, 100
antioxidants, 44, 108, 137–40
antipsychotics, 96
anxiolytics, 95
apnea (sleep), 35
apomorphine (Apokyn), 98
apples and apple juice, 127, 128
    Cashew Butter, 211
    Cell Support Juice, 367
    Cinnamon Apple Chips, 208
    Cran-Apple (juice), 361
    Cranberry, Carrot and Apple Teff Muffins, 203
    Curry-Roasted Squash and Apple Soup, 226
    Dandelion Slam Dunk, 365
    Moroccan Pumpkin Soup, 224
    Open-Face Salmon Salad Sandwich with Apple and Ginger, 291
    Orange Zinger, 362
    Slippery Beet (juice), 363
    Sweet Cinnamon Waldorf Salad, 242
    Turkey Apple Meatloaf, 314
Aricept, 95
aripiprazole (Abilify), 96
arsenic, 52
artichoke hearts
    Shrimp Risotto with Artichoke Hearts and Parmesan, 302
    Warm Green Goddess Dip, 213
asparagus
    Baked Cranberry Tofu with Creamed Asparagus and Leeks, 284
    French-Herbed Strata, 192
    Super-Easy Crab and Sweet Potato Sushi Rolls (variation), 294
astrocytes, 26, 34
atherosclerosis, 19, 30, 37–39, 40, 41
Ativan (lorazepam), 95
avocado, 136
    Avocado and Egg Breakfast Wraps, 186
    Avocado Salad, 245
    Chickpeas with Kiwi and Avocado Salsa, 256
    Chunky Guacamole, 212
    Kiwi and Avocado Salsa with Pomegranate and Red Onion, 257

Super-Easy Crab and Sweet Potato Sushi Rolls, 294
Azilect (rasagiline), 98

## B

*Bacopa monnieri* (brahmi), 103
bacteria (gut), 45
Baked Cranberry Tofu with Creamed Asparagus and Leeks, 284
Baked Risotto with Spinach, 339
Barbecued Lemongrass Pork, 315
Basic Ricotta, 199
basil (fresh)
    Couscous Salad with Basil and Pine Nuts, 252
    Insalata Caprese, 247
    Spaghetti with Sun-Dried Tomatoes and Broccoli, 286
    Tomato Basil Soup, 222
ba wei di huang wan (BDW), 102
BDNF (brain-derived neurotrophic factor), 121
beans and bean sprouts, 129, 135
    Fragrant Rice-Stuffed Peppers (variation), 278
    Green Bean, Pecan and Pomegranate Salad, 243
    Green Beans and Carrots with Aromatic Spices, 328
    Jerusalem Artichoke Stew, 260
    Minestrone, 230
    Pad Thai, 300
    Quinoa Chili, 275
    Rice Noodles with Spicy Spaghetti Sauce, 282
    Salmon over White and Black Bean Salsa, 289
    Three-Bean Chili, 276
    Three-Pepper Tamale Pie, 262
beef
    African Beef Stew, 317
    Beef and Quinoa Power Burgers, 321
    Beef with Broccoli, 318
    Minestrone (variation), 230
    Orange Ginger Beef, 319
    Peppery Meatloaf with Quinoa, 322
    Saucy Swiss Steak, 316
    Shepherd's Pie with Creamy Corn Filling, 320

# H

haloperidol (Haldol), 96
HDL ("good") cholesterol, 41
headache disorders, 21
health determinants, 60–61
 restoring, 115–23
Healthy Brian Diet Program,
 8–9
 goals, 108–10
 menu plans, 160, 164–66,
  168–77
 step 1 (nutrition), 115
 step 2 (determinants of
  health), 115–23
 step 3 (brain energizing),
  124–32
 step 4 (plaques prevention),
  132–34
 step 5 (inflammation
  reduction), 134–36
 step 6 (protection from free
  radicals), 137–44
 step 7 (detoxification), 144–48
 step 8 (omega-3s), 148–52
 step 9 (special nutrients),
  152–54
 step 10 (brain regeneration),
  154–57
 step 11 (care team), 158–59
 step 12 (making changes),
  160–62
herbal medicines, 101–3, 108
herbicides, 50, 148
herbs. See also basil; cilantro;
 parsley
 Baked Cranberry Tofu with
  Creamed Asparagus and
  Leeks, 284
 French-Herbed Strata, 192
 Gingered Beet and Quinoa
  Soup, 218
 Rice Noodles with Spicy
  Spaghetti Sauce, 282
 Rosemary Chicken Breasts
  with Sweet Potatoes and
  Onions, 304
 Saffron Mash, 336
 Sage and Savory Mushroom
  Frittata, 190
hindbrain (brain stem), 17–18
hippocampus, 17, 19, 59–60
histamine, 71
Hoffer, Abram, 65
Holy Smokes Pita Chips, 209
Home-Style Pancakes, 196
Home-Style Skillet Rice with
 Tomato Crust, 338

honey, 130
Hot Breakfast Cereal Mix, 183
hummus, 130
huperzine A, 103
hydration, 118–20
hyperglycemia, 57
hypermagnesemia, 88
hypoglycemia, 55–56
hypothalamus, 17
hypothyroidism, 86

# I

imipramine, 71
infections, 21
inflammation, 39–41, 150
 diet and, 134–36
Insalata Caprese, 247
insecticides, 50
insulin, 54, 56
iodine, 86
IQ (intelligence quotient), 149
iron, 86–88
ischemia, 19, 30–31

# J

Jerusalem Artichoke Stew, 260

# K

kale
 Cruciferous Chiller, 366
 Roasted Beet Tacos with
  Marinated Shredded Kale,
  261
 Simple Stir-Fried Kale, 329
Keshan disease, 90
kidneys, 48
kiwifruit
 C-Blitz, 359
 Chickpeas with Kiwi and
  Avocado Salsa, 256
 Kiwi and Avocado Salsa with
  Pomegranate and Red Onion,
  257

# L

lactic acid, 46–47
Lamb Tagine with Chickpeas
 and Apricots, 324
language (communication)
 disorders, 21
LDL ("bad") cholesterol, 41, 43,
 143
lead, 52–53
learning, 61

and brain health, 156–57
 DHA and, 150
 sleep and, 116
leeks
 Baked Cranberry Tofu with
  Creamed Asparagus and
  Leeks, 284
 Baked Risotto with Spinach,
  339
 French-Herbed Strata, 192
 Simple Stir-Fried Kale, 329
legumes, 131, 135. See also
 beans; lentils; peas
lemon balm (Melissa officinalis),
 102
Lemongrass Pork, Barbecued,
 315
lemons and lemon juice
 Refreshing Lentil Salad, 255
 Roasted Beet Tacos with
  Marinated Shredded Kale,
  261
 Tabbouleh, 251
lentils, 129
 Fragrant Rice-Stuffed Peppers
  (variation), 278
 Red Lentil Curry with
  Coconut and Cilantro, 271
 Refreshing Lentil Salad, 255
 Roasted Garlic and Lentil
  Soup, 231
 Tomato Onion Curry of Brown
  Lentils, 272
levodopa, 97, 98, 108
Lewy body dementia, 23, 26,
 96
lifestyle, 133, 134, 158–59
limbic system, 17
limes and lime juice
 Baked Cranberry Tofu with
  Creamed Asparagus and
  Leeks, 284
 Cherry Juice, 360
 Chunky Guacamole, 212
 Pad Thai, 300
linoleic acid, 151
linolenic acid, 149
lipids. See cholesterol
lipofuscin, 153
liver detoxification, 47–48
lorazepam (Ativan), 95
Lou Gehrig's disease. See
 amyotrophic lateral sclerosis
 (ALS)
Lumosity, 156
Lunch Box Peachy Sweet Potato
 and Couscous, 269
Lunesta, 100